Interaction and Relationships in Breastfeeding Families
Implications for Practice

DR. KEREN EPSTEIN-GILBOA PhD, MEd,

BSN, RN, FACCE, LCCE, IBCLC, RLC

HALEPUBLISHING

1712 N. Forest St. • Amarillo, Texas 79106 | © Copyright 2009 All rights reserved.

Interaction and Relationships in Breastfeeding Families:

Implications for Practice

KEREN EPSTEIN-GILBOA PhD, MEd, BSN, RN, FACCE, LCCE, IBCLC, RLC

© Copyright 2009
Hale Publishing, L.P.
1712 N. Forest St.
Amarillo, TX 79106-7017
806-376-9900
800-378-1317
www.iBreastfeeding.com
www.hale-publishing.com

All rights reserved. No part of this publication may be reproduced or transmitted in any form or by any means, electronic or mechanical, including photocopy, recording, stored in a database or any information storage, or put into a computer, without prior written permission from the publisher.

Library of Congress Control Number: 2009929521
ISBN-13: 978-0-9823379-0-5

Table of Contents

Chapter 1: Introduction

Personal Experience and Reasons for Researching Interaction in Nursing Families 1
Families Described in the Book 2
Summary 5

Chapter 2: The Clinician and the Nursing Family

Supporting Another's Perspective and Self-Awareness 7
Evidence that Clinical Bias Exists 8
Education and Enhanced Practice 9
Self-Awareness of Themes Interfering with Nursing 10

Chapter 3: Concepts and Theories

Nursing as a Physiologically Based Relationship 13
Behaviors Associated with Physiologically Based Nursing 18
The Psychological Development of Infants and
Children in Nursing Systems 24
Maternal Development through Nursing 28
Paternal Development in Nursing Systems 33
The Development of the Couple Relationship in
    the Nursing System 35
Family Systems Theory 39
Implications for Practice 41

Chapter 4 : Themes Affecting Perspectives of Nursing

The Significance of Themes for Practice 43
Long Standing Physiologically Based Nursing Patterns 43

Obstructed Nursing Patterns.. 44
Family Themes in the Twentieth Century Obstruct
   Physiologically Based Nursing... 48
Summary of Historical Family Themes and Nursing Behaviors 51
Present Day Family Themes and the Prevalence of Messages
   Obstructing Nursing...52
Healthcare Systems Convey Contradictory Messages...........................52
Messages Obstructing Physiological Nursing Patterns 55
Lay Literature and Academic Research on Families 73
Implications of Family Themes Associated with Nursing for
   Clinical Practice..74

Chapter 5: Family Development

Family Development..75
Prenatal Stage 76
Immediate Postnatal Period and Initiation 78
Establishing and Maintaining Exclusivity in the Nursing Unit................78
Summary of the Evolution of the Nursing Subsystem in the Prenatal,
   Initiation, and Establishment Phases of Development..................... 84
Clinical Implications.. 84

Chapter 6: Interactions in the Nursing Subsystem: The Development of Sensitive Mothering and Sensitive Interactions

Cue Based Interactions 89
Interactions in the Nursing Subsystem and Child Development 102
Interactions in the Nursing Subsystem and Maternal Development.......103
Clinical Implications...107

Chapter 7: Interactions with the Nursing Subsystem and the Development of Sensitive Fathering

Internalizing Sensitive Fathering 111

Challenges to the Trajectory of Sensitive Fathering 118
Resolving Ambivalence 122
Summary of the Interactions in the Nursing Subsystem and Paternal
    Development 123
Clinical Implications 124

Chapter 8: Interactions with the Nursing Subsystem, Couple Development and Parental Sensitivity

Complementary Interactions 127
Open Communication 128
Summary of Couple Processes Facilitated and Influenced by
    Interactions in the Nursing Subsystem 134
Clinical Implications 135

Chapter 9: Interactions with the Nursing Subsystem, Parents and Siblings: Children Reverberate Sensitive Behaviors

Trajectory of Sensitive Interaction 139
Experiencing, Observing, Learning, and Practicing Interactions
    with Siblings 139
Extending Themes and Patterns to Contexts Outside the Family ... 143
Clinical Applications 147

Chapter 10: Interaction between All Individuals and Subsystems: The Extension of Themes Associated with Nursing to the Family System

Family Interaction 149
Clinical Implications 156

Chapter 11: The New Breed of Nursing Families: Adult Focused Nursing

Adult-Focused Nursing 159
Clinical Implications 160

Chapter 12: Themes Promoting Physiologically Based Nursing Patterns and the Development of Sensitivity

Reverence for Physiology 163
Reverence for Children's Natural Needs and Cues 170
Nursing is an Encompassing Experience 171
Nursing is an Emotional Experience 172
Themes Interfering with Physiologically Based
   Nursing and Sensitivity 186
Summary of Themes Supporting the Development of Sensitive Interaction
   through Physiologically Based Nursing 190
Extension of Themes Promoting Sensitivity beyond Nursing 190
Sensitivity to Children's Needs for Proximity 191
Themes Promoting Sensitive Weaning and Separation Processes 198
Separation from Mother and Home 200
Respect for Children's Unique Needs, Rhythms,
   Cues, and Individuality 200
Recognizing and Meeting Parent and Couple Needs 201
Sensitive and Free Flowing Communication 206
Summary of Extension of Themes Promoting Sensitivity
   beyond Nursing 207

Chapter 13: Implications of Family Interactions in Nursing Family Systems

Implications for Nursing 209
Implications for Child Development 211
Implications for Maternal Development 214
Implications for Paternal Development 216
Implications for Couple Processes 218

Implications for Family System Theory 222
Implications for Existing Literature on Nursing Families 224
Clinical Implications 224

Chapter 14: Conclusions

Appendix A---Brief Synopses of Case Studies

Amit Family 239
Avir Family 240
Nightingale Family 241
Kinor Family 242
Forester Family 242
Morgan Family 243
Florence Family 244
Ford Family 245
Ginger Family 245
Mitchell Family 246
Peters Family 247
Stevens Family 248

Appendix B --- Example of One Case Study

Description of the Amit Family 249
The Process of Observations and Follow-up 249
Family Themes and Patterns 250
Present Nursing Subsystem 253
The Nursing Relationship and the Family 263
Conclusion 279

References 281

Index 305

Author Bio 311

Acknowledgements

There are so many that I would like to thank who have supported my efforts to write this book. Some of you have been around for many years.

I would like to thank all of you who were involved with my doctoral dissertation and the study this book is based on. I am most indebted to Dr. Richard Volpe who was my thesis advisor and on whom I continue to rely for his guidance and encouragement, for his calm and reassuring attitude, for stepping in to save the day on several occasions, and for his ability to reframe even the most distressing situations.

I am so grateful to Dr. Jack Newman for agreeing to be on my thesis committee, despite his extremely busy schedule, and for supporting and teaching me during the doctorate and in clinical practice over the years. I am thankful that I can continue to turn to you for support and advice, including guiding me to Hale Publishing.

I feel sincere gratitude towards Dr. Solveiga Miezitis for her extremely helpful insights, great direction, warm empathy, positive attitude, and ongoing encouragement, and for helping me find my own voice in the thesis. I will never forget how you helped me "birth" my dissertation when I was so afraid of "having another miscarriage."

And I am eternally grateful to Dr. Otto Weininger, for participating in my doctoral dissertation committee and in past projects. Sadly, Dr. Weininger passed away during the thesis process. His contributions to this dissertation and to my understanding of babies and families changed the way I think and work. I hope to do justice to the memory of Dr. Otto Weininger by reflecting these insights in my thesis, this book, clinical interactions, and future work.

Thank you to Dr. Marc Lewis for setting me on the right path as an academic, for supervising earlier research, and for his support.

Warm thanks to my former thesis group, close friends, and now post doctoral support group, Dr. Claudia Koshinsky Clipsham and Dr. Anona Zimmerman, for reading the document, for their encouragement and suggestions, and for teaching me the importance of good food for the body and soul.

Thanks to Christine Davidson for her editing skills, knowledge, extreme patience, and encouragement, and for continuing to work with me on new projects.

Thank you to Janet Rourke of Hale Publishing for her amazing editing skills and unbelievable patience, insights, and humor that helped me finally finish the book. Thanks to Dr. Kathleen Kendall-Tackett for reviewing the manuscript and for providing me with great insights that helped me make necessary changes.

My most sincere gratitude goes to all of the participants in the study this book is based on. I am so thankful to the families that kindly let me into their private lives and allowed me to tell others what I learned about them. I am indebted to the key informant interviewees who deepened my insights about nursing families and helped me make sense of the complex lives that nursing families live. This study would have never taken place without the generous help of these participants.

I am also very grateful to my family and friends for their patience, for listening to me as I formulated ideas, for encouraging me, and who continued to support me as I turned the dissertation into a book. I appreciate the efforts of some of you who also graciously agreed to act as key informants in this study. A special thank you to the "Amit" family.

Thanks to Jonathan Epstein for help with editing. Thank you to Dr. Raanan Gilboa for support and help, and for doing more than his share around the house so that I could concentrate on the thesis and then book. I will always remember Alex's unconditional love, and I appreciate the love I get from Joanna that has humored me through this process.

And, of course, I am most grateful to my former nursing child, Sari Gilboa, who is now a mature and beautiful adult, caring for children whose growth she sensitively fosters as a speech-language pathologist. I thank you, Inik, for your patience, understanding, advice, and amazing sense of humor. Thanks to Sari I learned how to mother, and I learned how precious nursing is for children, mothers, and families. It was this experience that triggered my interest in researching nursing families.

Chapter 1
Introduction

Breastfeeding has received immense attention in the medical community over the last three decades. Medical researchers and clinicians have followed women's cues and began to reintroduce nursing as a normal developmental task after decades of dismissing it as unnecessary. Most research focuses on the physiology of lactation. Studies have increased our understanding about the components of breastmilk, the physiological functions of lactation, implications of not nursing, and, of course, the significance of latching. However, the literature implies that the psychological aspects of nursing have not been investigated as deeply (Friedman, 1996; Marshall, 1995; Slade, MacPherson, Hume, & Maresh, 1993; Slusser & Lange, 2002). This imbalance in our understanding of nursing has left many nursing mothers and their families feeling unheard and alone.

Personal Experience and Reasons for Researching Interaction in Nursing Families

I have witnessed the implications of misunderstanding in my personal and professional life, and this prompted me to research the topic. I felt the personal frustration of not being understood when I was a nursing mother more than two decades ago. Most unfortunately, I saw other families experience the same frustration though my work as a nurse, lactation consultant, La Leche League Leader, childbirth educator, birth companion, psychotherapist, and researcher. I noted how hard it is for families to internalize a family style conducive to nursing when they are surrounded by misinformation about nursing and associated parenting. Family confusion is increased as they attempt to deconstruct the messages about nursing, infants, and weaning that are conveyed by the aggressive marketing of companies that profit from artificial baby milk and associated products. I experienced the strength of the union between these companies and their collaborators in the healthcare system and suffered from their wrath when I dared to challenge them.

I saw the misunderstanding of and interference in the physiological processes associated with nursing at all levels of interaction. I noted how families giving birth in hospitals were pressured to accept medical interventions without regard for the possible ill effects on the early nursing relationship. In the early postpartum period, I saw how babies were taken from their mothers for a variety of reasons lacking in evidence and given an artificial substance or oral apparatus that interfered with nursing and the infants' capacity to internalize the breast as the comforting object. I shuddered as I watched infants who had left their mothers' wombs prematurely lie alone in lonely isolates. It seemed that healthcare providers, focused on physical growth, were oblivious to the implications of loneliness and early interaction with breastmilk, or worse, artificial milk in a cold object rather than from a warm motherly breast. Subsequent nursing complications stemming from mishandling of birth, prematurity, separation, and interactions with artificial substances or an apparatus were usually handled technically, but without regard for the emotional meaning parents and infants attribute to this experience.

I also saw extreme disregard for the normal continuum of nursing, especially breastfeeding beyond infancy. I continuously heard about families' frustrated interchanges with healthcare professionals and psychotherapists who interfered with families' efforts to nurse, reprimanding them for the accompanying parenting style and family behaviors. Clinicians criticized frequent nursing, nursing beyond infancy, and maternal-child closeness. Parents were told that nursing and ongoing proximity are pathological and interfere with children's abilities to regulate their emotions and become independent. In addition, couples were told that nursing and closeness disrupt the marital relationship. I witnessed how parents, who refused to listen to professional advice, were called smothering and over protective. I heard the frustration that families felt when they told stories about not being heard, and that the nursing relationship was blamed for anything that went wrong in their families.

Along with noting the difficulties that nursing families' experience, I also observed their unique interactions. In my earlier research, I looked at the mother and nursing child dyad. I observed the lively and unique interactions that took place during nursing that seem to contribute to healthy interactions beyond breastfeeding. In my clinical work, I noted how instrumental fathers and siblings were and the influence they seemed to have on the nursing unit, and vice versa. I saw how families often worked together, ignoring diversity, immersing themselves in nursing and childcare, and bringing up healthy children. They had rich and interesting lifestyles that had not yet been investigated and described to the fullest. Training in family and couple therapy convinced me that I should extend the research and focus on the entire nursing family.

Families Described in the Book

The families described in this book are those who nurse in tune with the recommendations for nursing established by the World Health Organization

(WHO) (1981, 2001). According to the recommended practices, infants nurse exclusively for approximately the first six months of life and continue for at least two years. These practices are continually assessed and updated. They comply with normal female and infant physiological continuum; are congruent with the children's tasks of normal cognitive, physical, and emotional growth and development; and mirror historical practices. These recommendations also match those suggested by La Leche League for over fifty years and are resounded in updated medical policy statements (American Academy of Pediatrics (AAP), 2005; Health Canada, 2004). Accordingly, the families discussed in this book are those who nursed exclusively for approximately the first six months of life and continued nursing for at least two years. A few exceptions are made in cases of special circumstances, such as in adoptive families.

Information about the nursing families in this book is based on evidence gathered in a study I conducted on systemic interaction in nursing families. This study served as my doctoral dissertation (Epstein-Gilboa, 2006). This project followed earlier research on interactions between mother-infant nursing dyads (Epstein, 1993). The study on interaction in nursing families used a qualitative design and took place over a seven year period. The qualitative design enabled me to gather and analyze minute and intricate details over a period of time. The trustworthiness of the data is enriched by a triangulation of tools and the proportionally large group considering the qualitative design.

Twelve actively nursing families were observed, interviewed, and their data analyzed. One family was observed over a five year period. In addition, fifty-four key informants were interviewed and included professionals and lay people with experience with nursing or as nursing families. Some key informants had over thirty years experience working with nursing families. All key informants were carefully selected to ensure that they accurately represented breastfeeding families nursing in tune physiology as described earlier. Data from both groups were carefully analyzed and compared. The data analysis took into account individuality, while demonstrating several salient themes that characterize breastfeeding families.

Language Use: Nursing as the Term of Reference

Wiessinger's (1996) paper suggesting the importance of the use of language in breastfeeding discourse was taken seriously in the preparation of this book. This topic is of special interest to me as I write, investigate, and lecture about issues related to the impact of language on pregnancy, birthing, nursing, and parenting (Epstein-Gilboa, 1997a, 1997b; 1999, 2008; 2009). Hence, it was important to choose language carefully and ensure that the words used would imply the intended meaning.

The word used to describe breastfeeding in this book takes into account the physiological and, of course, psychological aspects of this behavior. Although breastfeeding is used intermittently, the readers will note that "nursing" is also used in the text. These words describe a multifaceted behavior. The term "nursing" is evident on multiple internet sites discussing breastfeeding, in the literature (Lauwers & Swisher, 2005), and also in La Leche League (2004) material, including their magazines for parents (New Beginnings, 1985-present) and lay counselors (Leaven, 1965–present). In addition, in my experience, nursing is commonly used in discourse between mothers and members of the nursing community.

The term nursing has a special connotation relevant for the issues discussed in this text. Nursing connotes the nurturing and caregiving aspects of breastfeeding and is devoid of references to feeding. Readers will come to understand as they read this book that nursing is an encompassing behavior and not a means of feeding. Moreover, an important discovery of this study (Epstein-Gilboa, 2006) is that referring to nursing as feeding reduces the encompassing nature of this behavior. Hence, nursing is used frequently in this text.

When the word "breastfeeding" is used, it is written as one word, as is the word breastmilk, again following the practice in nursing-friendly environments, such as in La Leche League (2004) texts. Breastfeeding shows the connection of the act to the maternal breast and contradicts the predominant themes of nursing as a mere and equal feeding choice.

Another issue that was taken into account was that breastfeeding is often defined inconsistently, leading to confounding results and interpretations (Harmon-Jones, 2006; Labbok & Krasovec, 1990). Attempts were made to define the style of nursing discussed as precisely as possible. Terms such as "physiologically based nursing patterns" are used, implying that the nursing patterns displayed follow physiological principles. There is a brief review of the physiology of nursing in chapter three.

The language and concepts used in this book reflect nursing as the norm and as the term of reference (Wiessinger, 1996), in contrast to other forms of infant feeding or pacifying. Behaviors that veer away from nursing have the preface "non" in front of them, as in "non-nursing." In addition, words for breastmilk substitutes are referred to accurately within a nursing mode (Epstein-Gilboa, 2002). The use of terms such as artificial feeding is commonly used by members of the breastfeeding community (author's experience). This practice is exemplified in the literature by material written by the Infant Feeding Action Coalition (INFACT, 2009a). These terms are used instead of the word "formula" that falsely designates this product as a superlative scientific substance (Baumslag & Michels, 1995; Minchin 1998; Palmer, 2009). Words associated with artificial feeding are generally written with two words, for example, bottle feeding.

Summary

This book was created for anyone who is interested in understanding more about how breastfeeding family members develop relationships and interact with one another. In addition, the book is meant to enhance one's interchanges with these families in all contexts, including healthcare, psychotherapy, social work, and lay services. All service providers will be referred to as clinicians or practitioners.

Some readers will have an in-depth understanding of the physiological function and mechanics of lactation. Others might have immense experience working with families, but only a minimal understanding of how breastfeeding works. This book is designed to meet the needs of readers from diverse backgrounds. The first few chapters will discuss theories that will help readers understand the family interactions described in the last few chapters. Different aspects of the background material will be more meaningful for some readers than for others. One might skim over parts of the background that are familiar and spend more time on areas that are less familiar. An in-depth reference list accompanies the book and will allow readers to focus on areas of interest.

This book uses evidence-based material, language, and accurate definitions of breastfeeding to bring clinicians closer to the reality of families nursing in tune with physiology and historically based patterns. This book will help clinicians understand why practitioners do not always provide optimal care to nursing families and how we can correct this and enhance our practice. The findings from this author's study on nursing families will be discussed and used to demonstrate salient themes and behaviors. Psychological theories will be applied to the discussion to give insight into the implications of nursing behaviors. The research presented in this book fills in the gap and provides clinicians with tools to understand and respond to the emotional meaning attributed to nursing and the psychological implications and behavioral patterns displayed in nursing families.

Chapter 2
The Clinician and the Nursing Family

Supporting Another's Perspective And Self-Awareness

In the introduction to this book, clinical misunderstanding of nursing families and the implications of misconstrued views on interchanges with families was discussed. In this chapter, the clinical process that enhance or deter us from hearing and then supporting families adequately will be addressed. Understanding family interchanges means that clinicians focus on the client's perspective, rather than on merely analyzing apparently objective information. This approach to clinical work is familiar to those trained in psychotherapy or in social work, but might be less known in medically aligned contexts. Practice based on client's narratives impels one to listen carefully to spoken and non-verbal messages and to follow family leads. Families are asked about their reality, the things they like, issues they want to work on, and what they feel they would like to see remain the same.

Looking into clients' realities helps us understand what makes nursing meaningful for them. We can use this information to enhance our practice with nursing families and to support them better. At the same time, we may also use novel concepts to increase our understanding of potential nursing families or those who seem conflicted about the experience. For example, how many clinicians have wondered why some families stop nursing despite adequate breastfeeding education, good enough latching, and apparently successful nursing? We can apply our enhanced understanding of what works and why to these more challenging situations.

An understanding of clients goes hand in hand with an increased understanding of our own feelings about nursing. Personal bias interferes with one's capacity to truly hear another person, especially when another's narrative negates our personal view. Medical and medically aligned professionals are often taught to ignore their feelings and to remain seemingly objective caregivers. Psychology recognizes that this feat is impossible and acknowledges that ignoring one's perspective may impair adequate service to the client.

In contrast to traditional healthcare models, the psychotherapeutic paradigm accepts that practitioners are whole people with life experiences that extend beyond the professional world. The term countertransference very briefly implies that the clients' issues affect the clinician and influence the quality of professional interaction. Within this paradigm, it is expected that the clinician acknowledge and understand the feelings that come up, and resolve issues in a way that advances interactions with the client. In other words, clinicians working with nursing families should evaluate how they feel about the narrative that the clients bring to their meeting.

Evidence that Clinical Bias Exists

The significance of self-awareness for work with nursing families cannot be overstated in light of evidence suggesting that clinicians seem to have trouble supporting nursing in the postpartum period, and that nursing beyond infancy and the lifestyle and parenting associated with breastfeeding are often criticized and blamed for any problems that arise in the family system (Epstein-Gilboa, 2006). The cycle of misunderstanding and insensitive interaction commences prior to giving birth when clinicians withhold information from families under the pretence of guarding them from guilt. The guilt myth is the false belief that providing parents with too much information causes parents to feel that they are being pressured. This apparent experience causes them to feel guilty when nursing does not go as planned. In actuality, parents (who also happen to be thinking adults) often feel very angry when they discover that information was withheld that might have helped them to make better decisions (Epstein-Gilboa, 1997a, 1997b, 1998a, 2000; Labbok, 2008; Lauwers & Swisher, 2005; Minchin, 1998; Newman, 1997, 1998; Newman & Pitman, 2009; Walker, 1993, 1998; Wiessinger, 1996).

The guilt myth continues to hamper clinical relationships following birth and is combined with additional forms of misunderstanding. Unnecessary maternal-child separation exemplifies another practice demonstrating insensitivity to the psychological aspects of nursing. This practice also contributes to breastfeeding problems and parents' dissatisfaction with clinical interventions (Benson Brown & McPherson, 1998; Blum, 1999; Elder & Gregory, 1996; Granju & Kennedy 1999; Newman, 1998). The emotionality of nursing is discarded further by false views that nursing may be duplicated through the bottle feeding experience (Danforth as cited in Shahar, 1990; Lamb & Kelly, 2000), and that there is no scientific proof that breastfeeding is linked to attachment (Eyer, 1996). Mothers who continue to nurse beyond infancy are severely pathologized, and according to Stein, Boise, and Snyder (2002) may be blamed, for example, for nursing in order to meet their own needs.

Misconceptions about nursing might have harmful implications for nursing dyads. The detrimental impact of clinical misconceptions are illustrated in Lamb and Kelly's (2000) portrayal of divorcing nursing mothers who refuse overnight visits and full day custody as hesitant, indecisive, and resistant. These theorists' suggestion that fathers give pumped milk to nursing children implies that breastfeeding is merely a food, erasing the unique relational meaning of nursing. In this case, clinical misunderstanding of the emotional experience of nursing hinders an existing, and likely strengthening, family relationship that is vital during the emotional devastation often associated with divorce.

Severe damage caused by misunderstanding is demonstrated in cases where clinicians intervene and harm seemingly pathological nursing relationships. The sensuality of nursing is not adequately understood in this culture and leads to negative attributions about nursing couples (Saha, 2002). Potential havoc to intact nursing families is exemplified in cases where the misunderstanding of the normal sensuality of nursing is misnamed as sexual abuse, and clinicians wrongfully apprehend nursing children from their mothers (Davidowitz, 1992; Owens, 2000; Saha, 2002).

The emotions, interactions, and behaviors associated with nursing are clearly misunderstood. Consequently, the actions of nursing families may be misinterpreted, scrutinized, and pathologized. At worst, this misconstrued view of nursing behaviors may lead to unjustified and perhaps irreparable damage.

Education and Enhanced Practice

One might propose that clinicians fail to support nursing families due to a lack of knowledge about the psychological meaning of nursing and associated behaviors. Data about the psychology of nursing is minimal in medical literature, and evidence relating to nursing is scarce in the psychological and social work literature. Based on this assessment, one might contend that the optimal means of enhancing care to nursing families is to provide more information to practitioners. However, while education will most certainly boost the quality of care in some instances, it is also important to remember the examples of ill regard in the healthcare system noted above. Despite the abundance of research available to healthcare providers working with nursing families, deficits in clinicians' knowledge base are apparent, subsequently reducing the quality of services and support provided to nursing families (Breastfeeding Committee for Canada (BCC), 2002; Brodribb, Fallon, Jackson, & Hegney, 2009; Lauwers & Swisher, 2005; Renfew et al., 2006). Moreover, many readers are certainly aware of situations where healthcare workers seem to fully disregard evidence. By the same token, many recall families who also ignore educational material and either refuse to nurse or nurse, but engage in behaviors leading to early weaning. These situations clearly indicate that the provision of education is not enough to alter behavior and help one get rid of a perspective that interferes with adequate practice.

Self-Awareness of Themes Interfering with Nursing

More insight into the predicament is gained when looking at the predominant culture surrounding nursing in western contexts. In western environments, non-nursing or, at most, short term nursing are the norm. Behaviors veering from the normal status are therefore considered abnormal. Within a therapeutic context, deviations require treatment.

Conceptualization of nursing, especially into early childhood, has not been accepted as a normal behavior for approximately the last century. Various cultural beliefs and practices, still relevant in the present context, obstruct nursing and facilitate the inception of artificial feeding as the norm. Furthermore, as this book will demonstrate, nursing into early childhood concurs with additional behaviors that are also regarded as repugnant in western settings. Considering that clinicians are whole people and are members of this culture, it can be expected that many are reviled by some of the issues associated with normal nursing patterns. It should also be noted that individual and family psychotherapists are not immune to the powerful influence of nearly a century of non-nursing, reverence for parent-child distancing, and associated issues. Therefore, all clinicians working with families in the transition to parenting and parents with young children should be aware of the impact of culture and history on their views and clinical interactions.

The likelihood that clinicians have views about issues implies that the first step to developing genuine client-focused interactions with nursing families is to accept that one does have these beliefs and feelings. One may become more receptive and helpful to nursing clients when one has this awareness. Stating one's views quietly or aloud to peers who validate the feelings facilitates the process. Understanding the root of one's personal philosophy might be enhanced by gaining insight into the history and politics of nursing, child rearing, and women in western culture, and of course, by exploring one's life experience in relation to these issues.

Once we have recognized our bias, we can begin the process of reflective listening and tuning into the client's reality. This step might be advanced by learning about nursing families in general and specific information about the client at hand. It is important to acknowledge individuality and to use apparent evidence only as a guide and no more. Again, it is the client's interpretation of the events that are central.

Finally, one may work on developing genuine positive regard for the family and their reality as a means of hearing the family from their perspective and finding suitable solutions. Clinicians may choose to work these feelings out with a friend, colleague, or professional psychotherapist.

The importance of self-awareness, accepting one's feelings, exploring one's own reality, and especially in the case of nursing, internalizing novel concepts is demonstrated by interactions between a family physician and a couple presenting with marital discord that have a nursing toddler who sleeps in their bed. This physician might have a hard time hearing the couple's underlying issues if she is influenced by her own experience of weaning her children early, has not read about normal nursing patterns, is convinced that nursing beyond one year of age is pathological, and feels that co-sleeping with children is unhealthy. The family's lifestyle might trigger the physician's sense of self in relation to her own child and her mothering if she nursed for a short period of time and if her mothering style differs from that presented by the clients. If these feelings are not recognized and worked through, the physician might focus on convincing the parents to wean their child from the breast and the parental bed, rather than noticing the couple's real issues and referring them to appropriate couple therapy.

In some cases, professionals will not be able to accept new ways of thinking about family life. This, too, is acceptable as long as the clinicians realize their limitations and refer clients to others who might be able to support nursing families better. Referring families to more appropriate sources in a respectful manner is another way of demonstrating genuine positive regard for the family. This is a means of recognizing that the client is worthy and has the right to the best service possible.

The next chapters will advance clinicians' understanding of nursing families. A discussion about novel concepts will enhance practitioners' cognitions about breastfeeding. Breastfeeding will be defined from a relational perspective and implications of this for individual and family development will be discussed. Family interaction and basic concepts of the family systems model will be described to help clinicians understand factors affecting the influence of nursing on the family and vice versa. Themes that have affected nursing family behaviors over the ages and in the present context will be reviewed. This will provide insight into the source of feelings that enable or disable us and families from supporting behaviors associated with nursing. And finally, the behaviors, attitudes, and recurring interactions that prevail in many nursing families will be discussed. Several case studies will be presented to clarify insights further and demonstrate how similar themes might be actualized differently in diverse family systems. This material will give clinicians an opportunity to practice accepting, coping, and altering their script to suit the reality of the nursing family, and help them form respectful relationships with nursing families.

Chapter 3
Concepts and Theories

This chapter will review theoretical concepts associated with nursing. First, an overview of breastfeeding will be presented, focusing on the relational implications and associated behaviors. Next, the implications of nursing for the individual and couple development will be covered. Finally, a discussion about a clinical tool used to understand family interaction will help us understand the role of nursing in the family and vice versa.

Nursing as a Physiologically Based Relationship

Nursing is an essential developmental task with physiologically based behaviors and patterns with immense implications for human development, including physiological, relational, emotional and psychological elements (American Academy of Family Physicians (AAFP), 2007; AAP, 2005; Heinig & Dewey 1996; INFACT, 1996b, 2003a; Lawrence & Lawrence, 2005; Oddy, 2001; Reynolds, 2001; Riordan, 2005; Slusser & Powers, 1997; United Nations International Children's Emergency Fund (UNICEF), 1998a, 1998c; WHO, 1981, 1998a, 2001, 2003; WHO & UNICEF, 1989, 1990; Zembo, 2002). Moreover, veering away from physiological patterns puts humans at risk for multiple health and developmental impairments (Chung, Raman, Trikalino, Lau, & Ip, 2008; Dewey, Cohen, & Rivera, 2001; Dundaroz et al., 2002; Hop et al., 2000; INFACT, 1992c, 1993a, 1999a; Walker, 1993, 1998, 2006, 2007a; US Preventive Service Task Force, 2008; WHO, 2003). Physiologically based nursing patterns reflect the developmental needs of the infant-child and change in accordance with the growing child's capacities and needs. A physiologically based nursing pattern commences within the first two hours following birth (WHO, 1998b; WHO &UNICEF, 1989), remains exclusive without any other substances for the first six months of life, and continues for at least the first two years of life (INFACT, 2002a; WHO, 1981, 2001, 2003). The evidence explaining the physiology of breastfeeding and supporting physiologically based patterns is important for clinicians to know. However, the immense amount of information on the physiology of nursing is beyond the scope of this book and may be found in numerous resources, including Lauwers & Swisher (2005), Lawrence & Lawrence (2005), and Riordan (2005).

Immediate Nursing Facilitates the Transition to Extrauterine Life

Family organization associated with nursing is initiated in utero where the mother and new family member engage in a unique existence; this existence excludes others and is accompanied by dyadic interaction (Chamberlain, 1997a, b; Montagu, 1978; Sullivan, 1972; Verny & Kelly, 1981). The joint existence prepares the mother for her future role as the external and sustaining mother. Symbiosis is interrupted prematurely before the human infant reaches a state of readiness for independent existence to allow the human head to travel through the maternal birth canal (Montagu, 1978).

Nursing plays a special role and eases the infant's transition into an external awareness by allowing the dependent newborn human to remain in touch with its former self, i.e., the mother, while concurrently introducing the infant to an autonomous sense of self. Similarly, maternal transformation (Rabuzzi, 1994) is eased as mothers let go of a sense of oneness with their fetal body part and begin to experience a modified form of infant embodiment through nursing (Schmied & Barclay, 1999).

Rejoining the mother at the breast continues the process of mutuality between the maternal-child dyad. During nursing, infants engage in a task that they have been well prepared for in utero through the sucking and swallowing of amniotic fluid (Hedberg Nyqvist, Sjoden & Ewald, 1999). The organized pattern of suckling that infants display (Koepke & Bigelow, 1997; Montagu, 1978), in addition to other physiological capacities, is enhanced by skin-to-skin interaction (Acolet, Sleuth & Whitelaw, 1989; Anderson, Moore, Hepworth & Bergman, 2003; Bergman, 2005; Hann, Malan, Kronson, Bergman & Huskisson, 1999; Ludington-Hoe et al., 1993; Ludington-Hoe, Morgan & Abouelfettoh, 2008; WHO, 1998b). Skin-to-skin interchanges between mothers and infants facilitate additional transactions that point to the continued interdependence between the formerly joined dyad. This is exemplified by the way that, following non-medicated births, naked infants placed on their mothers' chests independently find and latch on to their mother's breasts (Kennel & Klaus, 1998; Livingstone, 1996; Ransjo-Arvidson, et al., 2001; UNICEF Maharashtra, 2009; Widstrom, 1993; Widstrom et al., 1987; WHO, 1998a). It is fascinating that the secretion of the maternal hormone oxytocin is augmented through licking of the breast (Nissen, Lilja, Widstrom, & Uvnas-Moberg, 1995) and by the intricate way that newborns massage the breast with their hands (Matthiesen, Ransjo-Arvidson et al., 2001). Newborn behaviors facilitate the establishment of the unique relational feedback system that sustains the infant, mirroring interuterine symbiosis and helping mother and infant make the transition to extrauterine life.

Exclusive, Interdependent, and Infant Cue-Based Interactions

Infants continue to regulate the production and release of the essential life sustaining maternal substance through frequent infant initiated meetings at the breast that include appropriate positioning, attachment to the breast, and suckling. Maternal-infant physiological interdependence through nursing is regulated by maternal responses to infant initiated cues. Mothers answer their infants' cues by latching them to the breast. Appropriate latching and infant suckling initiates the maternal hormonal feedback loop, including the secretion of prolactin that creates milk and oxytocin that facilitates smooth muscle contraction ejecting maternal milk (Daly & Hartmann, 1995a, b; Lawrence & Lawrence, 2005; Livingstone, 1996; Mohrbacher & Stock, 2003; Riordan, 2005; Uvnas-Moberg, Widstrom, Werner, Matthiesen & Winberg, 1990; Woolridge, 1986a, b; WHO, 1998a). The efficiency of the maternal-infant nursing system is further suggested by the interdependence between the production of mother's milk and the infant's nursing behavior. Accordingly, when maternal nursing behaviors match infants' cues for closeness, maternal milk production reflects infants' needs for breastmilk (Daly & Hartmann, 1995a, 1995b). Nursing is a reciprocal and interdependent behavior that enables infants to develop the capacity to self-regulate their physiological needs. Furthermore, interference with this system puts infants at physiological and developmental risk (Anderson, 1989).

The high degree of bioavailability and accessibility of breastmilk (Lawrence & Lawrence, 2005; Riordan, 2005) leads to frequent and seemingly continuous infant regulated nursing sessions (Blaffer Hrdy, 1999) that are reminiscent of the constancy of the couple's former pregnant state. Unlimited meetings at the breast enrich infant health, milk production, and milk ejection, and increase the likelihood of lactation success (Alikasifoglu et al., 2001). It is interesting that frequent nursing enhances calmness due to the gastrointestinal hormone cholecystokinin (CCK), which increases absorption of fats and proteins, and enhances relaxation (Kennel & Klaus, 1998; Uvnas-Moberg, Widstrom, Marchini, & Winberg, 1987). In addition, frequent nursing affords infants temporary sole ownership of their mothers due to the pregnancy suppressant effects of a high level of prolactin that inhibits ovulation (Blaffer Hrdy, 1999; Quandt, 1995).

The interdependence of nursing mothers and children is demonstrated further by the biological impact of lactation on mothers. The influence of nursing on maternal biochemistry contributes to contextual and emotional issues and helps sustain the nursing unit. Most significantly, maternal physiology is enhanced by infant suckling, subsequently reverberating to the infant and enriching the nursing experience. First of all, nursing enhances maternal well being when infant suckling leads to the release of substances that enhance maternal digestion (Uvnas-Moberg et al., 1987; Widstrom et al., 1988) and the release of insulin (Widstrom et al., 1984). Next, the same hormones that create and eject the life sustaining breastmilk contribute to maternal behavior. Oxytocin is believed to have altruistic, caregiving, and attachment enhancing effects (Angier, 1991, 2000; Blaffer Hrdy & Carter, 1995; Kennel & Klaus, 1998; Klaus, Kennel & Klaus, 1995; Nissen et al., 1995; Nissen, Gustavsson, Widstrom & Uvnas-Moberg, 1998; Odent, 1999; Rosenthal, 1995; Small, 1998; Taylor et al., 2000). The hormone prolactin has an antianxiety effect on mothers (Nissen et. al, 1998). The efficiency of this hormonal feedback system is apparent in the early postnatal period, facilitating the development of mothering behaviors right from birth (Widstrom et al., 1990).

The hormonally based effects of nursing not only enhance basic mothering behaviors, but also protect mothers from extraneous factors, such as depression, that impede optimal maternal function. The physiology of nursing helps mothers modulate parasympathetic responses to stimuli, protecting them against severe responses to stress and depressive symptoms (Mezzacappa, 2004). The association between these factors is illustrated by the response of the immune system to stress. Accordingly, the immune system releases cytokines that cause an inflammatory response and neuroendocrine changes leading to depression. This system is exuberated further by additional stress. The calming effects of nursing, therefore, regulate the impact of stress on the immune system, protecting mothers against depression (Groër & Davis, 2006; Groër, Davis & Hemphill, 2002; Kendall-Tackett, 2005, 2007). Thus the impact of nursing on mothers indicates that breastfeeding is a circular act that sustains the infant while simultaneously ensuring the proliferation of reinforcing mothering behaviors that facilitate the continuation of the relationship at the breast.

Mutuality Impeded by Interference

Breaks in the physiological continuum of birth and breastfeeding may interfere with the establishment of normal nursing patterns, impeding exclusivity and duration (Kennel & Klaus, 1998; McLeod, Pullon, & Cookson, 2002; Riordan, 2005; Rogers, Emmett, & Golding, 1997; WHO & UNICEF, 1989). Medical interventions during birth and disruptions to maternal-infant closeness after birth may impede the establishment of nursing relationships

(INFACT, 2007a, 2009a; Righard & Alade, 1990; Torvaldson, Roberts, Simpson, Thompson & Ellwood, 2006; WHO & UNICEF, 1989; WHO, 1998b). Oral pacifiers (Fox & Schaefer, 1999; Kramer et al., 2001; Pollard, Fleming, Young, Sawczenko & Blair, 1999), artificial apparatus including bottles, and all substances other than breastmilk impede the development of normal nursing patterns, interfering with the unique way that infants latch on to and suckle at the breast, potentially impairing infants' suckling, damaging the nipple and breast, interfering with the hormonal feedback loop, and impairing the production and ejection of milk (Mohrbacher & Stock, 2003; Morton, 1992; Neifert, 1996; Newman, 1990, 1992a, 1992b, 1998; Newman & Sterken, 1992; Righard, 1998; Woolridge, 1986a, 1986b; WHO, 1998b). From a psychological point of view, infants may view artificial feeding or a pacifying apparatus as the giving object and refuse the actual maternal breast and mother (Epstein-Gilboa, unpublished document).

Nursing Enhances Mutuality in Adoptive Couples

The physiological mutuality of nursing is not limited to biologically related mothers and babies, but may also be enjoyed by adoptive mothers and children. Mothers can induce lactation without pregnancy and establish interdependent relationships with their babies through nursing. The nursing relationship facilitates the transfer of an infant's sense of symbiosis with the biological mother to the adoptive mother. Families with adopted children may also establish subsystems based on synchronized, mutual, and infant cue-based nursing relationships (Bouchet Horwitz, 2001; Cheales-Siebenaler, 1999; Gribble, 2006; Klaus & Klaus, 1998; Rogers, 1997; UNICEF, 1996b).

Maintaining Cue-Based Nursing Interactions

The oral exclusivity of the nursing relationship changes over time to reflect changes in infant oral, motor, immune, digestive, and cognitive development (La Leche League, 2004; Lawrence & Lawrence 2005; Riordan, 2005). At approximately six months of age, infants are developmentally equipped to gradually handle substances other than breastmilk as they continue to nurse (Slusser & Powers, 1997; WHO, 1981, 2001, 2003). Infants' growing motor and cognitive capacities enable them to gradually seek out interaction with other objects in their midst, while intermittently returning to the mother (Bowlby, 1987). For nursing couples, this includes frequent intermittent nursing sessions (Epstein, 1993). Recommendations that nursing continue for at least the first two years of life (WHO, 1981, 2001, 2003) suggest that the strong connection between nursing mothers and children remains a consistent aspect of the family. Initial exclusivity between the nursing unit changes gradually, allowing others to partake in increasing interactions with nursing children.

Physiological Continuum

The nursing relationship has a set pattern of behaviors reflecting the physiological development of infants and their mothers. The changes in nursing behaviors mirror the growth and needs of the evolving child. The physiologically based nursing continuum is reinforced by specific behaviors that facilitate the establishment and continuation of the interdependent nursing subsystem.

Behaviors Associated with Physiologically Based Nursing

The connection between specific behaviors, physiology, and the interdependent nursing relationship is demonstrated further by data showing that there is an association between proximity behaviors and physiologically based nursing patterns (Gorman, 2002; McKenna, 1996; Valsiner, 2000). Proximal strategies include constant holding, carrying, rocking in arms and co-sleeping (Ball, 2002; Dettwyler, 1995a; Hayes, Roberts & Stowe, 1996; Liedloff, 1985; McKenna, 1996; McKenna et al., 1994; McKenna, Mosko & Richard, 1997; Montagu, 1978; Small, 1998; Valsiner, 2000). Proximity behaviors enable mothers to consistently and frequently match infant cues with nursing (McKenna, 1996; Quandt, 1995; Small, 1998). The association between nursing frequency and duration (Vandiver, 1997) implies that proximity behaviors contribute to the development of physiological nursing patterns. Reviews of families over time and in diverse cultures show that maternal-infant proximity is associated with nursing beyond infancy (Baumslag & Michels, 1995; Blaffer Hrdy, 1999; Dettwyler, 1995b; Fildes, 1995; Fouts, Hewlett, & Lamb, 2001; Liedloff, 1985; Montagu, 1978; Quandt, 1995; Stein et al., 2002; Valsiner, 2000).

A review of anthropological literature indicates that cultures supportive of proximal strategies also display underlying beliefs and behaviors. Findings that proximity behaviors are facilitated in child-focused environments (Valsiner, 2000) indicate that parents' views of their child affect their capacity to be physically close to them on an ongoing basis. Data showing that child paced nursing seems to facilitate gentle child led weaning into childhood (Fouts et al., 2001) implies that allowing children continued and child regulated access to the breast facilitates the development of physiologically based nursing patterns.

Tactile Interaction

The association between positive child outcome, physiology, and proximity is demonstrated by touch in infant and child development. Tactile messages lay a template for healthy affect development (Montagu, 1978). It is significant that mothering behaviors are positively impacted by touch (Widstrom et al., 1990), an act that likely reverberates to the mother-infant system, maintaining optimal behaviors. Touch remains a salient component of the interactional repertoire displayed during nursing, enabling mothers and infants to experience and convey a wide array of messages and emotions (Epstein, 1993). Touch also enhances the paternal-child connection (Kennel & Klaus, 1998).

Tactile interactions between mothers and offspring take place even prior to birth. Humans are born earlier than they should be in order to help their proportionally large heads pass through the tight maternal birth canal. The gentle massage movements that infants experience as they endure birth and descend in the birth channel apparently enhance function much like the way animals trigger physiological function by licking their newly born offspring (Montagu, 1978). Touch activates suckling (Koepke & Bigelow, 1997; Montagu, 1978) and establishes the nursing feedback loop (Kennel & Klaus, 1998; Livingstone, 1996; Ludington-Hoe et al., 1993; Ransjo-Arvidson et al., 2001; Widstrom et al., 1987; WHO, 1998b).

Skin-to-Skin Interaction

Skin-to-skin interaction is an important tactile interchange that enhances development following birth. According to Montagu (1978), skin-to-skin contact increases the level of communication between mothers and infants. Fathers may also engage in skin-to-skin interaction, increasing their emotional connection to their infant (Kennel & Klaus, 1998). It is interesting to note the association between different beliefs, practices, and specific behaviors. In this case, skin-to-skin maternal-child interaction is prevalent in cultures allowing mothers and infants ongoing physical access to one another (Montagu, 1978).

Skin-to-skin interaction has growth enhancing and therapeutic implications. Kangaroo care, a behavior based on skin-to-skin interactions between a naked infant (dressed in diaper only) and another person wearing the infant on their bare chest, is used to enhance development in premature infants. This behavior is protective due to the positive influence of skin-to-skin interactions on infant and maternal development and on breastfeeding. Improved infant factors include enriched oxygenation, heart rate, breathing, temperature, digestion, and suckling. Through skin-to-skin interactions, maternal confidence and emotional state are enhanced. The increased contact also facilitates exclusive and frequent nursing sessions, augmenting breastmilk production and ejection. Increased nursing reinforces the cycle by augmenting immune and other functions (Bergman, 2005; Hedberg Nyqvist et al., 1999; INFACT, 2009b; Kennel & Klaus, 1998; Koepke & Bigelow, 1997; Ludington-Hoe et al., 1993; Ludington-Hoe & Golant, 1993; Ludington-Hoe et al., 2008; Mikeil-Kostrya, Mazur, & Boltrusko, 2002; Montagu, 1978; WHO, 1998b).

The same factors associated with skin-to-skin interactions that protect healthy development in premature infants are important for term babies (Anderson, 1989; Anderson et al., 2003; Bergman, 2005; Christensson et al., 1992; Gray, Watt & Blass, 2000; Kennel & Klaus, 1998; Montagu, 1978). Infants seem to cry less when they engage in skin-to-skin interaction (Kennel & Klaus, 1998). Skin-to-skin interactions in the early postpartum period enrich and increase duration of exclusive nursing (Mikeil-Kostrya et. al, 2002). In contrast, separating mothers and babies with clothing apparently reduces intercutaneous contact with long-term implications. Infants who spend most of their time clothed apparently develop a reduced sensitivity to touch that is sustained throughout their lives (Montagu, 1978).

Ongoing Closeness: Carrying, Holding, and Rocking

Skin-to-skin and other important interactions are enhanced by ongoing proximity between mothers and infants. Round the clock maternal-infant closeness facilitates a modified form of uterine protection by enabling mothers to watch, guard, and to respond to changes in their infants' behaviors and to regulate their immature physiological systems (Anderson, 1989; Bergman, 2005; Kennel & Klaus, 1998; Ludington-Hoe et al., 2008; Ludington-Hoe et al., 1993; Ludingon-Hoe & Golant, 1993; McKenna, 1996; Small, 1998). In contrast, separation interferes with mutual self-regulation of mothers and infants, placing infants at physiological and psychological risk (Anderson, 1989).

Ongoing holding is important beyond the newborn period. It is interesting that there are cultures that promote continuous holding and carrying of infants until they are mobile (Liedloff, 1985; Valsiner, 2000). Ongoing proximity behaviors are more prevalent in traditional societies and less common in urbanized industrialized societies, where tactile contact is reduced and reflects suppressed contact among adults (Valsiner, 2000). This finding once again reiterates that behaviors associated with childcare reflect underlying themes.

While one might guess that consistent and tactile interaction has benefits for young ones, it has also been suggested that this behavior has significance for maternal development. Liedloff (1985) calls the stage where infants are constantly held the 'in arms' phase, and suggests that this behavior helps mothers actualize impulses to provide for the offspring and enriches their capacity to understand and fulfill their infants' needs. Valsiner (2000) proposes that holding infants on laps enables mothers to demonstrate their ownership of the baby. It seems that holding and carrying behaviors enable mothers to internalize their novel tasks and define their boundaries to others outside the nursing unit.

The "in arms phase" behaviors have important developmental implications for infants. Messages of caring, loving, and tenderness are conveyed to infants through consistent gentle holding and rocking movements. Montagu (1978) suggests that maximal emotional benefits are reaped when holding behaviors persist on a twenty-four hour basis. Mothers carrying infants in western style baby carriers (slings) are apparently appropriately interactive and responsive to babies' cues, and when they also sleep with their babies, their children cry infrequently (Kennel & Klaus, 1998). This evidence implies that consistent responsive interaction enriches children's world-view, helping them feel fulfilled and emotionally content.

Insight into an infant's sense of contentment is provided by Liedloff's (1985) suggestion that ongoing contact helps infants learn how to signal their needs and rely on their mothers to meet these requirements. This author indicates that intricate maternal-infant games associated with this task take place in cultures supporting proximal strategies. Ongoing closeness enables infants to engage in sole interactions, even when they are surrounded by others (Valsiner, 2000). At the same time, infants' social development is enhanced by the social cultural experiences they experience as they accompany their mothers (Dettwyler, 1995b; Liedloff, 1985; Montagu, 1978; Small, 1998; Valsiner, 2000).

In addition, infants' experience of maternal movement provides them with unique vestibular experiences with likely positive implications for later motor skills (Liedloff, 1985; Montagu, 1978; Valsiner, 2000). The motion is calming (Valsiner, 2000) and, interestingly, is mirrored in lullabies and songs sang to children (Montagu, 1978). The salience of vestibular movement for calming is suggested by a study on one week old nursing babies that found that mothers used walking or rocking to soothe their infants (Hill, Humenick, & Tieman, 1997).

The sensations and notions that infants internalize through their experiences of constant holding provide the basis for the development of true independence from the mother when the child is ready to move out of the in arms phase of development (Liedloff, 1985). Several researchers indicate that children who are held eventually and independently move out of their mothers' arms and explore their environment (Liedloff, 1985, McKenna, 1996; Valsiner, 2000). Independence through constant dependence is an important concept in cultures supporting proximity behaviors and child led processes (McKenna, 1996). Moreover, Liedloff (1985) suggests that interfering with children's needs for independence and in arms behaviors may potentially impair development of healthy emotional well being.

Co-Sleeping

Cultures that enable infants to develop through in arms interactions also encourage mothers and infants to remain close during the night (Liedloff, 1985). Bedsharing enables infants to experience a sense of physical closeness and continued care from the mother, regardless of her state of sleep (McKenna, 1996; Valsiner, 2000). It is important to acknowledge false beliefs implying that co-sleeping is risky for infants and children (Nakamura, Wind, & Danello, 1999) and to note that research has demonstrated that these fears are unwarranted when bedsharing is part of related family practices (Okami, Weisner, & Olmstead, 2002) and when mothers' arousal states are not hampered by intoxicating or mind altering substances (Baddock, Galland, Bolton, Williams & Taylor, 2006).

Moreover, there are protective elements to co-sleeping. Maternal-infant bedsharing is an imperative survival strategy, allowing mothers to regulate infants' immature physiological systems (McKenna, 1996). Mothers who share their beds with their children touch, look, and check their infants more frequently than mothers who do not sleep with their offspring, even if the infant's cot is adjacent to the mother's bed. Bedsharing mothers also respond more quickly and more frequently to their infants than their solitary sleeping counterparts (Baddock et al., 2006).

The protective aspects of co-sleeping are strongly suggested by research implying that maternal-infant co-sleeping reduces the risk of 'Sudden Infant Death Syndrome' (SIDS) (McKenna, 1996; McKenna & Mosko, 1993; McKenna et al., 1997). The physiologically correct supine or side lying positions that infants are placed in opposite their mothers' faces protects babies by enabling them to breathe in their mothers' carbon dioxide, stimulating respiration. In addition, continued physical contact allows dyads to coordinate their sleep cycles, increasing the infant's level of arousal and decreasing periods of deep sleep. The contribution of co-sleeping to maternal regulation and infant physiology is also demonstrated by findings that shared sleeping quarters help mothers and children coordinate their arousal periods. These strategies protect infants by augmenting their capacity to remain oxygenated (McKenna, 1996; Pollard et al., 1999). Hence, closeness during the night increases the frequency of maternal cue reading and protective behaviors and guards infants from serious developmental life threatening impediments.

Maternal-child bedsharing has additional health implications, including facilitating frequent nursing sessions (Baddock et al., 2006; McKenna, 1996) and increasing the duration of nursing (Ball, 2002; Gorman, 2002; McKenna, 1996). Co-sleeping is also important for older nursing children, facilitating the maintenance of adequate milk production, even after the addition of solids after six months of age (Slusser & Powers, 1997; Stein et al., 2002). It is also important that although infants might cue frequently and children may nurse during the night long beyond infancy, nursing mates meet for short nursing sessions that do not usually require the dyads to fully awaken. It is most interesting that mothers nurse their children and engage in mutual touching with their children while both seem to be in a deep state of sleep (McKenna, 1996). Some co-sleeping nursing mothers claim that they never feel they wake up to nurse and find bedsharing a convenient way to cope with nighttime nursing sessions (Ball, 2002). Shared sleeping arrangements promote the duration and frequency of nursing and accommodate the nursing partners' sleep requirements.

Nighttime proximity plays a special role in enhancing children's emotional development by providing them with a sense of ongoing accessibility to the objects that signify security. In contrast, children who sleep in solitary conditions tend to have more complex bedtime routines and are more likely to have sleep aids, as well transitional objects, than children who co-sleep with their parents (Hayes et al., 1996). Co-sleeping may also act as a means of compensating children who are physically separated from their mothers during the day. Co-sleeping is promoted for children who spend time away from their mothers during the day, allowing them to make up for lost nursing time (Maher, 1995). Research shows that co-sleeping varies between families, and in some might also include the father (Ball, 2002), implying that the emotional well being facilitated by bedsharing may extend to other members of the family. In light of these findings, it is not surprising that research indicates that bedsharing is associated with positive child outcome (Okami et al., 2002). In addition to other benefits, co-sleeping enriches relational development and combines with other proximity behaviors to promote child development.

Implications of the Physiology of Nursing and Associated Behaviors for the Family

Physiologically based nursing patterns that match infant and children's physiological and emotional development are facilitated by proximity behaviors. At the same time, nursing in tune with physiology promotes proximity behaviors. The mutuality between these sets of behaviors points to their interdependence, and the essentiality of proximity behaviors for nursing. Hence, families nursing in tune with physiologically based principles likely arrange their families in a unique manner that facilitates closeness, interdependence, and exclusivity between members of the nursing subsystem.

The Psychological Development of Infants and Children in Nursing Systems

An important implication of the physiology of nursing and of the associated bidirectional proximity behaviors is that mothers and nursing children are involved in a relationship. Several of the behaviors that take place during the relationship appear to have emotional implications. Psychological theories help one decipher emotional components and understand how exactly nursing contributes to the building of healthy relationships, and the significance of this for child development.

There are various theories explaining relational development in children. Several of the models include attachment theory, object relations theory, separation-individuation theory, and models describing emotional regulation, the contribution of child temperament, parental attributions of child behavior, and the goodness of fit between parent and child. We will only look briefly at the paradigms that seem to provide the best explanations of physiology of nursing in psychological terms. Readers interested in learning more about additional theories may read Landy and Menna's (2006) book for more details.

There are differences between theories. However, most support the view that children's early relationships affect their ability to form relationships. Most theories imply that the quality of interactions that infants' experience with their primary caregivers, usually their mothers, help them formulate ideas about what to expect from and how to interact in relationships with others (Ainsworth, 1979; Ainsworth, Blehar, Waters, & Wall, 1978; Bell, 1974; Bowlby, 1987; Brazelton & Yogman, 1986; Crockenberg, Lyons-Ruth, & Dickstein, 1993; Fairbairn, 2002c; Fogel, 1993; Fraiberg, 1987; Fraiberg, Adelson, & Shapiro, 1987; Klein, 1997a, 1997b, 1998; Lyons-Ruth & Zeanah,

1993; Mahler, Pine & Bergman, 1975; Main, 1995; Oately & Jenkins, 1996; Scharff, 1997; Stern, 1974; Tronick, 1989; Tronick, Cohn & Shea, 1986; Weininger, 1984, 1989, 1992, 1993, 1996; Winnicott, 1957, 1958, 1964). In this section, the most prominent theories will be briefly reviewed, allowing clinicians to understand the contribution of nursing to healthy relational development.

Symbiosis and Individuation

Mothers and infants set the stage for dyadic mutuality during their symbiotic pre-birth existence (Chamberlain, 1997a, 1997b; Verny & Kelly, 1981). A few psychological theories acknowledge maternal-infant physiological symbiosis, although they do not refer specifically to physiology. These paradigms imply that infants initially experience a sense of oneness with the mother. The role of the mother is to patiently accept her infant's behaviors. In healthy relationships, children eventually understand that they are separate beings and individuate from the mother (Fairbairn, 2002b). It is interesting to note the similarity between the concepts of the infant's emerging sense of separateness, the moving away from the in arms phase described by Liedloff (1985), and the physiological based process of gradual weaning from the breast. The congruence between these concepts reinforces that there are developmental reasons for physiologically based mother-child closeness and gradual weaning, emphasizing the normalcy of this process.

Attachment Theory

Attachment theory discusses the psychological processes that help children formulate ideas about themselves in relation to others, often called internal models of relationships. This theory implies that infants have needs and that they inform others about their needs through cues. The quality of maternal responsiveness to infant cues, called sensitivity and attunement in attachment paradigms, determines how secure children will feel in their relationships. Mothers who sensitively respond to cues, and match their responses to the needs, help children develop a sense of security that enables them to trust and interact with others in a positive manner. Infants whose cues are answered intermittently, inconsistently, or ignored, or worse, infants who endure maltreatment, do not internalize this sense of security and are said to develop insecure, avoidant, ambivalent, or disorganized ways of relating to others. Children learn that they can depend on others when their primary caregivers – usually their mothers – match their responses to children's needs. The quality of sensitivity that children experience in their early relationships affects their interactions in relationships with others

(Ainsworth, 1979; Ainsworth et al. 1978; Bowlby, 1987; Cramer, 1986; Goldberg, 1991; Karen, 1990, 1994; Main, 1995).

Object Relations Theory

Object relations theory also refers to the importance of maternal behaviors and their impact on child development. The focus of this paradigm is on infants' interpretations of their experiences and the maternal capacity to emotionally support infant responses to events. Infants' subjective interpretations do not always mirror objective events. Suitably, these interpretations are called "phantasies" (correct spelling in object relations texts) (Fairbairn, 2002c, Fox, 1996; Greenberg & Mitchell, 2000; Isaacs, 1997; Klein, 1997a, 1998; Scharff, 1997; Scharff & Savege Scharff, 1991; Segal, 1992; Solomon, 1995; Sullivan, 1972; Weininger, 1989, 1992, 1993; Winnicott, 1958).

This theory implies that infants cope with their interpretations of the world by splitting their objects into parts. Infants see their mothers as a conglomeration of many part objects, including the breast part object. Similarly, feelings about part objects are also split, and objects are considered good, giving, and kind or bad, attacking, and withholding, depending on the quality of the infant's experience.

At first, the infant focuses on the part that gives comfort and relieves stress from hunger, thirst, and other experiences. The maternal breast is this part and the central context for "phantasies." It is important to note that this model does not refer to the physiology of lactation, but rather discusses the breast as a context for interaction. The breast object triggers emotions and thoughts about the relational world. From the infant's perspective, the breast is seen as a separate and fully functioning object. At times, the breast fills the child with pleasant feelings, and at other times, the infant might see the breast as damaging and hurtful. For example, an infant might interpret the breast as withholding when it flows slowly or attacking when it flows too quickly.

The role of the mother is to tolerate and patiently help the infant deal with their interpretation of encounters with objects. In this model, words such as patience, tolerance, acceptance, holding, and containing are used when referring to maternal behaviors that support optimal relational development. This model also reinforces the in arms concept (Liedloff, 1985) and implies that the all containing mother is everything for the infant until the child gradually develops an understanding that allows them to see others as important.

Winnicott (1958) indicated that maternal capacity was not perfect and that it was emotionally sufficient for mothers to be "good enough." This theorist indicated that the good enough mother and child are initially one unit. Initially, the good enough mother does and is everything for the young infant. This part of the theory is congruent with theories of symbiosis discussed previously. When mothers respond in a good enough fashion, infants feel emotionally contained or held by their mothers. Emotionally contained infants eventually realize that they and their mother are not one object. They cope with this loss and realize that the breast is part of the mother. They are able to see the mother as a whole object and gradually individuate. Infants transfer their feelings about interactions, internalized through interchanges with the breast, to their mother as a whole person, and similar to others theories, eventually to others (Fairbairn, 2002a; Fox, 1996; Greenberg & Mitchell, 2000; Isaacs, 1997; Klein, 1997a, 1997b, 1998; Scharff, 1997; Scharff & Savege Scharff, 1991; Segal, 1992; Solomon 1995; Sullivan, 1972; Weininger, 1984, 1989, 1992, 1993, 1996; Winnicott, 1957, 1958, 1964, 1994, 1997a; 1997b).

Emotional Development

Some theorists focus on children's emerging ability to understand and regulate emotional responses. From this perspective, mother-infant interactions facilitate transactions with others by enabling infants to learn to recognize and eventually to manage their emotional responses (Lyons-Ruth & Zeanah, 1993; Oately & Jenkins, 1996; Tronick et al., 1986). Infants copy elements of their interactions with their mothers in their interchanges with others (Bell, 1974; Brazelton & Yogman, 1986; Stern, 1974; Tronick et al., 1986).

Implications of Psychological Theory for the Nursing Relationship

Theories about healthy relational development emphasize the importance of answering infant and children's cues. Research on interactions between nursing mothers and children demonstrates that breastfeeding plays an important role in facilitating mutual emotional exchanges that contribute to the children's sense of being heard (Epstein, 1993). This research also suggests that nursing contributes to maternal development by allowing mothers to experience cue reading and feedback from children. It seems that nursing contributes to the development of internal models of relationships that facilitate interaction.

Healthy relational development through interactions with responsive, sensitive, patient, containing, and good enough mothers contributes to children's capacity to interact with others. The skills internalized are transferred to interactions with others, especially fathers, who may strengthen or alter the lessons learned. Diverse interactions will strengthen infant's relational capacities (Lamb, 1980, 1987). However, mothers are the primary object of interest, and it is common for infants and young children to retain a vision of the mother as the central comforting object in early childhood (Ainsworth et al, 1978; Bowlby, 1987; Fairbain, 2002c; Weininger, 1992, 1993; Winnicott, 1957, 1958, 1964).

Maternal Development through Nursing

The discussion on children's relational growth and nursing demonstrates that mothers' behaviors play an important role in child development. The information on maternal development implies that mothers' capacity to support healthy development is contingent on past experiences and events, such as mothering, in the here and now. Mothers mirror their internal models in all interactions, including those with children. Positive models are important resources for mothers, facilitating emotional availability (Ainsworth et al., 1978; Fraiberg et al., 1987; Main, 1995). Mothers' experience in the present is an important influence on mothering behaviors. Positive attributions of parenting and children's behaviors facilitate caring parenting behaviors (Grusec, Rudy, & Martini, 1997; Slep & O'Leary, 1998). In accordance with theories of perceived self-efficacy (Bandura, 1989), responsive caring is enhanced when mothers are confident and feel that they are efficient in their parenting capacities (Bugental, Blue, & Cruzcosa, 1989; Teti & Gelfand, 1991). Mothers' capacity to emotionally contain infants is enhanced when mothers feel that they are supported (Fish, Stifter, & Belsky, 1993; Unger & Wandersman, 1985; Winnicott, 1957, 1997a). The impact of maternal mood on parenting capacities is demonstrated by studies showing that depression decreases mothers' interactional capacities with their infants (Field, Hernandez-Reif, & Feijo, 2002; Fleming, Ruble, Flett, & Shaul, 1988; Korja et al., 2008; Persson-Blenow, Naslund, McNeil, Kaij, & Maimquist-Larson, 1984; Persson-Blenow, Naslund, McNeil, & Kaij, 1986). Hence, most of the traits affecting mothering indicate that mothers' perception of past and present experience influence their capacity to interact with their children.

Maternal Perceptions

Research dedicated specifically to the contribution of nursing to maternal development replicates the findings indicating that nursing is an important context for development. One salient finding is that mothers' feelings about breastfeeding affect their behaviors and these behaviors subsequently affect additional emotions and attitudes (Blyth et al., 2002; Bottorf, 1990; Ceriani Cernadas, Noceda, Barrera, Martinez & Garsd, 2003; Cooke, Sheehan, & Schmied, 2003; Dennis, 1999; Friedman, 1996; Gill, 1998; Leff, Gagne, & Jeffries, 1994; McLeod et al., 2002; Rabuzzi, 1994; Vandiver, 1997). For some mothers, nursing is perceived as part of the female continuum (Rich, 1986). Some mothers find nursing gratifying (Gill, 1998). This perception facilitates exclusive nursing (Ceriani Cernadas et al., 2003). The ability to reframe possible negative experiences (Cooke et al., 2003) and an understanding of the important outcomes of nursing helps mothers continue nursing when it is difficult (Creedy et al., 2003; Dennis, 1999; Torres, Torres, Parrilla Rodriguez, & Dennis, 2003). Previous accomplishments outside of nursing, feedback from others (Blyth et al., 2002), and the capacity to fulfill expectations of the nursing relationship also help mothers nurse (Hauck & Irurita, 2003).

The powerful impact of the nursing experience on mothers and their attitudes is evident in findings that mothers of older children describe nursing differently from mothers of younger infants (Blum, 1999). The good enough feelings that mothers internalize through nursing over time serve them well. These attributions help them cope with the negative cultural feedback associated with nursing a toddler in a western culture (Kendall-Tackett & Sugarman, 1995).

Confidence and Sense of Efficacy

One enduring implication of nursing for maternal development is the positive affect of nursing on maternal self-regard. Britton and Britton (2008) indicate that mothers who nurse exclusively likely come to nursing with intact self-concepts. Apparently, a positive self-concept determines mothers' capacity to nurse exclusively, and mothers with a positive sense of self in several domains are more likely to engage in exclusive nursing than mothers with negative self-concepts. Yet, these researchers also postulate that perhaps the experience of nursing also contributes to the development of a positive self-regard. One way that nursing enhances the development of maternal positive self-regard is by facilitating the development of a sense of efficacy (Epstein, 1993; La Leche League, 2004; Maclean, 1990; Rich, 1986; UNICEF, 1998b). Efficacy in this context means that mothers feel that they are capable of satisfying and meeting their infants' needs and are able to care for and protect their children through nursing. Some mothers focus on the amount of milk that they believe they produce, while others look for infant behaviors as feedback. Pridham, Schroeder, Brown and Clark (2001) suggest that mothers who are most attuned to their infants concentrate on their infants' behaviors rather than on their milk supply. Behaviors important to mothers include infant attachment and suckling, and signs that infants enjoy nursing. Some mothers respond to signs of infant satiety, such as falling asleep at the breast after nursing, as a means of gauging their efficiency. This last example suggests that in some cases mothers' perceptions of their milk supply and infant behaviors are interrelated variables providing information to mothers about their self-worth as nursing mothers (Ceriani Cernadas et al., 2003; Cooke et al., 2003; Hill, Hanson, & Mefford, 1994; Leff et al., 1994; Libbus & Kolostov, 1994). When mothers feel good enough about their ability to nurse or meet their infants' needs through breastfeeding, they continue nursing, including when there are difficulties (Cooke et al., 2003; Creedy et al., 2003; Dennis, 1999; Torres et al., 2003).

Regard for the Infant

Along with facilitating the development of confidence, nursing seems to endear infants to their mothers, and this also facilitates mothering behaviors (Benson Brown & McPherson, 1998; Blum, 1999; Buckley, 1992; Epstein, 1993; Kitzinger, 1979; Maclean, 1990; Rich 1986). For example, mothers are more likely to continue nursing when their infants' behaviors are similar to the mothers' expectations of how infants conduct themselves at the breast, and when they perceive that their children have an easy temperament. A sense of affection towards a baby also affects mothering, and nursing is facilitated when mothers believe that they feel attached to their infants (Ceriani Cernadas et al., 2003; Cooke et al., 2003; Matthews, 1991; Pridham et al., 2001; Vandiver, 1997).

Needs for Intimacy and Closeness

Infant behaviors contribute to mothering by meeting mothers' needs. Many mothers perceive that nursing provides them with a valuable sense of intimacy and bonding with their infant (Epstein, 1993; Kendall-Tackett & Sugarman, 1995; Rich, 1986; Schmied & Barclay, 1999). For some, this is accompanied by a highly valued sense of embodiment with the nursling (Saha, 2002; Schmied & Barclay, 1999), reminiscent of the infants' sense of oneness with their mothers. Mothers' reports of affinity towards other mothers' children whom they have nursed also attest to the sense of closeness and intense emotionality that mothers attribute to nursing (Angier, 2000; Benson Brown & McPherson, 1998; Blum, 1999; Giles, 2003; Kendall-Tackett & Sugarman, 1995; Kitzinger, 1979; Maclean, 1990; Saha, 2002; Schmied & Barclay, 1999).

Mothers' respect for closeness infers that mothers' feelings about their body and sense of self in relation to others also affect their perceptions of the nursing experience and behaviors. Mothers who enjoy nursing due to their belief that it is part of a natural continuum of natural processes illustrate the impact of this aspect of maternal meaning on nursing. Similarly, some mothers feel that nursing contributes to their body image and is integral to the mothering role, helping them nurture and form a bond with their infants. Mothers who enjoy nursing and revere the lifestyle associated with nursing also show how maternal perceptions of self in relation to others affect the nursing experience (Blum, 1999; Cooke et al., 2003; Leff et al., 1994).

Opportunities to Practice Sensitive Cue Reading

The good enough feelings that mothers seem to internalize about themselves and their infant through nursing likely contribute to their capacity to respond to the frequent nature of nursing. Frequent nursing sessions, the centrality of infant cues in the regulation of nursing, the intricate and intense interactions during nursing, and displays of positive infant affect seems to facilitate the development of sensitive mothering styles (Epstein, 1993). This study, like other research (Kuzela, Stifter, & Worobey, 1990), indicates that mother-infant interactions during breastfeeding are mirrored in between nursing sessions. Thus the sensitive mothering style apparently extends beyond nursing and has important implications for maternal and child development.

Facilitating Mothering in Compromised Situations

The facilitative features of nursing are also apparent for mothers in compromised situations, such as in depression. Mothers suffering from depression are less likely to nurse (Galler, Harrison, Biggs, Ramsey, & Forde, 1999). When they do nurse, mothers with depression breastfeed less often, wean earlier, and score lower on the breastfeeding confidence scale than mothers without depression (Field et al., 2002). Nevertheless, the same study found that non-nursing mothers with depression are less confident and more irritable than their nursing counterparts. This finding points to the significance of nursing in compromised situations. Accordingly, mothers suffering from depression who do not nurse are less emotionally available and attuned to their infants than they could have been if they had nursed. This information in combination with the research associating maternal depression with negative child outcome (Canadian Paediatric Society, 2004) emphasizes the importance of nursing for maternal and child development. Moreover, it is important to remember the physiologically based aspects of nursing that protect mothers from risk factors associated with depression (Groër & Davis, 2006; Groër et al., 2002; Kendall-Tackett, 2005, 2007; Mezzacappa, 2004).

Ambivalence and Weaning

The complexity of nursing for maternal scripts is also evident in the ambivalence associated with breastfeeding (First, 1994; Schmied & Barclay, 1999; Winnicott, 1997a). The literature suggests that maternal ambivalence about nursing contributes to early weaning. Blaffer Hrdy (1999, p. 491) suggests that some mothers see nursing beyond infancy as a binding experience and "fear that an infant attached means the mother enchained." Rabuzzi (1988) adds that some women in western cultures comply with patriarchal concepts that women's bodily sensations are irrelevant and should be disregarded. These authors' findings imply that many women deviate from a physiologically based nursing trajectory in order to avoid the negative connotations attributed to nursing beyond infancy. Mothers may also wean early when they focus on problems, don't identify with the role of the nursing mother, perceive that nursing is exhausting, and dislike the lifestyle associated with nursing (Cooke et al., 2003). Feelings of sensuality associated with nursing make some mothers uncomfortable with nursing (Rich, 1986; Rodriguez-Garcia & Frazier, 1995).

Loss and Grief

Early weaning may have persisting emotional implications for some mothers. Some feel emotional pain, grief, and negative self-perceptions following the loss of a desired nursing experience (Angier, 2000; Benson Brown & McPherson, 1998; Maclean, 1990; McLeod et al., 2002; Rich, 1986; Walker, 1993). Some mothers feel that they have failed when they wean earlier than expected, a sentiment associated with risk for postpartum depression (McLeod et al., 2002). Other mothers display negative attitudes and display a diminished sense of control (Dick et al., 2002). Mothers who were never able to actualize desired nursing relationships are believed to experience guilt and loss (Guttman & Zimmerman, 2000). It is hopeful, however, that mothers' subsequent nursing experiences may repair feelings of guilt and despair (Giles, 2003).

Implications of Nursing for Maternal Development

Nursing seems to contribute to mothers' capacity to develop sensitive mothering via relational experiences that add to the hormonal factors discussed in the section on physiology. This information emphasizes that nursing contributes significantly to maternal behavior and bidirectional development in breastfeeding families. Additional literature shows that these interactions between the nursing dyad (in some cases nursing triads) are influenced by the quality of support that mothers receive, especially from fathers (Blyth et al., 2002; Bronner, Barber, Vogelhut, & Resnik, 2001; Giugliani, Caiaffa, Vogelhut, Witter, & Perman, 1994; Heinig, 2001; Kistin, Abramson, & Dublin, 1994; Libbus & Kolostov, 1994). This information is consistent with family systems theories of mutual contingency and influence (Goldenberg & Goldenberg, 2007), and implies that in order to understand interactions in the nursing family, it will be helpful to also look at the development of fathers and their interactions with the nursing subsystem.

Paternal Development in Nursing Systems

Distinct Developmental Trajectory

There are several theories that facilitate our understanding of fathers in nursing systems. The literature reviewed above on the influence of internal models of interaction and parental attribution and cognition on mothering is relevant for fathers. However, at the same time, it is important to note that a salient finding of a review of the literature on fathers is that men follow distinct trajectories to fatherhood that differ from female development.

Differences between maternal and paternal paths to parenting are already evident in the prenatal period when, for example, women demonstrate more confidence about their future caregiving capacities than men do. The differences between mothers and fathers continue after birth. After an initial period of engrossment with the newborn, fathers tend to reduce their level of engagement and distance themselves from the intense mother-child bond. Research suggests that many fathers focus on their role as providers, engaging in playful exchanges and secondary caregiving roles during infancy (Griswold, 1993; Klaus & Klaus, 1998; Lamb, 1980, 1987; Lewis, 1986; Litton Fox, Bruce, & Combs-Orme, 2000; Pedersen, Anderson & Cain, et al., 1980; Pruett, 1997). Current and traditional psychological models also note that supportive tasks are another salient component of early fathering (Aldous, Mulligan, & Bjarnason, 1998; Lewis, 1986; Stern, 1985; Weininger, 1984; Winnicott, 1958, 1964). Fathers mirror infant development in their trajectory to fatherhood and increase their parenting tasks and engagement to reflect their children's increased interest in them as separate objects.

Fathers and Decisions about Nursing

Even though attention has been paid to paternal function in nursing systems, the information is inconclusive. Diverse views are apparent in the literature on paternal decision making. Some theorists indicate that men see nursing as a female task and allow mothers to make all of the decisions in this regard (Lewis, 1986). In contrast, several studies indicate that parents collaborate on decisions about nursing (Buckner & Matsubara 1993; Dick et al. 2002;

Giuglani et al., 1994; Jordan, 1990; Littman, Mendendorp, & Goldfarb, 1994; Sharma & Petosa, 1997). Some authors maintain that fathers influence decisions about the duration of nursing (Cohen, Lange, & Slusser, 2002) and others disagree with this view (Dick et al., 2002).

Paternal Perceptions and Support

A conclusion that one might come to from the information on paternal decision making is that fathers may play an important role in the development of the nursing unit. A salient concept in the literature is that fathers have the ability to support nursing relationships. The quality of paternal support is however contingent on fathers' attitudes and perceptions about nursing. Fathers may develop attitudes that help them support breastfeeding by attending educational programs about breastfeeding (Susin & Giugliani, 2008). Facilitative attitudes include a sense of involvement and the view that nursing promotes child health and welfare (Jordan & Wall, 1993; Pollock, Bustamante-Forest, & Giarrantano, 2002; Sharma & Petosa, 1997). Realistic perceptions of breastfeeding and associated behaviors help fathers encourage and sustain nursing (Losch, Durgy, Russell, & Dusdieker, 1995). In addition, paternal support is facilitated when fathers respect the nursing mother, perceive that they are efficient in their supportive tasks (Sharma & Petosa, 1997), and believe that they will have special time with the infant (Jordan & Wall, 1993; Losch et al., 1995; Pollock et al., 2002; Sharma & Petosa, 1997).

Fathers' supportive tasks and positive attitude may contribute to the development of healthy nursing relations. For example, paternal support contributes to the development of exclusive nursing (Ceriani Cernadas et al., 2003; Susin & Giugliani, 2008). In addition, supportive fathers may increase maternal self-esteem in relation to nursing and help mothers cope with nursing difficulties (Amper, 1996; Buckner & Matsubara, 1993).

Fathers, like their partners, also require support in order to sustain and encourage their partners and infants. Unfortunately, the research implies that fathers do not always receive adequate support, and this impairs their capacity to contain the nursing mother and child (Jordan & Wall, 1993). Fathers' ability to support nursing relationships are also impeded by disdain for and misconceptions about nursing, views that artificial feeding is easier and better than nursing, and views that nursing is mainly a means of feeding that excludes them from developing a relationship with their children. Paternal feelings of envy, exclusion, and subsequent resentment are notable aspects of the trajectory to parenting for some fathers, regardless of whether the child is nursing or not (Lewis, 1986; Litton Fox et al., 2000; Pruett, 1997).

These feelings disable fathers from supporting a nursing relationship (Freed, Fraley, & Schanler, 1993; Jordan, 1990; Jordan & Wall, 1993; Pollock et al., 2002; Saha, 2002; Sharma & Petosa, 1997).

Fathers' behaviors are also contingent on their relationship with the mother and their perception of couple issues. Some fathers find it difficult to support nursing when they perceive that mothers are frustrated with or ambivalent about breastfeeding. Paternal incapacity to simultaneously see partners and breasts as sexual and as motherly, as well as concerns that nursing disfigures sexual breasts, decrease fathers' ability to support nursing in some cases (Jordan & Wall, 1993; Sharma & Petosa, 1997). Similarly, some fathers have a difficult time supporting nursing when they believe that nursing decreases their partners' interest in sexual intimacy (Benson Brown & McPherson, 1998; Hyde, DeLamater, Plant & Byrd, 1996; Rodriguez-Garcia & Frazier, 1995; Sharma & Petosa, 1997).

Implications of Paternal Development for the Nursing Family

An important implication of paternal development in nursing systems is that parents have gender distinct trajectories to parenthood and different functions in the nursing system. Yet, there are also similarities between parents. Both mothers and fathers are affected by their perceptions and feelings. Paternal function may mirror fathers' feelings about their relationship with the mother. The quality of paternal functioning may affect the nursing relationship. Hence, a significant contributing factor to paternal function is the quality of the parental couple's relationship.

The Development of the Couple Relationship in the Nursing System

Mutual Influence

The influence of the couple relationship on fathers concurs with data showing that the parent-child relationship is part of a complex interactive system and that interactions between the couple affect the quality of parenting (Pedersen et al., 1980; Valsiner, 2000). For example, paternal support augments maternal caregiving capacities (Crockenberg et al., 1993) and the development of sensitive mothering styles (Parke, 1996; Winnicott, 1964). Mothers influence the degree of paternal involvement in parenting (Beitel & Parke, 1998; Doherty, Kouneski, & Erikson, 1998). These findings are replicated in research on breastfeeding (Litton Fox et al., 2000). Fathers suit their level of involvement to their perceptions of their partners' sense of confidence in their parenting skills (McBride & Rane, 1998). In addition, parents may affect one another's function as parents. For example, Feldman, Weller, Sirota and Eidelman (2003) demonstrated how fathers mirrored maternal proximity behaviors when they engaged in kangaroo care – a style of parenting where infants are worn on another's body in an ongoing manner.

Incorporation of Novel Roles and Tasks

The mutual affect of parents on one another is evident as parents attempt to redefine their roles and incorporate new tasks associated with the birth of a new baby. These transitional functions may challenge first time parents and those with older children. Transitions may be especially difficult when novel tasks interfere with existing interactions (Belsky & Hsieh, 1998; Belsky & Kelly, 1994; Carter & McGoldrick, 1989; Cowan & Cowan, 1999).

Shared Meaning and Communication Style

The transition is facilitated when couples have similar themes from their families of origin and like philosophies (Carter & McGoldrick, 1989). The capacity of couples to jointly support a nursing relationship, for example, might be affected by the degree of similarity in their views of closeness and intimacy (Combrinck-Graham & Kerns, 1989) and their perspectives of the significance of sexual relations for the parental couple (Benson Brown & McPherson, 1998; Rodriguez-Garcia & Frazier, 1995; Sharma & Petosa, 1997). Couple function is also regulated by the partners' communication style. An open communication style enables couples to state truthful feelings, accept differences and create joint philosophies, develop their unique trajectories to parenthood, and reciprocate one another's efforts. Hence, shared meaning facilitated by open communication facilitates the transition to parenting and the continuation of optimal couple function (Beitel & Parke, 1998; Belsky & Hsieh, 1998; Belsky & Kelly, 1994; Carter & McGoldrick, 1989; Cowan & Cowan, 1999; Crockenberg et al., 1993; Doherty et al., 1998; Galinsky, 1987; McBride & Rane, 1998; Parke, 1996; Pedersen et al., 1980; Satir, 1967).

Complementary versus Sameness Models of Task Allocation

Some theorists propose that couple function is enhanced when parents engage in similar parenting tasks (Cowan & Cowan, 1999; Goodrich, Rampage, Ellman, & Halstead, 1988; Held, 1984). For example, Cowan and Cowan's suggestion that fathers intermittently feed nursing infants exemplifies how equal task allocation is interpreted for breastfeeding families. The salience of this view is indicated by Blum's (1999) suggestion that some therapists are dissuaded from supporting nursing due to their perception that nursing interferes with equal task allocation and impairs healthy couple function.

Other theorists promote complementary task allocations. In this paradigm, partners reciprocate one another's efforts by engaging in different tasks that reflect their distinct qualities, including biological and gender differences. Apparently, complementary systems of task allocation strengthens the family and enhances the development of individual nurturing capacities and gender specific trajectories (Beavers, 1977; Ehrensaft, 1983; Goodrich et al., 1988; Held, 1984; Kelly, 1983; Silverman & Auerbach, 1999). Similar to other aspects of couple function, complementary interactions are facilitated by open discourse, mutual respect, and joint ownership of philosophies (Belsky & Hsieh, 1998; Belsky & Kelly, 1994; Carter & McGoldrick, 1989; Cowan & Cowan, 1999; McBride & Rane, 1998; Parke, 1996; Satir, 1967).

Clinicians influenced by feminist models that disagree with essentiality paradigms – models acknowledging biological and gender differences (Silverstein & Auerbach, 1999) – may have difficulty supporting clients displaying a complementary style of task allocation. This perspective is in line with feminist arguments that reference to female biology discredits women and their development and perpetuates hierarchical and patriarchal attitudes. Similarly, mothering and traditional female roles are believed to enslave and devalue women. Women are only equal when they are freed from traditional roles (Bassin, 1994; Chodorow, 1978; Dinnerstein, 1977; Eyer, 1992; Firestone, 1970; Silverman, 2003). However, while recognizing that there are valid aspects to this argument, it is important to note that this view ignores the positive contribution of biology to female development and, paradoxically, might actually contribute to the devaluation of the female experience. Their suggestions are reminiscent of biological eradication during the Middle Ages, when women were impelled to use wet nurses in order to service their husbands, rather than experience their womanhood.

Another school of feminist thought recognizes how biological experiences contribute to women's development. A maximizing approach validates women's biological experiences and presents motherhood as an important aspect of female development. Yet, nursing has not received the same attention as other female experiences, likely due to the perception that nursing impedes employment outside of the home, an apparent means of attaining equality. It is important to note, however, that in traditional cultures, women simultaneously mother and work at other jobs (Carter, 1995; Kitzinger, 1995; Maher, 1995; Palmer, 2009; Rabuzzi, 1994; Rich, 1986; Thurer, 1994).

Careful clinicians may refer to the attributes of the diverse feminist theorists and the developmental models discussed previously and apply them to the context of nursing. One may note that complementary models allow couples to integrate the physiological basis of the nursing relationship and associated gender specific tasks into their couple relationships. Lay literature shows that parental couples in nursing families complement rather than duplicate one another's tasks as described in *The Womanly Art of Breastfeeding* (La Leche League, 2004).

Research Specific to Breastfeeding

The research specifically on couple interactions in breastfeeding families is scarce in comparison to reviews of couples in non-breastfeeding families. The example of recommendations that fathers bottle feed nursing infants demonstrates the problems associated with applying terms of non-nursing to the context of breastfeeding. One interesting study on couples with breastfeeding infants concluded that although the quality of the parents' relationship affects paternal caregiving behaviors and support, it does not impact breastfeeding (Falceto, Giugliani, & Fernandes, 2004). However, this study looked at couples with young nursing infants who terminated nursing at a few months of age. It seems that this research might have come to different conclusions if the study had included parents of older nursing children.

Thus the information on the specific impact of nursing on couples over time is not readily available. Yet, the complexity of the nursing relationship and associated behaviors and our understanding of parents' mutual influence on one another seem to suggest that nursing beyond infancy would impact couple interaction. It is easy to understand how the lack of research might affect clinical work. Practitioners, especially those without personal nursing experience, might have difficulty understanding the issues presented by couples with children displaying physiologically based nursing patterns and require more information to advance their practice.

Implications of the Development of the Parental Couple for the Nursing Family System

Although the existing literature does not provide specific details about parenting couples in nursing systems, we can apply some of the concepts about couples in general to this context. We understand that couples have to alter their existing scripts to accommodate novel and gender-specific tasks. A complementary style of role and task allocation enriched by open communication and shared philosophies likely facilitates couple interactions and upholds the physiologically based nursing relationship. The influence of parents on one another, parenting experiences, and couple interaction seem to suggest that the nursing relationship affects the couple and vice versa.

Family Systems Theory

Review of the impact on individual and parental couple development points to an interdependence of growth among family members. For example, we noted that infant development is influenced by maternal perceptions, maternal nursing function is facilitated by paternal support, fathers' capacity to support nursing reflects their interactions with mothers, and the parental couple relationship is likely influenced by behaviors associated with nursing. In other words, family members mutually affect one another and their capacity to function. These concepts are congruent with a family systems model (Goldenberg & Goldenberg, 2007; Nichols & Schwartz, 2006).

Systems, Subsystems, and Circular Causality

Family systems theory is a paradigm used to understand and work with families. Within this paradigm, families are large units composed of interdependent individuals who are members of changing subsystems. Individuals and subsystems mutually affect one another. Development and change in families is circular and affects all parts of the system (Goldenberg & Goldenberg, 2007; Nichols & Schwartz, 2006). An ecological model (Bronfenbrenner, 1979) adds that external sources, such as cultural and societal influences, affect the circular changes in the family system and its components.

Family members may belong to several subsystems at the same time. For example, in a nursing family with three children, the subsystems include the mother-child nursing subsystem, the parental subsystem, both parents with each individual child, one parent with one or more children, the sibling subsystem, and then variations of the sibling subsystems. The interactions in each subsystem and between different subsystems and individuals affect the quality of interactions in the family as a whole and vice versa (Goldenberg & Goldenberg, 2007; Nichols & Schwartz, 2006).

Structure, Roles, and Tasks

Unspoken rules dictate how families organize their system, including the structure of relationships and boundaries between family members (Minuchin & Fishman, 1996). This aspect of family function is facilitated by the construction of roles and tasks. Membership, roles, and tasks change according to subsystem membership and are modified to reflect the changing needs of the family system (Epstein, Bishop, Ryan, Miller, & Keitner, 1993).

Family Themes

Family organization is influenced by salient themes. One may understand a family's themes by assessing recurring attitudes and behaviors displayed by the family. Attitudes might be apparent in members' narrative or interaction. Observed behaviors are the expressions of the theme. Themes are influenced by present events and may also reflect past events transferred from generation to generation (Beavers, 1977; Bowen, 1978; Framo, 1992; Goldenberg & Goldenberg, 2007; Kerr & Bowen, 1988; Kramer, 1985; Minuchin & Fishman, 1996; Satir, 1967).

Communication Style

Family themes affect and are influenced by the way family members communicate with one another. The communication style dictates the degree of emotional expression in the family. There are various communication styles, including open and closed styles. An open communication style promotes emotional growth by allowing members to voice their feelings in an accepting context, receive validation, and find means of resolving ongoing family challenges. A closed style will do the opposite and impair families' abilities to dispel tension (Beavers, 1977; Minuchin & Fishman, 1996; Satir, 1967).

Family Life Cycle

All family processes, including communication, family themes, and structure, are affected by and also influence the changes that families make as they develop through the family life cycle (Carter & McGoldrick, 1989). The family life cycle is composed of various stages of development that reflect specific milestones. As families make transitions to new stages of the family life cycle, they alter their roles and functions to reflect the novel developmental tasks of the system at the time. For example, when a first child is born, a wife and husband add the roles of mother and father to their existing scripts, and new parent-child subsystems are added to the existing couple subsystem. The capacity of the family system to adjust to transitions is contingent on the other aspects of family function, including family themes, communication style, and structure.

Transition to Parenting and Parenting of Young Child Stage of Family Development

Breastfeeding concurs with the transition to parenting and raising young children stage of family development. The family tasks associated with this stage of development include redefining relationships to include a new child, internalizing the parenting role, and reorganizing family duties (Carter & McGoldrick, 1989; Cowan & Cowan, 1999). Parents have to learn how to integrate the task of breastfeeding into existing family functions.

Implications of Family Systems Theory for Nursing

Family systems paradigm implies that nursing mothers and infants are a subsystem that is part of a larger family system. The nursing subsystem affects family interaction in other subsystems and vice versa. Interactions in the nursing unit affect and are also influenced by all aspects of family function, including family themes, recurring behaviors, communication style, interactions at all levels, the ability to internalize novel roles and tasks, and the ability to integrate the new member into the existing family system.

Implications for Practice

In this chapter, we reviewed concepts that help the clinician define nursing as a relationship and understand the impact of nursing on individual, couple, and family function. As clinicians, we can use this information to raise our awareness of the issues specific to nursing families. We will note that families nursing in tune with physiology might have specific interactions reflecting the impact of nursing on the system and vice versa. While it is hopeful that clinicians will be able to apply these notions to practice, it is also important to remember the role of personal bias in working with clients and to take note of our feelings as a means of increasing sensitivity to nursing families.

Chapter 4
Themes Affecting Perspectives of Nursing

The Significance of Themes for Practice

Clinicians' perspectives affect their interactions with clients. In this chapter, an overview of the themes that might impair or enhance our clinical ability to hear the narratives presented by families nursing in tune with physiology will be presented. It is interesting to note that many of the themes affecting present nursing behaviors are deeply ingrained with long standing historical roots. As readers go through the chapter, they might take note of the themes that have meaning for them. This initial awareness will hopefully lead practitioners to a path that will enable them to reframe their original connotation and become more open to families.

Long Standing Physiologically Based Nursing Patterns

A review of the literature that describes the history of nursing and childhood provides insight into family themes that have relevance for current nursing families. First of all, the literature shows that nursing behaviors are influenced by cultural beliefs and practices (Dettwyler, 1995a; Fildes, 1995; Rogers et al., 1997; Quandt, 1995; Stuart-Macadam, 1995). This view is consistent with systems notions that families are affected by external sources (Bronfenbrenner, 1979; Garbarino, 1976, 1977). A review of the history of nursing shows that behaviors varied according to the families' socioeconomic status, their geographic region, and their degree of urbanization versus agricultural setting (Benson Brown & McPherson, 1998; Dettwyler, 1995a; Fildes, 1995; Golden, 2001; Palmer, 2009; Rogers et al., 1997; Stuart-Macadam, 1995; Thurer, 1994).

Nursing into Early Childhood

The literature on the history of nursing shows that throughout the ages children commonly nursed into early childhood in most cultures (Benson Brown & McPherson, 1998; Blaffer Hrdy, 1999; Dettwyler, 1995a; Fildes, 1995; Maher, 1995; McKenna, 1996; Minchin, 1998; Palmer, 2009; Stuart-Macadam, 1995; Thurer, 1994; Valsiner, 2000). This behavior continued until the twentieth century (Stein et al., 2002; Thevenin, 1976). In some cultures, children nursed exclusively for the first two years of life (Small, 1998), and in many cultures children continued to nurse until six years of age (Dettwyler,

1995a; Stuart-Macadam, 1995). The information on long standing family patterns reflects the standards for nursing suggested by present healthcare professionals and organizations that use physiological principles to develop their policies (AAP, 1994; Dewey et al., 2001; INFACT, 1999b, 2002a; Slusser & Powers, 1997; WHO, 1981, 2001, 2003). Periods of exclusive nursing and nursing into early childhood follow physiological principles and have been a normal aspect of family interaction for most of history.

Proximity Behaviors and Reverence for Women and Children

The research on the history of nursing suggests that families that engaged in long standing and physiologically based nursing patterns also displayed proximity behaviors, including carrying and co-sleeping (Baumslag & Michels, 1995; Blaffer Hrdy, 1999; Dettwyler, 1995a; Fildes, 1995; Fouts et al., 2001; Kitzinger, 1995; Quandt, 1995; Stein et al., 2002; Valsiner, 2000). Various resources show that nursing and proximity behaviors occurred in families that valued mothers, motherly love (Bassin, 1994; Blaffer Hrdy, 1999; Clarke-Stewart, 1998; Dettwyler, 1995a; Eyer, 1992; Golden, 2001; Maher, 1995; Palmer, 2009; Thurer, 1994), children (Golden, 2001; Shahar, 1990; Valsiner, 2000), and child rearing (Blaffer Hrdy, 1999; Clarke-Stewart, 1998; Eyer, 1992; Ozment, 1983). In traditional hunting and gathering societies where women's work was revered, mothers and children nursed freely for unlimited periods of time. Children were carried and co-slept with their mothers (Dettwyler, 1995a; Palmer, 2009; Stuart-Macadam, 1995). Similarly, women and children engaged in nonrestricted nursing relationships during the Neolithic Period when peace and sexual equality reigned and in medieval Germanic societies where married couples were viewed as equals. In these cultures, women owned property and children were not swaddled (Thurer, 1994). Thus evidence shows an association between physiologically based nursing patterns, proximity behaviors, and respect for women, mothering, children, and child rearing.

Obstructed Nursing Patterns

Patriarchy, Devalued Women and Children, and Mixed Messages

The likelihood that families that engage in physiologically based nursing patterns also display specific behaviors and themes is supported by literature on the history of families that veered from common nursing patterns. Families who deviated from natural nursing patterns were ruled by patriarchal systems that controlled women and children (Maher,

1995; Palmer, 2009; Thurer, 1994). Authoritarian figures interfered with families' capacity to engage in nursing by conveying mixed messages that simultaneously promoted breastmilk as superior while implying that the behaviors associated with nursing were wrong (Angier, 2000; Benson Brown & McPherson, 1998; Golden, 2001; Maher, 1995; Palmer, 2009; Shahar, 1990; Thurer, 1994; Wolf, 2001).

Couple Precedence, Distancing, and Wet-Nursing

A view that coincided with patriarchy that interfered with nursing was that conjugal relations were more important than the mother-child relationship (Benson Brown & McPherson, 1998; Blaffer Hrdy, 1999; Maher, 1995). This view was presented together with the long standing myth that sexual intimacy harms breastmilk (Benson Brown & McPherson, 1998; Blaffer Hrdy, 1999; Golden, 2001; Maher, 1995; Shahar, 1990; Thurer, 1994). In order to enable mothers to fulfill their duties as wives, while simultaneously ensuring that children received human milk untainted by sexual relations, children were sent to wet nurses (Benson Brown & McPherson, 1998; Blaffer Hrdy, 1999; Golden, 2001; Fildes, 1995; Maher, 1995; Minchin, 1998; Palmer, 2009; Shahar, 1990; Thurer, 1994; Valsiner, 2000; Wolf, 1999).

Distancing and Status

The degree of distancing from the maternal breast varied. In Puritan families, women, mothering, children, and child rearing were valued, but women were subordinate to their husbands. Mothers nursed their children, but were culturally pressured to wean their offspring at two years of age in order to resume sexual relations with their husbands, even though they felt that weaning children before they were ready was wrong for the child (Ozment, 1983).

Other families distanced children from their mothers' breasts altogether. Families of means in central Europe during medieval times viewed women and children as chattel. Wives were obligated to fulfill their husbands' needs and produce heirs. To guarantee that children received untainted superior breastmilk, while also ensuring that women fulfilled their duties as wives, mothers disregarded their biology, often to the detriment of their physical health, sending their infants to the breasts of other women (Benson Brown & McPherson, 1998; Blaffer Hrdy, 1999; Eyer, 1992; Fildes, 1995; Golden, 2001; Maher, 1995; Minchin, 1998; Palmer, 2009; Shahar, 1990; Thurer, 1994; Valsiner, 2000; Wolf, 2001).

The practice of wet nursing varied according to the family's status in society. It seems that the degree of distancing between mothers and children associated with wet nursing was proportional to status of women and children in a culture. The prestigious children of royalty, for example, were wet nursed by women who resided in their homes (Shahar, 1990), just as American children in the eighteenth century were who were considered worthy enough to be educated (Golden, 2001; Shahar, 1990; Valsiner, 2000). In contrast, the disregarded children in the aforementioned upper class families in medieval Europe were wet nursed for many years far away from their mothers and homes (Benson Brown & McPherson, 1998; Blaffer Hrdy, 1999; Fildes, 1995; Maher, 1995; Minchin, 1998; Palmer, 2009; Shahar, 1990; Stuart-Macadam, 1995; Thurer, 1994).

Extreme Disdain and Artificial Feeding

The association between status and distancing is also demonstrated by cases where children were refused human milk. Artificial feeding occurred in cultures, such as Iceland during the Middle Ages, where infants were ignored, never held, swaddled (Thurer, 1994), and fed the milk of other animals, often dying as a result (Maher, 1995). The most disdained members of society, such as the children of destitute women, were placed in orphanages and were provided with substandard artificial concoctions that often culminated in their untimely deaths (Blaffer Hrdy, 1999; Minchin, 1998; Palmer, 2009; Riordan, 2005; Thurer, 1994). In contrast, other than in cases of maternal sickness or death (Riordan, 2005) or in a few reported cases of dry nursing among aristocracy in the eighteenth century (Fildes, 1995), the more revered upper classes had the lowest rate of artificial feeding throughout history (Riordan, 2005).

Distancing, Envy, and Contempt

Male Envy of Female Biological Capacities

A review of the literature on the history of mothering implies that a possible source of disdain for women, children, and nursing is unresolved male envy of female capacity (Epstein-Gilboa, 2009). Male envy of female capacity is recognized in the literature (Rabuzzi, 1988; Thurer, 1994). Envy makes sense in light of the psychological explanation that envy occurs when one is unable to obtain a desired object. Unresolved envy results in contemptuous behaviors that include attempts at belittling envied qualities (Klein, 1998). It most certainly seems that forcing mothers to forgo their natural capacity to nurse and interfering with the mother-infant relationship shows evidence of unresolved envious behavior, especially since the superiority of breastmilk has been recognized throughout cultures and the ages (Epstein-Gilboa, 2009).

The abuse that seems inherent to distancing behaviors is further proof of the contemptuous nature of these behaviors. For example, the powerful way that fathers banished their offspring to distant wet nurses, often without regard for their welfare (Palmer, 2009; Shahar, 1990; Thurer, 1994), seems to match the definition of child maltreatment as a misuse of power (Volpe, 1995). Contemptuous behaviors in the ancient Greek and Roman societies that practised wet nursing included infant exposure, child prostitution, and hateful attitudes towards wives and mothers (Blaffer Hrdy, 1999; Thurer, 1994).

Female Self-Disdain

The literature demonstrates that contemptuous behaviors were not limited to men. Examples are reports that mothers envied the wet nurses who replaced them (Golden, 2001; Wolf, 1999). On the one hand, some mothers perceived that wet nursing helped them fulfill their duties as wives, while ensuring that their children received supreme breastmilk (Benson Brown & McPherson, 1998; Blaffer Hrdy, 1999; Golden, 2001; Fildes, 1995; Maher, 1995; Minchin, 1998; Palmer, 2009; Shahar, 1990; Thurer, 1994; Valsiner, 2000; Wolf, 1999). Mothers apparently perceived that they were able to uphold their social standing (Shahar, 1990), fulfill social duties, pursue their own interests, and ensure that their physical attributes were not impaired by nursing (Benson Brown & McPherson, 1998; Golden, 2001). On the other hand, evidence suggests that some mothers suffered and missed their children (Blaffer Hrdy, 1999), enduring social sanctions when they dared to act on this and nurse them (Benson Brown & McPherson, 1998). In light of these ambivalent feelings, it is not surprising that some mothers felt and expressed scorn, anger, disdain, and outright disgust towards nursing, breastmilk, and wet nurses (Golden, 2001; Shahar, 1990; Thurer, 1994; Valsiner, 2000; Wolf, 1999). Mothers' expressions of contempt were illustrated by practices of hiring wet nurses of lower socioeconomic status than themselves (Golden, 2001; Fildes 1995; Palmer, 2009; Shahar, 1990; Thurer, 1994; Valsiner 2000; Wolf, 1999). Belittling behaviors also included forcing wet nurses to abandon their natural offspring in order to nurse the children of those considered more worthy (Blaffer Hrdy, 1999; Giles, 2003; Golden, 2001; Palmer, 2009; Shahar, 1990; Valsiner, 2000).

Envy and Patronizing Behaviors

In the nineteenth and early twentieth century, a new form of contempt for female capacity arose with the advent of women's disdain for their own biology (Golden, 2001; Wolf, 1999). Dissimilar from earlier displays of outright scorn, contempt was displayed subtly through apparent caring and patronizing behaviors that reduced the value of the envied object (Silverman, 2003). Accordingly, physicians reinforced middle and upper class women's lack of confidence in their capacity to nurse (Blum, 1999), portraying them as weak vessels whom they medically sanctioned not to nurse, seemingly for their own good (Golden, 2001). They also justified women's growing disgust with wet nurses and nursing (Golden, 2001; Wolf, 1999). Consequently, women lost their confidence and were revolted by their physiology. This ushered in a new form of mother-infant distancing.

Family Themes in the Twentieth Century Obstruct Physiologically Based Nursing

Patriarchy, Reverence for Science, Mixed Messages, and Artificial Feeding

The themes and behaviors of families in the early twentieth century were similar to those described earlier and provide insight into present family practices. At the beginning of that century, physicians' relationships with mothers helped them evolve into central authoritarian figures that ruled family life (Golden, 2001; Wolf, 1999, 2001). Like their authoritarian predecessors, physicians contributed to the move away from nursing by conveying mixed messages that simultaneously praised and obstructed nursing (Angier, 2000; Benson Brown & McPherson, 1998; Eyer, 1992; Golden, 2001; Kitzinger, 1995; Palmer, 2009; Thurer, 1994; Wolf, 2001). The concurrent admiration of and disdain for human milk was hastened by the growing worship of science and the germ theory (Eyer, 1992; Golden, 2001; Maher, 1995; Minchin, 1998; Palmer, 2009; Ryan & Grace, 2001; Saha, 2002; Thurer; 1994; Wolf, 1999, 2001). Human milk was used as the prototype for the creation of seemingly cleaner and more scientific concoctions that physicians prepared with chemists (Golden, 2001; Wolf, 1999, 2001), and these were named "formulas" as a means of designating their higher scientific value (Minchin, 1998; Palmer, 2009). The alliance between chemists and physicians fortified the growing reliance of families on these sources, helped found the new speciality of pediatrics (Eyer, 1992; Golden, 2001; Wolf, 1999, 2001), and instituted artificial feeding as the norm for all families (Baumslag & Michels, 1995; Minchin, 1998; Palmer, 2009).

The fortitude of the messages conveyed by the new speciality of pediatrics altered age old patterns of reserving artificial feeding for the disdained. Instead, artificial feeding became synonymous with privilege (Golden, 2001; Wolf, 1999, 2001). The internalization of artificial feeding as a norm in all classes was advanced by the industrial revolution and urbanization that led to the decrease in maternal nursing among the lower classes (Dettwyler, 1995a; Golden, 2001; Minchin, 1998; Palmer, 2009; Riordan, 2005). Under the facade of health promotion, the introduction and aggressive promotion of artificial substances coincided with additional family behaviors that separated mothers, babies, and the rest of the family from one another (Saha, 2002).

Medicalization, Distancing, and Rigidity

Broken nursing patterns concurred with additional disrupted physiology, indicating again that family themes facilitating or impairing physiologically based nursing patterns are part of a continuum of beliefs and actions. The medicalization of all physiologically based family behaviors was also apparent during the birthing process, where women became secondary to the physicians who managed their births, often while mothers were anesthesized (Arms, 1994; Eyer, 1992; Harper, 2005; Rabuzzi, 1988; Rich, 1986). Fathers were vanquished to lonely waiting rooms, could not touch their infants due to germ theories, and were patronized by hospital staff (Lewis, 1986). Infants were separated from their mothers and whisked off to sterile nurseries where their development could be manipulated and measured (Minchin, 1998; Palmer, 2009; Riordan, 2005; Wolf, 2001). Natural nursing processes were blocked and eventually replaced with artificial feeding. The efforts of those who still attempted to nurse were obstructed by instructions that they "feed" their infants in a scientific manner based on strict regiments set by medical experts (Benson Brown & McPherson, 1998; Blum, 1999; Eyer, 1992; Golden, 2001; Maher, 1995; Minchin, 1998; Palmer, 2009; Riordan, 2005; Ryan & Grace, 2001; Saha, 2002; Thorley, 2003; Wolf, 1999, 2001). As a result, nursing became an activity based on timing, measurements, and quantity rather than quality, and the spontaneous nature of nursing based on infants' signals for closeness began to disappear in young families (Minchin, 1998; Quandt, 1995; Winnicott 1958, 1964).

The misunderstanding of the unique physiology of nursing led to nursing problems and a reduction in the incidence of long term nursing, as mothers searched for ways to quantify their children's growth in a manner deemed as scientific (Benson Brown & McPherson, 1998; Blum, 1999; Palmer, 2009; Wolf, 2001). The downfall of nursing as the norm is demonstrated by the low rates of initiation in the second decade of the twentieth century (Maclean, 1990; Saha, 2002; Wolf, 2001). By the middle of twentieth century, most families – even those who attempted nursing after birth – were artificially feeding their children (Blum, 1999; Eyer, 1992; Golden, 2001; Minchin, 1998; Palmer, 2009; Riordan, 2005; Quandt, 1995; Thurer, 1994; Wolf, 2001).

Experts, Distancing, Rigidity, Self-Control, and Devalued Mothers

The weakened stance of mothers during birth and regarding nursing was extended to parenthood. Mothers relied on expert advice rather than on their own wisdom or feelings for mothering (Bassin, 1994; Blum, 1999; Clarke-Stewart, 1998; Eyer, 1992; Kitzinger, 1995; Maclean, 1990; Thurer, 1994; Wolf, 2001). Experts reflected an increased interest in children's psyche and the attitude that early childhood education was important (Blum, 1999; Clarke-Stewart, 1998; Eyer, 1992). Tender love was deemed unscientific, and parents were advised not to spoil their children and to abstain from hugging, rocking, or showing other forms of physical love towards them (Clarke-Stewart, 1998; Montagu, 1978; Valsiner, 2000; Wolf, 2001). Mothers were advised to periodically take breaks from their children and to go out without them (Wolf, 2001). Distancing behaviors concurred with efforts to instill a sense of self-control in children through strict schedules, including regimented feeding practices (Clarke-Stewart, 1998; Eyer, 1992; Wolf, 2001) and early toilet training procedures (Wolf, 2001). Self-control as an ideal was also evident in the advice that dissuaded parents from picking up crying babies (Montagu, 1978). Maternal self-debasement was evident in the way that mothers were convinced of their reduced capacities to educate their own children. Consequently, they put their children in nursery schools as early as eighteen months of age in order to ensure that their offspring received superior education from experts who apparently could do a much better job at educating their children than they could (Clarke-Stewart, 1998).

Couple Precedence and Sexualized Breasts

While mothers were encouraged to remain distant from their children, they were advised to give attention to their spouses. This idea was accompanied by notions that the couple relationship was built on romance, sexual relations were conducted for mutual pleasure, and breasts were sexual objects owned by the father (Wolf, 2001). Like earlier times, male ownership of female physiology coincided with women's lack of confidence and disrespect for their bodily functions, including disgust with lactation and nursing (Giles, 2003; Wolf, 2001). Women reiterated their physicians' instructions and advised one another to artificially feed their infants (Wolf, 2001). By the middle of the twentieth century in the western world, nursing had all but disappeared (Blum, 1999). Women no longer participated in or witnessed their natural processes (Wolf, 2001).

Women Reclaim their Bodies

Gradually, changes occurred in the 1970s when women began to reclaim their rights to natural processes (Blum, 1999; Eyer, 1992; Maher, 1995; Rabuzzi, 1988; Ryan & Grace, 2001; Wolf, 2001). Nursing, however, was not a central interest to feminist groups (Blum, 1999; Carter, 1995). The true impetus for the resurgence of nursing was instituted by La Leche League, which evolved from a small support group of nursing mothers in the 1950s into a worldwide organization (Blum, 1999; La Leche League, 2004; Maher, 1995; Wolf, 2001). To retain their central status, healthcare providers promoted nursing in the United States beginning in the 1970s, albeit in a manner that disregarded physiologically based nursing behaviors, such as nursing beyond four to six months (Saha, 2002). Although nursing had slowly become fashionable again, themes that interfered with the implementation of family behaviors associated with nursing over the ages not only remained, but were rejuvenated through novel concepts.

Summary of Historical Family Themes and Nursing Behaviors

A review of family breastfeeding behaviors over the ages reaffirms that themes associated with nursing concur with beliefs and practices that either help or hinder parents' ability to establish physiologically based nursing patterns in the family system. First, we note that nursing behaviors do not occur in isolation, rather that several factors influence the way that families integrate nursing into their system. Mixed messages are conveyed about nursing and related behaviors by patriarchal leaders that reflect cultural attitudes. The application of psychological theory to cultural and micro perspectives suggests that deep-set feelings, especially envy, influence behaviors. Cultural and family feelings about females, wives, mothers, children, childrearing, and mothering affect nursing behaviors. Physiological nursing patterns are most likely to take place when women are valued at home and in society, and any form of deviation from normal nursing patterns implies the opposite. We also note that equality and physiological nursing concur with maternal-child closeness, an association that becomes more apparent in an analysis of family behaviors in the twentieth century. The last century was marked by additional salient themes that impaired nursing, including patriarchal medical control, devalued female physiology and status, negative views of closeness and spontaneous cue-based interaction, and reverence for scheduling and apparent independence. A review of present themes demonstrates that many of these early themes continue to affect how nursing is applied now. This information is significant for the family and the practitioner.

Present Day Family Themes and the Prevalence of Messages Obstruct Nursing

The review of the history of nursing clearly reinforces that family behaviors related to nursing reflect salient cultural perspectives. The salient themes in the last century moved families away from nursing and associated proximity behaviors, and left a mark on current societal views of nursing, women, infants, children, childrearing, and family life. The likelihood that remnants of earlier themes remain and continue to impair the establishment of physiological nursing patterns is suggested by findings that despite increasing rates of nursing initiation, families continue to stray from physiology, introducing substances other than breastmilk prematurely and fully weaning early (Blyth et al., 2002; Bolton, Chow, Benton & Olson, 2009; Chung et al., 2008; Dick et al., 2002; Feldman-Winter, Kruse, Mulford & Rotondo, 2002; Forste & Hoffman, 2008; Haiek, Gauthier, Brosseau & Rocheleau, 2007; INFACT, 2002a; Matthews, Webber, McKim, Banoub-Baddour & Laryea, 1998; Sheehan, Watt, Krueger, & Sword, 2006; Walker, 2007a). For example, 84.5% of Canadian women initiated nursing at birth, only 48.3% of Canadian mothers were still nursing at four months, and by six months only 38.7% of mothers were still nursing. Statistics also demonstrate that only 38.4% of the mothers who continue to nurse at four months are doing so exclusively, and that by six months, only 18.7% of Canadian mothers nursed their infants in an exclusive manner (Statistics Canada, 2003). Studies on families in the United States (Li, Ogden, Ballew, Gillespie, Grummer-Strawn, 2002) and in the UK (Kelly & Watt, 2004) demonstrate similar findings.

Healthcare Systems Convey Contradictory Messages

Insight into the current confounding context where breastfeeding behaviors contradict evidence pointing to the essentiality of physiological breastfeeding is clarified when one recalls that historically patriarchal leaders conveyed contradictory messages to families lauding nursing, while simultaneously promoting practices that impeded maternal and physiological nursing. Unfortunately, present patterns mirror history. Like in the past century, the health care system remains a central patriarchal body responsible for services and for disseminating information about breastfeeding. The salient message that breast is best is conveyed alongside practices that interfere with the establishment and continuation of normal physiologically based nursing patterns. These practices include providing inaccurate information about nursing and encouraging parents to supplement nursing infants with additional substances, destroying breastfeeding exclusivity (Baumslag, & Michels, 1995; Feldman-Winter et al., 2002; Minchin, 1998; Labbok, Wardlaw, Blanc, Clark, & Terreri, 2006; Levitt, Kaczorowski, Hanvey, Avard,

& Chance, 1996; Newman, 1998; Palmer, 1991, 2009; Tender et al., 2009; Valaitis et al., 1996; Walker, 2007a). Destroying nursing exclusivity at this early stage often leads to partial versus exclusive nursing (Bolton et al., 2009). Mothers who intermittently provide their infants with substitutes for breastmilk are more likely than mothers who nurse exclusively to wean their children early (Bodnarchuk, Eaton, & Martens, 2006). These examples indicate that practices that interfere with the establishment of the physiological continuum often impair the development and duration of physiological nursing patterns. Hence, despite proclaiming admiration for nursing, the health care system impedes physiology.

The hypocrisy inherent to destroying a desired behavior is clarified by ecological models indicating that development and behavior are the function of interactions between multileveled sub-units in a mutually influential system (Bronfenbrenner, 1979). This implies that multiple sources influence the quality of services provided and the interactions between health care clinicians and nursing families. A review of the special role that health care providers and their systems play in transferring messages to families seems necessary when one recalls that the purpose of this chapter is to help clinicians gain insight into personal themes impacting work with nursing families. The relevance of this section for all clinicians is suggested by an ecological perspective that implies that even though the majority of research is on the health care system, other agencies working with families are also influenced by and affect themes associated with nursing. This suggestion is reinforced by documents, such as the *Global Strategy for Infant and Young Child Feeding* (WHO & UNICEF, 2003), that attempt to educate community and government agencies about optimal practices associated with breastfeeding.

Alliance with Companies Profiting from Artificial Feeding

Like in the last example, the ecological model reinforces the concept that interactions between families and their direct service providers are influenced by and affect interchanges with larger systems that may not come into direct contact with clients. The historically based alliance between the healthcare system and companies that profit from the sale of artificial baby milk remains an influential force impeding physiology. These companies promote their products directly to families through media, advertising, and marketing disguised as gifts. The strong alliance with the health care system provides businesses with indirect access to the target population by influencing clinicians working with breastfeeding clients. Several ingenious tactics include advertising products to health care providers through sessions disguised as education, donating free artificial milk and apparent gifts, and funding materials and programs aimed at nursing families. These tactics normalize and endear products to the service providers and obligate the health care system to follow conditions set by the artificial baby milk company (Baby Milk Action & Baby Feeding Law Group, 2009; Baumslag & Michels, 1995; Breastfeeding Committee of Canada, 2002; Brady, 2009; Chetley & Allain, 1998; Heinig, 2001; Humenick & Hill, 1996; International Baby Food Action Network (IBFAN), 1999; INFACT 1993c, 1997b, 1998; 1999c, 2007b; Minchin, 1998; Newman, 1998, 2009; Palmer, 2009; Peddlesen, 1998; Richter, 2002; Saha, 2002; Valaitis et al., 1996; Van Esterik, 1995; Walker, 2001, 2007b). Collaboration between health institutions and these companies often lead to the creation of tempting programs for families that have been compared to "ginger bread cottages" that draw families in and ultimately lead to corporate financial gain (Epstein-Gilboa, 1997a, 1997b, 1998b, 2003). The messages used to draw families to ginger bread cottages and to products are altered to reflect changes in salient attitudes, behaviors and nursing patterns. A press release by an artificial baby milk company (Abbott Laboratories, press release, 2003) confirms research showing that these companies study nursing patterns. Whereas, originally artificial baby milk companies strived to convince healthcare providers and the public that their "formulas" were better than nursing, present messages mirror the pattern of increased breastfeeding initiation and apparent adoration of breastfeeding as best. Accordingly, messages used to sell artificial baby milk now imply that the unique features of breastmilk are replicated in the new and improved product (INFACT, 2002b). In addition, companies reflect the increased rates of breastfeeding initiation by focusing on prompting early weaning to their products, for example, by producing apparent educational packages or websites on breastfeeding that direct families to their products (Mead Johnson, 2009). The information on breastfeeding always starts off with breast is best and is often spiced with subtle hints about nursing difficulties. There are references to the possibility of and positive attributes of partial feeding. This tactic in combination with other methods familiarizes families with the product, contributes to early weaning, and ensures that the company's products will be chosen over others (Baby Milk Action, 2006; Baby Milk Action & Baby Feeding Law Group, 2009; Brady, 2009; Drazin, 1991; Frank, 1989; INFACT, 1993c, 1994, 2002b; Newman & Pitman, 2009; Reddy, 1995; Snell, Krantz, Keeton, Delgado, & Peckham, 1992; WHO 1998b).

Many readers are likely aware that the healthcare institutes create measures and continue to update programs aimed at reducing the influence of artificial baby milk companies and enhancing services associated with breastfeeding

(Chetley & Allain, 1998; Richter, 2002; Van Esterik, 1995; Walker, 2007a; WHO 1981, 1998b, 2003; WHO & UNICEF, 1989, 1990). The significance of these programs and initiatives is indicated by findings showing an association between enhanced baby friendly practices–activities supporting physiologically based breastfeeding – in medical institutes and increased exclusivity rates (Labbok et al., 2006). However, it is also significant that ongoing monitoring of clinical practice is necessary to ensure compliance even in institutions deemed baby friendly (Merten & Ackermann-Liebrich, 2004). In other words, it seems that some clinicians do not fully internalize the importance of physiological nursing and that impeding themes exist despite improvements. The limited research on nursing beyond infancy is one indication that detrimental themes still reign and that physiological patterns are not yet the norm (Stein et al., 2002).

Messages Obstructing Physiological Nursing Patterns

Artificial Feeding is the Term of Reference

The continued discomfort with the physiology of nursing is upheld by messages reinforcing existing themes. Decades of artificial feeding have established a non-nursing culture that refers to artificial feeding as a normal and expected aspect of infancy, childhood, and parenting. Messages about the normalcy of artificial feeding are conveyed by concepts, language, images, and symbols, implying that bottles and pacifiers, for example, are synonymous with early childhood. These concepts are applied to nursing and impede the establishment and duration of physiological nursing patterns. The use of artificial feeding as the norm in the context of breastfeeding is exemplified by the application of measurements and scheduling to nursing instead of cue-based interactions (Baumslag & Michels 1995; Dettywler, 1995b; Henderson, Kitzinger, & Green, 2001; INFACT, 1995, 1998; Minchin, 1998; Newman, 2009; Palmer, 2009; Piper & Parks, 1996; Scott & Mostyn, 2003; Stuart-Macadam, 1995; Thurer, 1994; Wiessinger, 1996).

Nursing is a Feeding Choice

The use of artificial feeding as the template for nursing is also evident in discourse pertaining to breastfeeding. Aspects of artificial feeding are the variables used for comparison. Given that artificial feeding is a method of feeding and no more, nursing is portrayed similarly (Dettywler, 1995b). This view of nursing erases the unique emotional and physiological features of breastfeeding, reducing it to a mere commodity. The reduction of nursing to the level of artificial baby milk is attained further by grouping the concept of food together with the popular cultural concept of choice. The salient message is breastfeeding and artificial feeding are interchangeable feeding choices (Baumslag & Michels, 1995; Dettywler, 1995; INFACT 1992b, 1993a, 1993c, 1996a; Wiessinger, 1996).

It is important to review what the term choice really means in the present context. This term was originally intended as a means of enabling clients to make well informed decisions. However, the word choice is often used in the healthcare system without actually offering clients options or real information. The façade of providing choice when there is none enables the system to abuse the rights of clients to true informed decision making (Epstein-Gilboa, 2009).

The abuse of the term choice specifically regarding nursing is exemplified by a website (http://www.babyfeedingchoice.org/index.html) apparently set up by artificial baby companies. The site poses artificial feeding and nursing as two feeding choices. They imply, for example, that laws disabling companies from providing mothers with free samples of their products impairs mothers' ability to receive information, infringing on their right to "choose the best feeding option for their babies."

The salience of positioning breastfeeding and artificial feeding as interchangeable feeding choices is apparent in lay and medical discourse, and surprisingly, also in psychological discussions pertaining to relational development. One would expect relational theorists to paint a different picture due to their focus on micro details in interaction. Yet, the habit of seeing nursing and artificial feeding as interchangeable are long standing, evident in the period when artificial feeding was first posed as the norm. For example, Freud (1905, as cited in Montagu, 1978, p.95) stated, "It was a child's first and most vital activity, his sucking at his mother's breast, or at substitutes for it (author's italics), that must have familiarized him with this pleasure..." It is also most interesting to note that the phenomena of exchanging artificial feeding for nursing is also apparent in object relations theory, despite the centrality of the maternal breast in these models (Klein 1997a, 1998; Winnicott, 1958, 1964). However, it is important to remember that object relations was formalized during the time period when medical experts, medically controlled birth, artificial feeding, and scheduled parenting were ushered in and becoming the norm.

Nursing is a Superlative Behavior

The concepts of artificial feeding as the norm and breastfeeding as a mere interchangeable feeding choice are fortified further by misconstruing messages about the essentiality of nursing. In view of the fact that artificial feeding is the normal method of feeding, breastfeeding becomes the abnormal way. Within this framework nursing is nice, but not necessary (Walker, 2007a). Another related and more potent message is that nursing is supreme and unattainable (Saha, 2002; Wiessinger, 1996).

Many readers likely recall presenting nursing as best and believing that this helped them promote breastfeeding. However, compare this to other body functions. We rarely think that we have to promote or encourage other bodily functions, such as breathing or digesting. Moreover, we most certainly do not present these normal functions as supreme. They are simply normal physiological functions. Breastfeeding is the same, and yet, it is presented as ideal, better, and the best way. Views of nursing as best imply that it is idealized and beyond the reach of parents who strive for normalcy (Wiessinger, 1996). The association between normalcy and parenting is reinforced by the salient concept of good enough parenting (Winnicott, 1994).

The message that nursing is supreme rather than necessary is strengthened when information about the risks of not nursing appropriately and the risks of artificial baby milk are omitted, usually under the pretext of sheltering parents from guilt (Epstein-Gilboa, 1997a, 1997b, 1998a, 2000; Labbok 2008; Lauwers & Swisher, 2005; Minchin, 1998; Newman, 1998; Newman & Pitman, 2009; Walker, 1993, 1998; Wiessinger, 1996). The guilt myth dissuades clinicians from providing mothers with accurate information. Artificial baby milk companies in the United States successfully used this myth to stop a Health and Human Services campaign that had intended to provide families with the truth about the risks associated with not breastfeeding (INFACT, 2004; Petersen, 2003).

The combined messages that families internalize are that nursing is a superior feeding choice, likely better than what they want. Moreover, there are few risks to artificial feeding. Thus while nursing might be best, it is less desirable than familiar baby milk. By providing artificial baby milk, they perceive that they are parenting normally and in a good enough fashion.

Parents' perspectives of normalcy in relation to nursing in a context of breastfeeding as supreme change and take on different meanings and expressions according to the stage of development of the nursing relationship. In the prenatal stage, some parent's desire for normalcy may lead them to refute nursing altogether (Wiessinger, 1996). Parents who initiate nursing, but introduce artificial feeding early may be holding on to their idealized views of parenting from the prenatal stage, while gradually reconciling themselves to the idea that they might not be perfect parents. Other parents who dispose of breastfeeding and fully wean might see artificial feeding as the normal way when they replace prenatal views of themselves as ideal with the desire to be good enough as they cope with the challenges of parenting. The last example demonstrates how messages about the complexity of nursing, the importance of apparent free choice, and the desire for apparent normalcy subtly implied in advertisements about artificial baby milk encourage early weaning.

Disregard for the Unique Features of Nursing

Views of artificial feeding as normal are also apparent when terms associated with bottle feeding are applied to the unique features of nursing, including the anatomy and physiology of breastfeeding. Using wrong terms disables one from nursing correctly, contributing to early weaning. For example, the correct anatomical and physiological descriptions for breastfeeding include areola, breast, asymmetric latch, wide mouths, and suckling (Fisher, 1984; Koepke & Bigelow, 1997, Matthews, 1993; Mohrbacher & Stock, 1997; Newman & Sterken, 1992; Renfrew, 1989; Renfrew, Fisher, & Arms, 1990; Riordan, 2005; Woolridge, 1986a, 1986b). However, it is common to see nursing discussed as if it was bottle feeding using terms such as "nipple", "suck", and "feeding" (exemplified in Isaacs, 1997; Kaplan, 1978; Klein, 1997, 1998; Sullivan, 1972; Valsiner, 2000). Mislabelling impairs teaching, leads to missed assessment and interventions, and impairs parents' ability to nurse correctly.

The prevalence of describing nursing with artificial feeding in mind is also suggested when nursing and non-nursing populations are grouped together in research studies. Failing to note the unique qualities of nursing populations erases the distinct impact of nursing on development. The disregard for the distinct impact of nursing on behavior impairs the quality of research, clinical judgment, and intervention, and also disables parents from making good enough decisions.

Indifference to the specificity of nursing is also evident in discussions about child development. For example, Winnicott (1989, pg. 499) attributed breast refusal in a four-month-old infant receiving supplemental bottles to maternal attitude, without looking into the possible impact of obstructive devices on nipple preference. Sullivan's (1953) suggestion that breastfeeding infants require other forms of oral stimulation when their needs for hunger and thirst are fulfilled, reflect the common view of nursing as merely feeding, ignoring the emotional meaning and calming aspects of nursing. Bowlby's (1987) suggestion that nursing is not a necessary aspect of the attachment process disregards the unique cue-based system and interactional components of nursing. The lack of regard for the unique features of nursing impairs our ability to provide accurate nursing information and assess nursing problems accurately, and fails to excite parents about nursing.

Disregard for Physiological Patterns

Disregard for the unique features of nursing is also exemplified in the misunderstanding of the physiology of nursing, contributing to early weaning patterns. Language used to describe nursing is one means of pressuring parents to wean early. For example, nursing beyond infancy is often called "extended nursing," implying that it is prolonged and not customary. A coexisting view is that nursing is a method of feeding that loses its nutritional value over time, and it is therefore pathological to nurse when there is no nutritional significance. It is not surprising that those continuing to nurse beyond acceptable periods experience societal negativity and ambivalence. Many conceal that they are nursing despite the increasing number of like families (Dettwyler, 1995a; Stein et al., 2002).

The concept of limiting nursing to a short period of time is deeply ingrained and was already evident during the era when nursing was being eradicated. Klein (1998) advised parents to wean their babies by eight or nine months. The salience of themes of limited nursing in this context is demonstrated by references to this pattern as the norm in the breastfeeding literature. For example, one study on interaction and nursing implied that the normal weaning period is at approximately four to six months of age (Gerrish & Mennella, 2000). Our discomfort with nursing beyond the elected boundary is exemplified by severe negativity towards those who dare to nurse beyond early infancy. Mothers nursing a young child are pathologized and described as unable to set limits and to separate from the child. Others contend that mothers use nursing as tool to delay the resumption of a sexual relationship. At the same time, children's perspective of nursing as a comfort object is unrecognized (Stein et al., 2002).

Broken Physiological Continuum

Naturally, one can't help but wonder what causes clinicians and families to voice contempt towards nursing and to ignore research demonstrating the essentiality of physiologically based patterns. We can use our earlier analysis of historical nursing patterns for insight in this case. It is important to remember the historical association between disregard for female physiology, broken breastfeeding patterns, and unresolved patriarchal male envy leading to the destruction of desired but unattainable female processes (Epstein-Gilboa, 2009). Unresolved patriarchal envy and resulting contempt is identified in present context by the reduction in women's life cycle events to medical and reproductive experiences ruled by technological interventions. Any doubt about the relevance of this concept to the present context is ruled out when one notes the high rate of unnecessary medical intervention in pregnancy and birth, including surging cesarean rates (Block, 2007; Cassidy, 2007; Harper, 2005; Kroeger, 2003; Wagner, 1994) and the prevalence of nursing problems. Research demonstrates that there is a connection between interventions during birth and difficulties with nursing (Beck & Watson, 2008; Kroeger, 2004; Walker, 2006). Disregard for nursing is part of a pattern of devaluing and interfering with female physiology. Women's envied capacity to give birth and nurse are impaired and reframed as pathological processes requiring the aid of medical specialists (Epstein-Gilboa, 2009).

Another implication of reducing female physiology to medical processes is that abnormal birth and sequel are viewed as normal (Davis-Floyd, 1994; Wagner, 1994). The redefinition of nursing problems as expected occurrences interferes with adequate assessment of early nursing, leads us to accept inappropriate intervention, and disables the establishment of normal nursing patterns. Once again, we are using abnormality rather than physiology as the term of reference.

Let's look at existing practices in postnatal units. Here again we can see that rather than recognizing and fixing broken parts of the continuum, some healthcare practitioners and families use conceptualizations of artificial feeding to guide them. Healthcare providers might teach mothers inaccurate nursing technique based on positions associated with artificial feeding and accept subsequent pain as normal (Newman, 2009). It is important to remember the discussion earlier in the chapter that referred to how healthcare providers may advise parents to supplement newborns with substances or to use feeding tools or pacifiers that impede the establishment of nursing. These practices trigger health problems in the present and, more commonly, in the distant future (AAP, 2005; Lawrence & Lawrence, 2005; Riordan, 2005; Newman, 2009; Walker, 2006, 2007a), increases the risk for early weaning (Blomquist, Jonsbo, Serenius, & Persson, 1994; Bodnarchuk et al., 2006; Bolton et al., 2009; Levitt et al., 1996; Newman, 1998; Newman & Pitman, 2009; Tender et al., 2009), and puts infants at risk for nursing problems, inclusive of latching and suckling difficulties (Newman, 1990; Neifert, Lawrence, & Seacat, 1995; Riordan, 2005; Walker, 2006). From a psychological point of view, the feeding tool becomes the "good and giving breast" and often the slower flowing maternal breast becomes the withholding and bad breast, leading infants to reject mothers' breasts (Epstein-Gilboa, 1999, unpublished manuscript). Families entrenched in a predominantly artificial feeding culture internalize the medically endorsed and harmful practices as normal and move away from physiological nursing despite earlier intentions.

Confusing Views of Breasts

Cultural misnaming and misunderstanding of the nursing breast is another problem contributing to the clinician's incapacity to support and to families' inability to internalize physiologically based nursing patterns. A central problem is the inability to see the breast as a multi-purposed organ, with the capacity to function in different ways at the same time (Angier, 2000; Saha, 2002). The multiple and simultaneous roles that breasts have (Bartlett, 2000) were noticed throughout history, suggesting that present views of the breast are socially constructed. For example, biblical Hebrews saw breasts as erotic (Song of Solomon 4:5 Tanukh, Hebrew Bible) and motherly (Song of Solomon 8:1, Tanukh, Hebrew Bible; Thurer, 1994).

Sexual Breasts

A salient perception in western culture is that breasts are only sexual objects (Angier, 2000; Blum, 1999; Baumslag & Michels, 1995; Dettwyler, 1995b; Rodriguez-Garcia & Frazier, 1995; Saha, 2002). Perspectives of sexuality are historically and culturally constructed (Baber & Murray, 2001; Maher, 1995). One might remember that the view of the female breast as a sexual object was established in the early twentieth century, along with reverence for romantic love and sexual enjoyment (Wolf, 2001), and coincided with the long standing perspective that husbands own their spouses' breasts (Blum, 1999; Thurer, 1994). These feelings are expressed through concerns that nursing might disfigure the sexual breasts (Saha, 2002). Male uneasiness about sharing the treasured breasts with the infant impedes nursing and may contribute to couple discord (Benson Brown & McPherson, 1998; Jordan & Wall, 1993).

Male ownership of the sexual breasts implores mothers to conceal their nursing breasts (Bartlett, 2000; Stearns, 1999; Valsiner, 2000) from everyone except the husband (Maher, 1995; Sharma & Petosa, 1997. Bartlett proposes that hiding nursing breasts interferes with mothers' ability to speak openly and proudly about breastfeeding and that (Bartlett, 2000) if men nursed, they would not be asked to conceal their breasts. Women who dare to defy cultural norms and nurse openly in public often suffer displays of hostile sexism (Silverman, 2003), and are subject to harassment (Benson Brown & McPherson, 1998; Brooks, 2001; Guttman & Zimmerman, 2000; INFACT 1996c, 1997a; Maher, 1995; Saha, 2002).

Motherly Asexual Breasts

Breasts may also be seen as solely motherly objects. All evidence of sexuality is removed from these breasts; they are not erotic and are owned by the infant. Motherly breasts are reinforced, for example, by sexless nursing apparel and by calling nursing breasts by childish names (Angier, 2000; Bartlett, 2000; Giles, 2003; Stearns, 1999).

However, denying that there are sexual aspects of the nursing breast may interfere with nursing and negates important aspects of the female experience (Saha, 2002). Separating the sexual breast from the maternal breast increases women's disdain for their own physiology (Maher, 1995) and distances women from their own body functions (INFACT, 1992a, 1993b; Rabuzzi, 1988; Rich, 1986). When women distance themselves from the bodily feelings associated with nursing, they may deny the sensuality (Saha, 2002) associated with intense tactile and intimate interactions with the nursing child (INFACT, 1992a, 1993b; Maher, 1995; Montagu, 1978; Rabuzzi, 1988; Rich 1986; Saha, 2002).

The lack of acknowledgement of sensuality associated with nursing mothers causes confusion for some mothers and impairs their ability to nurse (Rodriguez-Garcia & Frazier, 1995; Saha, 2002). The similarity between feelings associated with oxytocin release during nursing and sexual arousal may contribute to maternal confusion. However, it is important to note that the physical feelings are neither directed towards nor associated with the child (Bartlett, 2000; Saha, 2002). Mothers' feelings of aberration are justified by cases where women who dare to disclose their feelings face severe sanctions due to cultural revulsion and disgust with the apparent sexuality of nursing (Davidowitz, 1992; Saha, 2002).

It seems that rather than celebrating female physical sensations, western cultural themes and practices neutralize women's sensual experiences (Maher, 1995). Women's life cycle events are reduced to medical and reproductive affairs (Kleinplatz, 2001). For example, the natural processes of birth are replaced by technological interventions that often lead to nursing problems (Kroeger, 2003; Kroeger & Smith, 2003; Lothian, 2005; Reddy, 1995; Smith, 2007) and predispose mothers to terminate nursing (Bourgoin et al., 1997). Breastfeeding counselors may ignore mothers' emotions, including sensual feelings (Giles, 2003; Saha, 2002). Often the only reference to sensuality pertains to women's marital relationships (Maher, 1995; Saha, 2002). In addition, discussions on the physical implications of nursing center on maternal weight loss, a concept that fits into cultural adoration of thinness (Benson Brown & McPherson, 1998; Saha, 2002). Nursing is mainly poised as an optimal and scientific form of infant feeding (Giles, 2003; Saha, 2002; Wolf, 1999, 2001). Consequently, the sensual aspects of the nursing relationship are repressed and replaced by thoughts about the maternal-child bond, the extraordinary properties of breastmilk, or pleasant memories of love from childhood (Angier, 2000).

One can't deny that views of breasts as motherly reflects their physiological function and facilitates nursing (Dettwyler, 1995b). However, posing breasts as solely motherly objects may complicate the nursing experience for some mothers. It is important to remember that prior to motherhood women's breasts likely had other meanings for women and their partners, especially sensual and sexual attributions. For some women, views of breasts as only motherly implies that they must give up their former selves, definitely a disheartening implication of nursing contributing to the complex process of novel role internalization. Self-denial and apparent sacrifice also counters some mothers' desire to be normal and good enough.

Hence, denying that nursing breasts are multifaceted organs interferes with the maternal experience. Exclusively sexualized breasts distance women from their experience by giving ownership over to men and forcing women to conceal nursing. Solely motherly breasts distance women from themselves and their relationships. Both versions reinforce historically instated themes of female self-disdain and distances women from their body functions.

Contradictory Feminist Contributions

One may wonder whether feminist theory provides some clarity to confused mothers and to those trying to support them. Surprisingly, the information on nursing breasts is not as elaborate or as easy to find as material on other female body functions in of the feminist literature. In addition, the material on breastfeeding is contradictory. On one hand, theorists impel women to distance themselves from their physiological continuum and motherhood in order to advance their status (Bassin, 1994; Chodorow, 1978; Dinnerstein, 1977; Eyer, 1992; Firestone, 1970; Silverman, 2003). When one bears a historical perspective in mind, it is easy to understand that there is validity to this view in certain contexts. However, on the other hand, one cannot help but note that the view that women ignore their physiology reflects a male perspective and exemplifies the phenomena where females internalize and express male views of women (DeBeauvoir, 1989). In this case, devaluing female physiology is reminiscent of unresolved patriarchal envy that requires women to reduce their own value by cancelling out the uniquely female activity of nursing or women who engage in the process (Epstein-Gilboa, 2009). Impelling women to give up physiological processes is an expression of female self-disdain and is reminiscent of the biological eradication and devaluation of women during the Middle Ages that was actualized through wet nursing. Female self devaluation contributes to present day scorning of women supportive of physiology. Point in case are examples where women advocating for nursing and discussing hazards of artificial feeding are vilified (Minchin, 1998) and described as "breastfeeding police" (Eyer, 1996, pg 72). Hence, although there are valid components to the noted feminist arguments suggesting that women distance themselves from physiology, they ignore the actual contribution of biology and, paradoxically, seem to contribute to the devaluation of the female experience.

In contrast, essentiality paradigms (Silverstein & Auerbach, 1999), female physiological processes, and motherhood are validated as important aspects of female development in maximizing feminist discourse (Blum, 1999; Carter, 1995; Eyer, 1992; Guttman & Zimmerman, 2000; Kitzinger, 1995; Lindberg, 1996; Maher, 1995; Palmer, 2009; Rabuzzi, 1994; Rich, 1986; Thurer, 1994). Women-focused theorists are increasingly looking at the immense potential of nursing as an enhancing experience for women. Discussions refer to the multifaceted breast, sensuality, and the positive impact of nursing on women's sense of self (Bartlett, 2000; Giles, 2003). These views reflect those expressed by early feminists who longed for suffrage in the beginning of the twentieth century. These mothers felt that their breasts were multifaceted objects and expressive tools that enabled them to display their passion (Silverman, 2003).

Devaluation of Women's Bodily Experiences in Healthcare

In contrast to maximizing feminist views of breasts as multifaceted organs, abundant with sensual, sexual, and emotional components, the healthcare system seems to retain a singular view that discards the complex emotionality surrounding nursing. Breasts are seen mainly as lactating organs that produce the superlative breastmilk. Concepts of motherly breasts may enter the equation; however, female sensuality and sexual breasts are clearly absent from medical images. One might propose that as members of western culture, healthcare providers attempt to rid themselves of predominant sexual images of breasts in an effort to provide optimal and ethical care to clients. Consequently, in their commitment to solely lactating breasts, healthcare providers deny the sensuality and emotions associated with nursing.

Ignoring the multifaceted roles of the breast and the nursing experience reduces the quality of services provided to nursing families. Much like in earlier history when the authoritarian figures focused on breastmilk rather than on the mother-infant relationship (Maher, 1995; Palmer, 2009; Shahar, 1990; Thurer, 1994), the present tendency to focus on lactation and breastmilk, in the absence of references to the psychology of nursing (Saha, 2002), obliterates the relational aspects of nursing (Maher, 1995). Moreover, the focus on breastmilk implies that the nutritional product is the central factor and is consistent with the themes that nursing and artificial feeding are feeding choices (Baumslag & Michels, 1995; Dettywler, 1995b; INFACT, 1993c; Wiessinger, 1996).

Reduction of the Nursing Relationship to a Product

Medical ownership of lactation turns emotional, sensual, and relational nursing into an optimal and scientific form of infant feeding. This act contributes to female disembodiment, a condition where mothers are removed from their bodily feelings and decentralized. Instead, breastmilk is the main ingredient of nursing (Angier, 2000; Benson Brown & McPherson, 1998; Blum, 1999; Bourgoin et al., 1997; Giles, 2003; Kleinplatz, 2001; Kroeger, 2003; Maher, 1995; Reddy, 1995; Saha, 2002; Wolf, 1999, 2001). The present focus on milk is exemplified by the suggestion that when professionals say "breastfeeding is best," they actually mean "breastmilk is best" (Maher, 1995; Saha, 2002, p.66). This phenomenon is reminiscent of earlier authoritarian figures' focus on breastmilk and disregard for the maternal-child relationship that impelled families to wet-nurse.

A review of present research on breastfeeding validates the supremacy of milk over relationship. There is an overwhelming biomedical focus on the components of breastmilk that overrides studies, such as the ones used in this book, that look at the relational aspects of nursing. One cannot deny that the study of human milk has contributed to the reintroduction of breastfeeding, has enabled clinicians to take breastfeeding seriously, and has validated mothers' desire to return to nursing. However, dangers of this focus were voiced over a decade ago when theorists noticed the growing biomedical orientation of research on breastfeeding (Beasley, 1991) and warned that the intensifying medicalization of nursing and introduction of breast pumps would demote the relational aspects of nursing (Palmer, 2009).

Pumped Breastmilk versus Maternal Nursing and the Nursing Relationship

The growing popularity of breast pumps and the aggressive marketing tactics of breast pump companies (Heinig, 2003) justify earlier concerns. Some of the tactics used to market nursing pumps resemble the marketing techniques of companies that sell artificial baby milk. This is exemplified by a package called M.O.M. (Mother's Own Milk Program), with the logo "Helping mothers to nurse longer" (Playtex, 2003), that shows jovial pictures of infants, bottles, and a mother bottle feeding her infant with apparent pumped breastmilk. Pictures of infants nursing at the breast are conspicuously absent, fortifying the message that breastmilk, not the nursing relationship, is central.

Pumps may be necessary tools that facilitate breastfeeding under certain limited conditions. For example, pumping may be used when infants demonstrate extreme difficulty nursing at the breast, such as in cases of severe prematurity or illness. Maternal reasons may include separation due to employment, for example, and pumps may be used to enhance milk supply prior to and sometimes during adoptive nursing. Pumps also enable women to donate milk when necessary. And of course, pumping enables one to obtain an optimal substance to provide infants when it is essential to supplement nursing. However, there are many examples of the over use of pumps. For example, the pump may be used when fathers strive to "feed" their babies and fulfil the cultural myth that feeding an infant is necessary for paternal bonding (Happy & Healthy Pregnancy, 2009). The seeming over use of pumped milk, rather than maternal nursing, is also suggested by the practice of providing pumped milk through cups, feeding tubes, finger feeding, or bottles as corrective measures. Overwhelmed clinicians attempting to cope with anxious mothers and infants displaying difficulties nursing may use these interventions in the absence of, or after a very short trial at maternal nursing, and with the central focus of providing the infant with a substance (writer's experience). While pumped milk seems to resolve the acute apparent feeding problem, it adds to the existing iatrogenic issues that follow birth (Kroeger, 2003; Kroeger & Smith, 2003; Lothian, 2005; Reddy, 1995, Smith, 2007), and according to this writer's experience, in many cases have long term implications. Many readers will identify with the difficult task of helping a mother with an older baby attempt to relatch as she copes with a sense of rejection and the frustrations of pumping, while simultaneously meeting the needs of her offspring. Considering that the aim of this chapter is to help clinicians clarify the themes that direct their practice, open minded clinicians might ask themselves whose agenda they meet when they focus on getting a substance into a baby, rather than establishing a nursing relationship.

Focusing on ensuring substance intake rather than on the unique physiological connection between mother and child is also an expression of artificial feeding as the term of reference that was discussed earlier in this chapter. Within this mindset, we use pumped milk to try and correct problems, rather than prevent problems in the first place or correct them using a nursing model. Giving infants pumped milk means that one is providing a substance, not an interaction. This act distances us from the physiological continuum and helps us remain consistently loyal to the medicalization of this process. Using artificial feeding as the term of reference breaks the normal physiological continuum and nursing cycle, and hampers the nursing relationship.

Infants also play a role in the sequelae. Applying object relations psychological concepts to these practices provides one with insight into infants' possible perspective of substitute nursing objects. Accordingly, aside from causing latching and suckling problems, these tools may represent the mother object. In some cases, infants will perceive the artificial feeding tools as good breasts, providing relief more efficiently than the actual maternal breast. This will decrease the likelihood that the infant will accept the actual maternal breast and will increase maternal frustration, perpetuating a negative cycle (Epstein-Gilboa, unpublished manuscript). Thus the use of mother's milk without the mother decreases maternal confidence and competence at nursing, erasing further the relational component of nursing.

Devaluing the nursing relationship breaks the normal physiological continuum and nursing cycle, alters physiologically based maternal-child contingence and interactions, and demotes women, destroying their confidence. This concept has historical value. One might say that the breast pump is the modern wet nurse, allowing others to express their contempt for unresolved envy of mothers and to take over the motherly role (Epstein-Gilboa, 2009). Like our foremothers, women are encouraged to give their children the milk, while distancing themselves from their offspring and their physiology. It is important to remember that disregard for female physiology has deep historical roots, likely stemming from unresolved envy (Epstein-Gilboa, 2009). Contempt leads us to demote and change the female continuum into something controllable by external elements. The primary means of control over female capacity is medical and commences long before nursing is initiated, fortifying the claim that one must fix pregnancy and birthing disruptions if one wants to instill physiologically based nursing patterns. Demoted physiology facilitates existing views of artificial feeding as the norm and alters the acknowledgement of the unique features of nursing into reverence for the milk substance alone. Pumping in place of mothering through nursing is essentially weaning, albeit not from breastmilk, but most certainly from normal maternal and child physiology, and the nursing relationship. In other words, using the pump in place of the mother not only denies the physiological connection, but also points to a desire to separate mothers and infants. Focusing on breastmilk separates the mother from the child and follows historically set themes where broken physiology concurred with mother-child distancing.

Reverence for Distancing, Separation, and Autonomy

It is important to remember that physiological patterns are facilitated by other behaviors. Proximity behaviors play an important role in this process, enabling mothers and children to engage in cue-based nursing exchanges. It is not surprising then to note that messages obstructing physiological nursing patterns concur with concepts that interfere with maternal-child closeness. This pattern has deep historical roots.

Separation as a Revered Developmental Milestone

Like earlier times, broken physiological patterns concur with parent-child distancing. Historical themes associated with parent-child separation, including patriarchal prominence, adult and couple precedence, and female and child devaluation (Palmer, 2009; Shahar, 1990; Thurer, 1994), contribute to distancing in the present context. The concept that parent-child distancing enhances child development that was added to historical themes in the past century is salient in the present context. It is important to remember that at the time, apparent scientific experts implied that parents helped their children build good character through strict schedules, processes that apparently instilled self-control, and distal strategies (Clarke-Stewart, 1998; Montague, 1978). These concepts evolved into the leading themes that guide present developmental paradigms. Salient themes stress individualism over interdependence (McKenna, 1996), disregarding child-led cues for closeness and encouraging early separation. An important rationale upholding the historically based association between broken physiology and distancing is that maternal-child separation is essential to healthy development.

Reverence for Distancing Behaviors

Psychological models contribute to the perspective that apparent independence and parent-child distancing is integral to healthy child development. Individuation and processes of separation are referred to in bidirectional relational models that otherwise emphasize maternal-child attunement, and acknowledge infants' needs for closeness (Ainsworth et al., 1978; Bowlby, 1987; Kaplan, 1978; Klein, 1998; Mahler et al., 1975). The expectation that normally developing infants and toddlers tolerate distancing is exemplified by the use of a reunion segment as the means of assessing the quality of attachment in a tool called the Strange Situation (Ainsworth et al., 1978). It is important to note that this assessment tool does not emphasize separation, but focuses on how children interact with their mothers following separation. Nevertheless, using reunion as a means of assessing healthy development, rather than, for example, observations of ongoing maternal-infant interaction, implies that emotionally typical infants and young toddlers are able to tolerate intermittent separation.

Moreover, what one might infer from these models is that closeness is healthy, as long as the degree of proximity alters over a specific time and children are able to tolerate some distancing. It is easy to see how nursing and proximity behaviors that persist into early childhood might be pathologized within these contexts. However, readers acquainted with cultures where young infants are consistently carried and young children rarely leave their mothers' side likely see the problematic aspects of this presumption. Within this framework, children seeking closeness beyond parameters deemed normal and who are involved in separation processes that do not mirror cultural expectations might be falsely labelled and pathologized within contexts revering early distancing.

Reverence for distancing within psychological frameworks is indicated further by references to dysfunctional closeness in family systems models. Like bidirectional paradigms, family systems models that emphasise optimal interactions and closeness also refer to separation as an important part of family development. Individuation is seen as a sign of health and apparent overt closeness is referred to as enmeshment and as a symptom of family dysfunction (Kerr & Bowen, 1988). It is easy to see how families with a diverse meaning of closeness, for example, those practicing continued maternal-child proximity and bed sharing, might be misconstrued as dysfunctional by some clinicians using family concepts related to separation.

Separateness, Independence, and Autonomy

One implication of being separate from others is that one functions alone. Not surprisingly, autonomy is highly respected alongside reverence for distancing, and individualism is emphasized as more important than interdependence (McKenna, 1996, Valsiner, 2000). Within this context, independence framed as a lone function is a primary goal of optimal developmental trajectories. Furthermore, it becomes imperative that the child learn how to function alone as quickly as possible, disregarding child-led processes. Like earlier times, parents are advised to control children's actions through strict schedules. Parents are also told that picking children up too often is over indulging, impeding the development of good character and independence (Liedloff, 1985; McKenna, 1996; Stein et al., 2002; Valsiner, 2000).

The perspective that children should learn how to become independent from an early age is also evident in some current psychological discourse and is suggested by the measures used by some theorists to assess emotional self-regulation in very young children. Self-regulation is an important developmental task that evolves gradually through reciprocal interactions with sensitive parents who help children understand their emotions and internalize means of resolving the feelings that they experience. The task of self-regulation involves the gradual capacity to understand one's and others' emotions and to express feelings appropriately in response to varied situations (Landy & Menna, 2006; Lyons-Ruth & Zeanah, 1993; Oately & Jenkins, 1996; Tronick, 1989; Tronick et al., 1986).

Self-calming and the ability to fall sleep alone exemplify some of the behaviors measured in the assessment of self-regulation in early childhood (Greenspan & Wieder, 1993). These behaviors differ greatly from those associated with the processes of ongoing nursing and maternal calming into early childhood and might lead some clinicians to label developmentally appropriate children as unhealthy.

Similarly, the highly active maternal cue reading and calming associated with proximity strategies and nursing into early childhood might also be misconstrued as pathological by some clinicians. For example, Tronick (1989) suggests that children's capacity to develop self-regulatory processes may be hampered when interactions between mothers and infants are overly coordinated due to exaggerated maternal monitoring. Comparably, theorists suggest that some mothers are unable to differentiate between their needs and their children's requirements, causing children to adapt to their mothers' needs and impairing their capacity to individuate (Silverman, 2003). On one hand, one might understand that theorists are implying that over monitoring is another expression of inaccurate cue reading, a justifiable argument. In addition, one cannot dispute the importance of allowing children to resolve issues for themselves (Weininger, 1992). However, one might wonder how these theories might affect clinicians' perspective of the closeness, interdependence, and mutuality associated with nursing. It is easy to see how some might doubt nursing parents' ability to support the development of self-regulation when one compares distancing strategies, inclusive of child versus parental calming, to a parenting style that includes nursing into early childhood, ongoing child carrying, and co-sleeping.

Self-Focused versus Self in Relation to Others

Naturally, one can't help but wonder why models that cherish closeness and sensitive interaction simultaneously infer, albeit as a secondary goal in some paradigms, that separation is nevertheless important. What is the reason that closeness is limited and distancing is respected in these models? Feminist theory provides insight into this paradox and suggests that relational models that emphasize independence and separation are influenced by patriarchal principles in comparison to feminist models that stress connection in relationships (Gilligan, 1993). This argument is validated by the review of the literature on the history of nursing and childhood that demonstrates that patriarchy often interfered with maternal-child closeness (Maher, 1995; Palmer, 2009, Thurer, 1994). In addition, most of the theories of bidirectional development were formed during the twentieth century when patriarchy, science, distal strategies, scheduling (Golden, 2001; Maclean, 1990; Maher, 1995; Minchin, 1998; Ryan & Grace, 2001; Wolf, 2001) and self control (Clarke-Stewart, 1998) prevailed. It seems that these concepts influenced the formation of psychological models that still play a primary role in our understanding of relationships. Consequently, present views of self in relation to others reflect these historically based precepts that contradict the interdependence and closeness associated with nursing. Patriarchal predominance that altered nursing and mothering throughout generations is still very much ingrained and impedes support for the interdependence and closeness associated with nursing.

Interestingly, the review of literature on the history of nursing and childhood demonstrates that patriarchal concepts ruled family relationships and interfered with physiologically based nursing patterns (Maher, 1995; Palmer, 2009; Thurer, 1994). Many theories of bidirectional development were formed during the twentieth century when patriarchy, science, distal strategies, scheduling (Golden, 2001; Maclean, 1990; Maher, 1995; Minchin, 1998; Palmer, 2009; Ryan & Grace, 2001; Wolf, 2001) and self-control (Clarke-Stewart, 1998) prevailed. It seems that present views of self in relation to others reflect these historically based precepts that contradict the interdependence and closeness associated with nursing. Patriarchal predominance that altered nursing and mothering throughout generations is still very much ingrained in most of us and impedes support for the interdependence and closeness associated with nursing.

Respect for apparent autonomy and lone function concurs with and supports parent-child separation and vice versa. While the central rationale is that distancing advances child development, McKenna (1996) suggests instead that parents use their children's best interests as an excuse to use distal strategies. In reality, these strategies help them advance their desire to separate from their children.

Couple and Adult Precedence

Also similar to earlier times, messages associated with distancing children from mothers concur with the devaluation of children's needs. An adult focused parenting philosophy conveys this message and is identified by practices where parents' needs precede children's requirements. The propensity of parenting books set on training infants to sleep and to act in accordance with set schedules, rather than using child cues and developmental milestones, exemplify the adult centeredness that prevails in western culture. Adult precedence explains reverence for apparent equality in parenting tasks, even when these strategies disable parents from meeting their infants' needs and impair nursing. The adult centered philosophy is evident in research on maternal reasons for disliking nursing, including beliefs that breastfeeding interferes with their schedules and personal freedom, and impairs their employment availability (Blum, 1999; Guttman & Zimmerman, 2000; Libbus, Bush, & Hockman, 1997; Lindberg, 1996).

Couple precedence is a historically based practice demonstrating adult centered philosophy. The high degree of reverence for conjugal relationships is demonstrated by references to this practice in breastfeeding books that encourage mother-child closeness. Accordingly, nursing mothers are reminded to fulfill their sexual duties to their husbands and to pump their milk in order to go out alone with their husbands (Maher, 1995).

Distancing at Night

Couple precedence is often used as an excuse to discredit parent-child co-sleeping, and many believe that a child in the parental bed interferes with the cherished private marital relationship. The perspective that the night belongs to romantic couples impels some parents to end night time nursing sessions prior to signs of readiness from the child (Maher, 1995; McKenna, 1996; Palmer, 2009; Small, 1998; Thurer, 1994; Valsiner, 2000). Apparent child centered reasons are also used to dismantle parent-child co-sleeping. Klein's (1998) advice that parents and children sleep separately in order to guard children from parental sexuality exemplifies the misconceptions about the apparent sexual nature of parent-child co-sleeping. Other reasons include injury prevention, such as a study published in a medical journal that claims that children under two years may suffocate if they sleep with their parents (Nakamura et al., 1999). This view is contradicted by other research and contradicts the protective elements of co-sleeping that were reviewed earlier in this book (Ball, 2002; INFACT, 2003b; McKenna, 1996; McKenna et al., 1997; Okami et al., 2002; Valsiner, 2000). It is important to remember that children have slept with and woken up beside their parents and others for most of history. It seems more likely that our discomfort with closeness, desire to appear independent and alone, and the sexual connotations of sleep may force some clinicians and families to pathologize co-sleeping and the comforts it affords families with busily nursing children.

Lay Literature and Academic Research on Families

Nursing in Tune with Physiology

It is most encouraging that several interesting dissertations accompany an ever growing body of lay literature and Internet resources that provide insight into families that nurse in congruence with physiological principles and standards set by the WHO (1981, 2001, 2003). These sources show that these families display behaviors that mirror historical and anthropological themes of physiologically based nursing and proximity patterns (Bar Yakov, 2002; Bumgarner, 2000; Gorman, 2002; Green, 2001; La Leche League, 2004; Sears, 1988; Thevenin, 1976). According to lay literature, children nurse exclusively for approximately the first six months of life and continue to nurse for a few years. Children approach their mothers for nursing in a comfortable manner, using nursing as a means of comfort and security (Green, 2001). Full weaning occurs gradually and is child-led, full weaning occurs at approximately 36 months (Bumgarner, 2000; La Leche League, 2004; Sears, 1988; Stein et al., 2002; Thevenin, 1976).

Both parents are very involved in parenting; fathers and mothers engage in gender-specific tasks, especially in early infancy (Bumgarner, 2000; Granju &Kennedy, 1999; Kitzinger, 1979; La Leche League, 2004; Sears, 1988). Children's need for closeness is central and families engage in proximity behaviors, including co-sleeping (Ball, 2002; Bar-Yakov, 2002; Bumgarner, 2000; Green, 2001; La Leche League, 2004; Sears, 1988; Thevenin, 1976). Families engage in child-led behaviors (Bar-Yakov, 2002; Bumgarner, 2000; Green, 2001; La Leche League, 2004; Sears, 1988.) Lay literature calls the style of parenting that includes allowing children to nurse at will and to remain physically close to their parents as "attachment parenting" (Sears, 1988, 1990; Granju & Kennedy, 1999). According to the literature, this family style has a positive effect on parental development. The centrality of parenting in the scripts of these mothers and fathers is suggested by the way that they use little or no substitute childcare and go on joint family outings facilitated by shared wearing of the infant (Ball, 2002; Bar-Yakov, 2002; Green, 2001; Sears, 1988).

Implications of Family Themes Associated with Nursing for Clinical Practice

The discussion about interaction in breastfeeding families began by clarifying the role of bias in clinical practice. By reviewing the themes associated with nursing, clinicians can note how some of these themes have meaning for them, and how these attributions might affect the quality of their interactions with clients. Many themes associated with nursing are deeply ingrained in our culture and thus in clinicians. Views of closeness, couple precedence, and of course, breastfeeding in our families of origin, throughout our childhood, during university, in clinical training, and during our interactions in professional settings have likely been internalized. Similarly, nursing families have internalized meaning throughout their lives, and this will affect how they experience and tolerate nursing and associated behaviors.

The salient prevailing themes affecting families' ability to implement and our ability to support physiologically based nursing patterns include: artificial feeding as the norm; confusion about the female breast, disdain for natural female biology; reverence for separation, distal strategies, and apparent independence; adult centered attitudes; and couple precedence.

The salience of these themes contributes to our understanding of why many families in western contexts initiate nursing, but quickly stray from physiological patterns. The association between these themes and non-nursing implies that physiologically based nursing patterns concur different themes and behaviors. This proposal is validated by a growing body of literature indicating that there are families who nurse in tune with physiology and whose behaviors suggest that they hold themes that differ from the salient themes in western culture. The rest of this book will discuss these families and provide insight into their prevailing themes. Hopefully, clinicians' newfound awareness of themes affecting their practice will enable them to hear families better and will enable them to support families engaging in physiologically based nursing and associated behaviors.

Chapter 5
Family Development

The data in this chapter and those that follow reflect the findings of the study described in the introduction to this book (Epstein-Gilboa, 2006). The participating families are called families, mothers, fathers, children, and case study group. The other group of participants in the study is referred to as key informant interviewees. Several terms are used to describe those providing services to families including clinicians, practitioners, counselors, and services providers.

In this chapter, the evolving nursing family is described and the focus is on stages of development leading up to the maintenance stage of family development. The maintenance stage is the most complex and enduring aspect of family interaction and nursing. Several of the following chapters will be devoted to the evolution in each subsystem, showing the contribution of each unit to the sensitive family interaction. Please note that clinicians should only use the descriptions of these families as a guide. Remember that families are individual, and it is important to focus on individual narratives above all else.

Family Development

Families nursing in tune with physiologically based patterns went through several stages of development. Like all families in the transition to parenting and parenting of young children (Carter & McGoldrick, 1989), the families reflected events that took place prior to breastfeeding. Specific preparation for nursing was evident prior to giving birth. Themes related to nursing were firmly established at this stage and remained salient aspects of interaction as the family evolved. Following birth, parents in the initiation stage actively commenced breastfeeding. In the postpartum period, parents established the exclusive nursing subsystem. Families altered their roles and tasks to facilitate exclusivity. When exclusivity was firmly established, parents entered the maintenance stage and continued to engage with one another in a complementary style, while altering some of the tasks to suit the evolving exclusive nursing unit. The maintenance stage of nursing included exclusive nursing patterns, with gradual weaning commencing at six months when substances other than breastmilk were slowly added to the infants' diet. During the maintenance stage, families engaged in a variety of interactions and behaviors reflecting and influencing the creation of salient themes associated with nursing. Their interactions led to the creation of sensitive family interactions that reflected the cue-based interchanges associated with nursing. Most families continued to maintain nursing and associated behaviors for the first few years of life until children gradually weaned. While nursing and associated behaviors disappeared, the associated themes remained salient aspects of family interchanges over time.

Prenatal Stage

Establishing Themes

The themes that affected interactions in nursing families were formed prior to the birth of the nursing baby. Parents shared a perspective of nursing as a natural, normal, and developmentally enriching behavior. Nursing was seen as essential for maternal and child health. Many families also talked about the dangers of not nursing. One father's statement exemplified the couple's views of nursing as natural. The father explained how he and his wife thought about nursing prior to giving birth saying, "I never even thought that it was a decision to make. It is just a normal thing to do."

Respect for natural processes corresponded with many families' overall appreciation of normal physiology. For some, this idea was present prior to becoming nursing parents, and in other cases, breastfeeding contributed to this perspective. Many couples actualized their respect for natural processes through non-medicated births. Some families had home births with at least one of their children.

Mothers' and Fathers' Distinct Trajectories

It was interesting that mothers and fathers reached conclusions about the normalcy of nursing in different ways. Mothers researched nursing and associated parenting in the prenatal stage. They read material, took classes, learned about nursing in their academic lives, and for some, the knowledge about nursing stemmed from their professional background. However, the most efficient and valued means of learning stemmed from the pregnant mothers' relationships with nursing women. One reason that interactions with other mothers were most efficient was that mothers-to-be were able to learn tangible information and insights about nursing beyond infancy. Information through interaction helped mothers make plans for the future initiation and duration of nursing.

Fathers had a very different trajectory to nursing. Interestingly, fathers were also influenced by experiences with other nursing women and with prenatal preparations. Yet, in contrast to mothers, many fathers, regardless of their level of education, did not read material about nursing and parenting. One father, who was an educator with years of experience with nursing families, suggested that most material was woman focused and did not speak to men. However, it seemed that many men also ignored information packages that were apparently male focused.

One father of several formerly and presently nursing children summed up how many fathers felt about decisions about nursing when he talked about how he felt before the birth of his first nursing child. He stated, "I didn't have any knowledge about it one way or the other. Whatever she (his wife) felt, I went with her lead. I was supportive. It was the natural way to go." Like this father, many dads indicated that they saw nursing as a female responsibility and followed the mother's lead.

Exceptions to this rule were fathers who had learned about nursing in their families of origin. These fathers were more active in decisions regarding nursing, while at the same time they claimed that they respected the mother's right to make final decisions about nursing and associated parenting.

Fathers implied that they took a secondary position due to their perception that nursing was a female physiological task. This view was exemplified in one father's remarks, "At the time (prior to birth), it was her decision. She is the one who is willing to spend the time and do that. If she is willing to do that, more power to her!" An adoptive father expressed similar support for his wife as she attempted to induce lactation. He said, "It was completely Amy's decision because she had to do so much. She had to wake herself up in the middle of the night sometimes to just pump. But I was really glad that she was doing it!"

Mothers validated their partners' positions and seemed quite comfortable leading the way towards nursing in the prenatal period. One first time mother with previous professional experience working with new parents explained how new parents act to her partner and gave him instructions about what he was supposed to do for her after she gave birth. She emphasized strongly that he was not allowed to provide her with any artificial feeding substances and was to encourage her to nurse under all circumstances.

There were some fathers who found it difficult to follow the mothers' leads. One father of a formerly nursing school aged child and a nursing toddler implied that he felt left out and angry when his wife made decisions about nursing without him. The father's tone was angry when he said, "Me? Not much say in the matter (about decisions regarding nursing). Whatever she wanted was fine. I don't think that I said let's do it that way. I certainly didn't put up a fight. There was no reason to. It's natural. There is nothing is wrong with it. There was never a problem. I didn't say I don't want you to do it that way." The distinct difference between the father's angry tone and his apparently accepting words implied that like the other fathers, he revered nursing as the natural sequel to birth, and yet he felt angry when he perceived that he had been excluded from making decisions about nursing. This father remained ambivalent throughout both of his children's nursing relationships.

Immediate Postnatal Period and Initiation

It seemed that fathers continued to follow their partners' leads in the immediate postnatal period. Mothers often initiated the first nursing session while their partners looked on in awe. A key informant with many years experience working in a birthing unit stated, "They (fathers) begin to love their infants as they watch the mother nurse." Mothers and fathers described their first nursing experiences from different perspectives, yet with the same level of intensity and wonder. For example, parents of an actively nursing toddler described the first time their son nursed. The mother said, "They put him on my tummy immediately. It was incredible! He nursed like a pro right from the start!" Similarly, her partner said, "I thought that it was cool; I was surprised."

Establishing and Maintaining Exclusivity in the Nursing Unit

Following initiation of nursing, the parents' primary goal was to ensure physiological interdependence between the nursing dyad-triad. Several key informant interviewees reflected family reverence for exclusivity in their descriptions of the mother-infant relationship, including calling it a "sacramental relationship." Another said, "Mothers and newborns are in a magic circle, anyone who comes too close is intruding."

Complementary Parenting Task Allocation

Parents reorganized their system to allow mothers to nurse without interference and to ensure that all of the babies' needs were met. Mothers focused on their infants and nursed almost constantly. They seemed mesmerized by their infants while they attempted to learn about them, their needs, and how to respond to those needs. At the same time, mothers were busy with self-care and efforts to integrate the birthing experience into their sense of self. Mothers with perceived positive birthing experiences seemed to incorporate their new sense of self with great ease and pride, and continued nursing with ease. These mothers also seemed to overcome nursing difficulties if they should arise. Mothers with complicated birthing experiences more commonly had nursing problems, due to both physical and psychological reasons. Previous commitment to nursing, including themes of reverence for physiology and paternal support, helped them overcome obstacles and facilitated the transition to cue-based mothering.

During the early postpartum period, fathers took care of the newborns' basic needs outside of nursing, for example, bathing the infant and changing diapers. The active fathers also engaged in many different complementary tasks, including physically and emotionally supporting mothers, cooking meals, and looking after the household. These tasks also included childcare when there were older children in the home. Fathers helped mothers rearrange formerly singular nursing relationships when the birth of a new child created a tandem nursing situation (nursing more than one child). For example, one father tempted an older nursing child with a game when mom wanted to nurse the newborn alone for a few moments.

Parents of two young children demonstrated the joint efforts that mothers and fathers made to ensure exclusive nursing through a system of complementary task allocation. The mother recalled how she felt following the birth of the couple's first child saying, "I was totally out of commission. I did my first diaper change when Jeffrey was two or three weeks old. Steve (her husband) had to take control for the first two or three weeks. I nursed him and that was all that I did." Her husband's comments also demonstrated their shared efforts and the positive sense of self fathers internalized at the same time. In a proud voice, the dad said, "Here is my son and I had to kick into action mode. I had to take care of him... I had never looked after a baby before and I was on my own. I was thrown into parenthood without any experience. I had never even held a small baby before, other than the one time that I had held the neighbor's baby. ...Our families live out of town so I was on my own. I took a two week vacation and I fully cared for my wife and baby. I did everything, except breastfeed the baby."

Fathers and Protective Tasks

Protective tasks were an integral aspect of the fathering role during the establishment of the exclusive nursing relationship. When infants were newly born, fathers defended the nursing system against potential threats to the establishment of the essential nursing functions. The protective actions reflected the complementary interactional style.

At times, mothers instituted the protective actions. For example, a mother recalled how she had been despondent when her newly born second child had been removed to a nursery due to apparent medical reasons. The father reinforced her feelings. He physically helped her take the baby and leave the hospital prior to official discharge, amidst threats from the healthcare staff. In another case, a second time mother directed her husband to immediately retrieve their newly born infant from the nursery where she had been taken against the mother's wishes.

Fathers often initiated protective steps based on the information they learned from their partners prior to their children's birth. In one case, a father without any practical experience with infants prior to the birth of his first son implemented information that his wife taught him prior to giving birth. She had a difficult birth and was unable to function as well as she had expected. He followed her earlier advice and ensured that artificial feeding and pacifiers were not introduced. The insights that she provided him also helped him recognize his limitations, and he brought in additional resources when needed.

Like the father described above, many fathers stepped in and protected exclusive relationships when mothers were physically or emotionally incapacitated. The tasks they fulfilled demonstrated their mutual ownership of nursing. The strong role of the protective father, guarding the exclusive nursing relationship, was poignantly demonstrated by a father whose wife lay comatose following a horrific birthing experience. He persevered in his quest to initiate nursing despite the extreme negativity that he faced on the part of the health team, including the hospital lactation consultant. This father persisted due to his belief that he was fulfilling his wife's desire to nurse upon recovery.

The father above demonstrated how fathers can initiate the creation of an exclusive nursing relationship without their partner's assistance. This important role was also demonstrated by an adoptive father who initiated the first nursing session in his family. This father learned about nursing from his wife and mirrored her strong desire to nurse. He actualized this shared view by initiating the first nursing session immediately following their child's birth. He told the biological mother about his wife's intentions to nurse and asked if his wife could nurse the one-day-old baby as soon as possible. His wife was aghast and anxious about the biological mother's reaction. Much to the couple's joy, the surprised biological mother was overjoyed about their decision to nurse and invited the adoptive mother to initiate nursing right away.

Challenges to Paternal Support and Implications for Nursing Mothers

There were conditions that interfered with the father's ability to consistently ensure that nursing was initiated and remained exclusive. In the early postnatal period, some fathers seemed to have difficulty coping with what they perceived as maternal discomfort. Furthermore, maternal pain seemed to be more important to fathers than infant difficulties. It is interesting that when fathers looked back on earlier experiences, they tended to focus on the mothers' emotions, or less commonly on their own emotions, and rarely described the infant's feelings during the crisis. This is in contrast with the intense fascination fathers displayed towards their newborn children that was often apparent in the same narrative. These examples indicate that in some nursing systems, in the initial period, fathers' prioritized the mothers' needs over those of the infants.

Fathers who perceived that their partners experienced pain seemed to have difficulty supporting the establishment of the nursing relationship. This seemed to be especially true for fathers who believed that their partners had suffered unduly during birth. These fathers appeared less capable of coping with nursing difficulties than their counterparts who held more positive views of the birthing experience. It was also interesting that fathers expressed more anxiety regarding the apparently painful birthing experience than their partners did. Yet, true to circular interactions, paternal distress often triggered negative responses in the mothers, subsequently impeding the establishment of nursing.

The significance of maternal pain was demonstrated further by the centrality of this topic in fathers' narratives of previous nursing experiences. For example, the parents of three children described their first nursing experience that had taken place a decade earlier. Along with describing the positive aspects of the nursing experience, the father recounted his wife's pain vividly and in detail. He said, "The first two weeks were hell...They were so difficult, physically more than anything. Angela (the mother) was having more and more pain. ...It was bleeding, it was raw, it needed some time to heal." In contrast, the mother, although admitting that her nipples had been sore, used humor to tell the same story, recalling a few anecdotes that occurred at the same time. Her husband countered her humorous tales with, "It wasn't funny at the time!"

Fathers' perceptions of pain seemed to decrease their ability to effectively guard the nursing relationship and ensure exclusivity. Again, fathers' capacity to tolerate their perceptions of pain related to their views of the entire situation, including the birth preceding nursing. The difficulty that men had withstanding their wives' apparent discomfort was demonstrated by one father who, believing that his wife had endured what he felt was undue pain, said that his baby was taking too much from the mother. In another case, a father said that it was difficult for him to see his wife "sacrificing" so much for the infant. In both of these cases, the fathers pressed their wives to provide their infants with other means of comfort. In both of these cases, the mothers stated that they were irritated by their partners' attempts to interfere with nursing exclusivity.

The capacity of mothers to withstand their partners' tension and to nurse in an exclusive manner depended on the mother's emotional state, their perception of their partner's opinions, and the relationship between the couple. Some mothers were unable to sustain exclusive nursing when fathers pressured them to interrupt exclusivity. Mothers in systems with open communication styles seemed to be able to cope more successfully with their partners' anxiety than mothers in systems with contrasting communication styles.

Sense of Efficiency Restores Supportive Function

There were some important factors that helped fathers overcome their anxiety and return to a supportive stance. Fathers encouraged nursing when they found solutions to the problem that caused them anguish. They were especially relieved when the solution was tangible and when they could participate in repairing the problem. Some fathers felt relief when they were able to help their spouses latch (attach) and position the baby at the breast. Others enjoyed assessing suckling technique and providing mothers with instructions that enhanced nursing. For some in more complex situations, tangible help included placing feeding tubes at their wives' breasts in order to help reluctant babies latch onto the breast.

Shared Ownership of Nursing and Mutual Support

Fathers also turned to their inner convictions about the essentiality of nursing and used those feelings to help them support mothers' efforts. Dads seemed to overcome anxiety and support nursing when they received reinforcement from mothers. Mutual support while parents worked together to resolve nursing issues had positive effects on the couple beyond nursing. For example, mothers proudly recounted the help they received from their partners in the present and in earlier nursing relationships. An important point that mothers reiterated in their narratives of paternal support was that the fathers understood and supported their quest to nurse in tune with physiology. This made them feel validated. Fathers internalized a sense of efficacy and pride when they perceived that they helped fix a damaged nursing relationship. The pride was evident in one fathers' voice as he proclaimed, "I helped with the latching!"

The good enough feelings that fathers internalized gave them a sense of importance that enriched further their commitment to reinstate the exclusive nature of the nursing relationship, even in difficult situations. Fathers with this positive sense of self were able to encourage mothers to induce lactation or to relactate, to overcome sore nipples and other maladies, to help babies with latching problems, and to save nursing relationships in situations that seemed hopeless. For example, one father encouraged and physically assisted his wife to nurse from one breast alone, without supplements, after it became apparent that her other breast had been irreparably damaged by prior surgery. In another case, an adoptive father tried to help his spouse cope with the reality that she was unable to fully sustain her newborn adopted child with her milk in the same way that she had exclusively nursed their older adopted child. This dad drove all over the city everyday to retrieve donor breastmilk. The donor milk was fed to the baby in a tube at the breast and not only complemented his wife's existing milk supply, but also enabled the mother-infant dyad to continue their nursing relationship in the most natural way possible. This father downplayed his role and said, "But I can't imagine who wouldn't do that. It's not like it is her baby, it is our baby that I am helping out here. ..."

Respecting Exclusive Tasks of the Nursing Subsystem

Fathers' commitment to nursing was evident in the efforts they made to not interfere with tasks that were specific to nursing; fathers refrained from artificially feeding or providing their infants with oral comfort. The few fathers who fed their infants in emergency situations implied that they had done this reluctantly, were uncomfortable about their actions, and looked forward to reinstating normal nursing. In addition, these fathers claimed that feeding had not affected their relationships with their children. One key informant interviewee, a father of several former nursing children, several of whom were now adults, was puzzled by fathers who wanted to feed their babies and stated emphatically, "Why would a father want to feed a nursing baby?"

In circular fashion, paternal support of exclusivity enabled mothers to internalize the cue-based behaviors associated with nursing, enriching their skills and strengthening themes as they interacted with infants at the breast. Increased maternal confidence and competence reverberated back to fathers. Fathers reduced their direct care and protective activities, increasing these tasks when necessary. Mothers retained the central role as primary cue respondent, answering most infant cues through nursing.

Summary of the Evolution of the Nursing Subsystem in the Prenatal, Initiation, and Establishment Phases of Development

Mothers and fathers entered the nursing relationship with shared views; however, their trajectory to nursing was different. Mothers taught their partners about nursing and fathers followed. The distinct parenting paths continued while parents initiated and established nursing. Mothers nursed while fathers supported and protected the nursing unit. Paternal protection was challenged at times when fathers were overcome by feelings of helplessness that were triggered when fathers perceived that mothers endured hardships. Most fathers overcame obstacles when they sensed that they were efficient and able to repair damage. When the nursing system was fully established, fathers complemented mothers' work as the central figure meeting most of the infants' cues through nursing. Once nursing was established, fathers reduced their level of protective and supportive actions, stepping up these tasks when they perceived it was necessary. The system arranged their roles and tasks to allow the nursing subsystem to engage in initially exclusive, unique, and evolving interactions. The nursing subsystem remained intact until gradual weaning took place a few years later.

Clinical Implications

The information on nursing families demonstrates that the changes that take place in these systems are congruent with the principles of a changing family life cycle. This implies that a central clinical task is to support families as they make the transition to parenting or to the addition of another child into the family system. Optimal practice includes knowledge about the general issues associated with the transitions at this stage of family growth and alteration of tools to suit the presenting family's specific phase of development. However, it is important to note that the information provided in this and other chapters is a guide to interactions with families. While using this guide, one should simultaneously focus on clients as individuals. The meaning of the nursing experience might not be the same for all families encountered in clinical practice. Practitioners should be open to families' diverse interpretation of the nursing experience and not try to fit families into a set cast. Naturally, the type but not the style of interaction between the clinician and the family will vary depending on one's clinical focus. In all cases, the most important factor guiding practice is using one's knowledge of the impact of nursing on family development and vice versa, while listening and responding to individual narrative.

Healthcare professionals working with couples in the prenatal stage, such as childbirth educators and lactation consultants, should optimally take a couple's gender specific learning styles into account and rethink the tools we use to transfer information. For example, while mothers might cherish handouts, the data seem to indicate that this educational tool might not be relevant for fathers. Our understanding about maternal leading and educating in the prenatal stage implies that we need to find ways to reinforce mothers' scripts and provide them with a means of teaching their partners. In the population described, maternal tutoring was a natural part of the couple interchange, except in cases where fathers felt excluded. Anticipatory guidance, including helping couples learn about gender specificity, will normalize this apparent imbalance and facilitate the internalization of novel concepts. In addition, fathers may benefit from group sessions where they can hear about their male counterparts' feelings and experiences, once again normalizing the events at hand. The obvious connection between broken physiology and nursing difficulties implies that clinicians should follow ethical principles and provide families with truthful information about physiological birth and implications of medical interventions during the birthing process for nursing and other postpartum behaviors. It is also important to provide parents with information about the feelings they might experience following birth, for example, a mother's desire to be with the infant and issues that might hamper a father's capacity to support nursing.

Clinicians working with families in birthing and postpartum contexts may also facilitate couple growth and enhance the exclusivity of nursing. Birth attendants from all professional backgrounds may support parents' efforts to birth without intervention and refine their skills to help those who are less committed or knowledgeable about normal birth. It is important to recognize the impact of paternal perceptions of pain and to assist them to see maternal perspectives and strengths during birth. Ensuring optimal conditions for the initiation of maternal-infant exclusivity are part of clinical service at this stage.

Following birth, clinicians should find ways of enhancing couples' attempts to develop shared themes enabling nursing and establishing exclusivity. The transition to parenting is often complicated when couples have different perspectives and goals. Through discussions, one might enhance parents' abilities to listen to their partner and formulate novel joint concepts.

Understanding the impact of maternal pain on paternal capacity to support nursing means clinicians need to find ways for fathers to express their distress and obtain validation, while at the same time encouraging fathers to find ways to repair perceived damage. Healthcare providers can facilitate reparative processes by teaching fathers practical ways of helping with nursing and providing positive feedback to fathers for their efforts. Psychotherapists might be able to help fathers verbalize this problem in greater depth than healthcare professionals; however, all clinicians can help fathers understand the process that they are experiencing. Assisting mothers to tell fathers about their needs for exclusivity and validating this feeling might also help fathers realize that simply by encouraging their partners they are repairing perceived harm. In addition, healthcare providers can encourage mothers to state their appreciation for partners who help them meet goals. This intervention seems to facilitate increased paternal support.

At this stage of development, as with all stages, clinicians in the field of individual or couple psychotherapy can help couples enrich their growth by providing a means of processing the experience and enriching communication skills. In addition, one can reinforce existing strengths by validating feelings and reframing difficult situations. An empathetic clinician can point out what is working, rather than what is not, and help couples celebrate each small step.

It is important to recall the significance of countertransference in clinical practice and recognize that our own feelings affect our interactions with clients. The birth, initiation, and establishment of exclusivity stages are often difficult stages for clinicians to tolerate. In some cases, clinicians might find it hard to support clients whose reality negates their own perspective and lifestyle. Some situations may seem overwhelming. It is easy to get caught up in parents' feelings of helplessness and hopelessness and to mirror their tension in interactions with them. In addition, it is important to remember that all clinicians are members of a culture that uses artificial feeding as the norm. Practitioners might have trouble supporting a couple's desire for exclusive nursing when it negates their primary view of health. For example, clinicians feeling overwhelmed by couple distress and infant signs of discomfort might feel that letting go of nursing exclusivity might help the family return to homeostasis and benefit the system more than reinforcing exclusivity. In this case, it is important to try and differentiate between the clinician's feelings about nursing and personal sense of being overwhelmed, and the real issues presented by the client.

A clinician's awareness of their own scripts, stress levels, and efforts to decipher these difficult feelings are the first step to enhancing practice. Like with clients, one has to remind oneself about normal processes, the impact of broken physiology on couple function, and then, most importantly, remember that these situations usually work when reframed. One can focus on the strengths in each couple while helping them make the transition to parenting a nursing child and the maintenance stage of nursing.

At times, one might feel that despite all of their good enough efforts, they have not been able to help a couple overcome issues. Or a clinician might feel that they have tried to accept the clients' reality and desire for nursing exclusivity, but are unable to accept that perspective. This is a good time to seek support from colleagues and accept that the responsibility for growth ultimately lies in the hands of the couple. One should also remember that referring clients to other resources when necessary is an ethical and kind act.

Chapter 6: Interactions in the Nursing Subsystem: The Development of Sensitive Mothering and Sensitive Interactions

In this chapter, interactions in the breastfeeding family after nursing has been established and until full weaning takes place will begin to be reviewed. It is important to remember that family systems are composed of subsystems that affect and are influenced by one another and the family as a whole. The impact of breastfeeding on the system and vice versa is the focus, so we start by looking at interactions in the nursing sub-unit. The interactions during and in between nursing will be described, and then possible development implications of the nursing relationship for children and mothers will be addressed. Similar to the last chapter, examples from the study of nursing families are interspersed throughout this chapter and in following chapters.

Cue-Based Interactions

Mothers persistently watched and interpreted infants' signs, usually responding with nursing. In infancy, mothers initiated nursing when infants awakened, whined, looked at the mother, looked at the breast, opened their mouths and moved in the direction of the breast, tensed their muscles, and grimaced. The least frequent cue was crying. As with all cues, crying was responded to immediately. Infants reinforced the interactive cycle by calming down when they were put to the breast. The positive reinforcement that infants provided to mothers was demonstrated by a mother of a two-month-old baby who watched her infant latch on and said, "That's what you want isn't it. Now you are happy."

As babies grew and developed, they added other cues for nursing to their repertoire. Young and non-verbal children used many physical and direct cues to show their mothers that they wanted to nurse. For example, babies moved closer to their mothers and touched their mothers' breasts. Mobile children tended to periodically venture away and return to their mothers, whom the children used as a safe base from which to explore their environment. Children intermittently interrupted their play and crawled, or older children walked, to their mothers, climbed up on their mothers' laps, pulled up the mothers' blouses, and latched on to the breast independently.

Similar to early infancy, mothers of older children used nursing to console their children in moments of need. For example, a mother picked up her two-year-old daughter in response to the child's sudden and unprovoked aggressiveness towards an older sibling. As she held her obviously tired child in her arms, she asked the child if she wanted "mommas" (name for nursing). As the mother latched her daughter onto the breast, she gently touched the little girl's head and repeated, "You are so tired; you are so tired, aren't you?" Her comments demonstrated how a mother may interpret a child's feelings and respond with comfort through nursing. The little girl immediately calmed down and reinforced her mother's actions.

Cue Names for Nursing

Children's cues for nursing became more complex and more coherent when their acquisition of language skills increased with age. One of the earliest uses of language in cueing for nursing was in the form of special names for nursing. In many cases, the mothers created the name based on the sounds that children used to cue for nursing. In other cases, mothers made up usually childish sounding names for nursing that children repeated. Children asked for nursing by using the cue word, and similarly, the mothers asked children if they wanted to nurse by asking them if they wanted "bubbas" for example. One key informant interviewee had researched this aspect of child development and verified that naming nursing was a common occurrence, and names often reflected children's linguistic capacities.

The developmental process associated with naming nursing was exemplified by twin nurslings, who were observed from the age of five and a half months to over four years of age. During infancy, family members joined the mother in calling nursing "tzi tzi" (this family did not speak English and "tzi tzi" meant "titty" in their language) when the boys were infants. It seemed that this was the name the older daughters had used when they nursed. Later on, the name for nursing became "et zeh" that mirrored the way the twins had pointed to the breast and said "et zeh, et zeh" (meaning "that," "et zeh" is the word for "that" in their native tongue). When the twins were approximately two years old, one of the little boys made up a name for nursing that sounded like "ima," the word for mother in their language. The name composed by the toddler was "imi." In addition, he also made up the name "ibi" for his mother that sounded like "imi," but with a "b" rather than an "m." His twin brother followed suit, and then the whole family referred to the act of nursing as "imi." Soon both boys initiated nursing sessions by calling out "Imi, imi, imi..." as they came over to their mother, crawled on her lap, and latched on to nurse, either at the same time or in sole sessions. They continued to call nursing "imi" until they weaned at approximately four and a half years of age.

It is interesting that, like this family, other families in the study used names for nursing that sounded like the name for mother. Two families, for example, called nursing "momma" or "mommas." When these families used words sounding like mother for nursing, they were able to distinguish the name from the other word they used for the actual mother, and use them accordingly.

Other families used words that resembled common names for the breast, nursing, and even breastmilk as their designated nursing cue name. However, they created a warmer connotation for the name by changing it to a more childish and cuter sound. For example, one family called nursing "booby." Similarly, another family used the word "bubbies" or "bubba," which also sounded somewhat like momma. Yet, another family used the word "a little titty." One family called nursing "nurse." Two families used the word "milky" when they talked about intentions to nurse or in their discussions of nursing. Most interestingly, in one family, nursing had been called "nuni" for several years; however, the mother claimed that she changed the name to "nursing" when she began to realize that calling nursing by any other name was, in essence, disguising an activity that she was actually proud of. Another interesting example of a cue word with deep underlying meaning was the use of the word "Pa" for nursing. The family explained that this was short for pacifier and implied that they saw the breast as a comforting object.

Exchange of Emotional Messages during Nursing

Mothers and children continued to read one another's cues and engage in reciprocal interactions during nursing sessions. Nursing partners exchanged emotional messages in many forms as they looked, smiled, and touched one another as the babies suckled. Infants vocalized and children later spoke to their mothers as they nursed at the breast. Mothers mirrored their actions.

One mother with a nursing toddler exemplified the complex interchanges between nursing couplets. The little toddler and her mother smiled at one another intermittently while the little girl nursed. They gently touched one another in a synchronized manner. Like many other children, while this toddler nursed on one breast, she touched her mother's other breast. Also similar to other cases, the mother reported that she withstood this type of touching, although she said that it was not always a comfortable feeling, especially when the baby did this in a public place.

Some children touched their mothers with their whole bodies while they nursed. Some moved their feet and hands on their mother's stomach and chest as they nursed. In one family, a little eighteen-month-old boy liked to stroke his mother's long blond hair as he suckled peacefully. The mother stated that she had purposely grown her hair in response to his interest.

Interactions during nursing changed as children grew and mothers suited their responses to their children's nuances. An eighteen-month-old boy, for example, intermittently walked over to his mother for brief nursing sessions in between playing with objects that he found in the room. His mother sat on the floor. He came over to her, touched her breast, pulled up her blouse, leaned his head towards her breast, and remained standing as he latched on. He stood with his feet firmly set on the ground as he nursed. His mother commented that he usually preferred standing while he nursed. In addition, the toddler moved his head back and forth between the breasts and nursed on each one for short periods. As he continued this pattern of alternating between the breasts, his mother smiled, gently massaged his back, and spoke to him calmly in a loving tone. He finished nursing, climbed off his mother, and continued his explorations.

As with this child, most nursing sessions were terminated in response to children's cues. In early infancy, babies demonstrated satisfaction by falling asleep, reducing the intensity of their suckling, looking away, and pulling off the breast. Older children often moved away from the breast and continued with other activities. Some verbal children announced happily that they were finished for the moment. Sometimes mothers with nursing children over the age of two years intermittently prompted their children to end nursing sessions. Study participants indicated that they sometimes had less patience for long nursing sessions with their older children, especially if their child nursed very frequently and seemed to linger at the breast. However, they also emphasized that mothers watched their children's cues and only asked them to finish if they were exhibiting signs that the mothers perceived as signs of readiness for a break.

Frequent, Encompassing, and Flexible Nursing Sessions

Mothers interpreted most of their children's signals as cues for nursing. Nursing was ongoing, regardless of the children's age, sometimes occurring several times an hour. Key informants described nursing dyads as "symbiotic," and their function as "oneness." Symbiosis was exemplified in a mother's description of her nursing relationship with her daughter who had nursed for several years. She said, "I would never let her be alone for a moment. I nursed her all day and all night long. When she wasn't nursing, I would be with her."

The capacity of the mothers to continually respond patiently to their children's cues for nursing was also suggested by the existence of changing and unpredictable nursing patterns in the majority of nursing families. The needs of the study infants and children for nursing changed in frequency and intensity in a non-linear fashion. The unpredictable nursing patterns were exemplified by the nursing pattern of an infant at four weeks who cued for nursing every hour and a half, and nursed for about twenty minutes. In contrast, at nine weeks, she displayed short, continuous, intermittent nursing segments with small breaks between the nursing sessions. In keeping with the parental theme of responding to natural cues, the mother responded to the infant's self-initiated signs by gently placing her on the breast.

Maternal versatility was suggested by mothers' capacity to cope with both structured and flexible nursing routines. Structure often coincided with meeting the needs of additional children. For example, a mother of three children attempted to nurse her youngest daughter earlier in the afternoon in order to be free when her older children's school was dismissed. Yet, this dyad altered their set nursing session and included additional nursing sessions when the older child intermittently demonstrated an increased need for nursing.

Mothers coped with flexible and unpredictable nursing patterns in all contexts and took their children with them when they went out. Many mothers nursed in public almost right from birth. New and inexperienced mothers found it difficult initially due to reasons of modesty. Mothers increasingly gained a sense of comfort with nursing in public, and most experienced mothers indicated that they felt at ease nursing in public places. Most mothers concealed their breasts. Exceptions to this rule were exemplified by one experienced mother who, after nursing four children, refused to conceal her breasts when she nursed in public. She emphatically declared that, "I will not cover up my breasts when I nurse! My children can't breathe when I do that and their needs are more important than anything else!"

Mothers' ability to nurse in an ongoing and flexible manner was facilitated by a belief that nursing meets many needs for their children and was essential for their development. The encompassing nature of nursing was illustrated in one mother's discussion of her six-year-old daughter's former nursing patterns. This happy and very independent little girl had weaned a year earlier. Her mother described the former nursing relationship by saying, "She (the daughter) would nurse just for life in general. She was an "everything" nurser. Nursing was for everything!"

According to the key informants, one of the many functions encompassed by nursing was comfort. While mothers of young infants often focused on the way nursing met their infants' physical needs, like their more experienced counterparts, they also spoke about comfort in their narratives of nursing. Maternal appreciation of children's needs for comfort through nursing seemed to contribute to the frequent nature of nursing in both infancy and early childhood.

Challenges to Cue-Based Nursing

Mothers who disregarded the encompassing nature of the nursing relationship, even intermittently, missed important cues for nursing. Their lack of sensitivity to cues was especially prominent when they focused on nursing as primarily a means of nutrition. One mother nursed her older child into early childhood, suggesting that she believed in the holistic value of nursing. In addition, she fervently defended the comforting aspects of nursing in her arguments with her husband. Yet, she frequently referred to nursing as a means of feeding in her descriptions of nursing and her daughter's behavior. For example, she called nursing "food," named her daughter's needs as "hunger," and described her daughter's behavior in terms of feeding saying, "she just wants to suck and she doesn't want milk." The focus on food in her narrative appeared to limit her capacity to understand her infant, and consequently, she missed many of the infant's cues to nurse. Instead, she gave her finger to the baby to suck when she felt that her "baby was not hungry." Impaired responsiveness was aggravated further when the mother reluctantly began to use non-nursing comfort measures, including a pacifier and an infant swing, to appease her daughter's apparently persistent cues. It is important to note that these steps were initiated by the father who seemed resolute in his opinion that nursing was mainly a way of feeding babies.

Older children who nursed frequently despite full diets reinforced the idea that children do not see nursing as merely food. For example, one two-year-old climbed on her mother to nurse in between playing. Following this nursing session, she ate a large meal, and then finished her older brother's dinner. After dinner, she played for a short while with her brother, and then verbally and physically indicated to her mother that she wanted to nurse again. Her mother pleasantly complied, and the little toddler nursed until her evening bath.

Cue-Based Interactions in between Nursing

The ongoing focus on meeting children's needs in a cue-based manner continued in between the flexible and frequent nursing sessions. Mothers seemed determined to meet their children's needs for closeness at all times. These mothers held, carried, and wore their infants in infant carriers close to their bodies in between frequent nursing sessions until the children were independently mobile. Toddlers and older children frequently returned to their mothers for nursing, hugs, warm tactile interactions, or verbal reassurance in between their independent activities. Carrying and closeness were extended to outings, and mothers took their children with them when they went out. Children remained physically close to their mothers, including at night, and mother-child co-sleeping was common for the first few years of children's lives, an act that facilitated nursing during the night.

The ongoing proximity between mothers and children was exemplified by a mother who proclaimed, in a positive and proud tone, that the only time that she was not holding or nursing the baby was when the father held him for short periods of time. She said, "...I don't have to feel guilty for not breastfeeding (when her husband held the baby in her place). It was fifteen minutes that I knew that I was not needed!"

It appears that nursing and closeness in between breastfeeding contributed to mothers' cue reading capacities. One first time mother of a young toddler explained, "It (nursing) helped me build up my relationship with my son...I am very aware of his needs and I am very perceptive to his cues. There is the closeness and the bonding. When you are breastfeeding, you have to be with the baby. You have to have that typical closeness with the emotional closeness. You can't just drop your baby off with somebody else. He was with me all of the time. I could sense the differences in his cries. I could tell even before he was going to cry, he must need to nurse. He was only two weeks old. Having him close, you can see the changes. I carried him all of the time. He was held everywhere, while I was preparing dinner he was held, while I went for walks."

Tandem Nursing

The sensitivity, flexibility, openness, and reciprocity that the mothers demonstrated in dyadic nursing relationships was also apparent when mothers nursed more than one child at the same time – tandem nursing. Tandem nursing was commonplace in nursing families with twins or when older children were not yet ready to let go of the breast following the birth of a new sibling. The prevalence of tandem nursing was suggested by the finding that half of the families in the study group had engaged in tandem nursing at one time.

Children of Different Ages

Sometimes tandem nursing subsystems contained children of different ages. It seemed that although tandem nursing reduced opportunities for sole interactions between mothers and each nursing child, it decreased sibling rivalry and enriched the relationships between the siblings. Mothers' behaviors and narratives indicated that they tried to be fully responsive to each child, despite the challenges, and they tried to match nursing to individual nursing needs. Younger children nursed more frequently than their older siblings, and the breast played a more central role in their relational script than it did for older siblings. At times, siblings nursed separately; at other times, they nursed together. In addition to warm interchanges between nursing siblings, intermittent aggressiveness also took place at the breast.

Twins

Nursing twins exemplified tandem nursing of children at the same developmental stage. It was interesting that various families organized twin nursing in diverse ways. For example, one mother nursed her twins at the same time since their birth. This mother also answered individual cues when they were elicited. She said, "I let them nurse whenever, some days they are teething and they might nurse quite a bit. Other days, they could care less." Another mother tried to nurse her sons separately when they were infants; however, she altered this pattern to suit her children's needs that fluctuated over time.

The second mother was a member of a family that was observed over a four year period. Initially, the twins appeared oblivious of one another, and each one nursed as if he was alone at the breast. Both nursed frequently throughout the day and night, and sometimes their meetings at the breast coincided. During their second year of life, the twins began to notice one another, and this affected their interactions regarding nursing. Often one twin followed the other to the breast, as they continued to nurse frequently in an almost equal manner. At times interactions at the breast seemed to exclude the mother, as the twins played or pushed one another aggressively while nursing at the same time. They copied one another's antics at the breast and, for example, when one brother invented a new cue name for nursing, his twin imitated him. Another example of the complexity of the twins' interchanges at the breast was the way the twins switched breasts in the middle of a nursing session. This game was initiated by one of the twins at eighteen months of age, and it was believed that he did this in order to enjoy both breasts at each nursing session. His brother initially gave in and switched upon his brother's command. Eventually, this changed and both cued the other to switch.

Following the twins' second birthday, the nursing pattern changed again. One twin continued to nurse very frequently during the day, while his brother reserved his nursing for almost hourly sessions during the night. At age three, the twins no longer ran after one another to the breast, often nursing separately and demonstrating very different nursing patterns. They enjoyed talking about nursing and did not demonstrate any interest in weaning. The significance of nursing for the boys was illustrated by an event that took place when they started preschool towards their third birthday. One of the twins was severely insulted by a preschool teacher who suggested that he was a big boy and that he needed to stop nursing. He refused to go back to the school. His sensitive parents understood him, validated his feelings, and resolved the problem. He then returned to preschool, and his teacher learned to be more sensitive about nursing.

Both twins continued to nurse on their fourth birthday. However, one twin was much more interested in nursing than the other twin. The more interested twin was also the more outgoing twin. They continued their pattern where one twin nursed more frequently during the day, while the other nursed at night. The twin who nursed more frequently at night had seriously reduced the frequency of his nursing. The twin who nursed more frequently during the day stated clearly that he did not intend to wean and said, "I need to nurse." Nevertheless, like his brother, he gradually reduced the frequency of nursing. The apparently less interested twin weaned fully at approximately four years and four months of age. His brother followed him and had weaned by the age of four and a half years. According to the mother, the twin who had been more interested in nursing continued to put the breast in his mouth about once a week, although he did not actually suckle. Both boys continued to talk about nursing and to play with their mother's breasts after they weaned. At the age of four and a half, the twin who had weaned first proudly declared to his mother, "Mommy I almost never play with your breasts anymore!"

Child-Focused Weaning Patterns

Similar to the case with the twins, weaning seemed to be a long and gradual process in most nursing relationships. Weaning began during the second half of the first year of life, when complementary foods were slowly introduced. Most infants in the study population nursed exclusively without additional substances for at least the first six months of age, some for longer periods. Mothers actualized their respect for natural developmental processes by withholding solids until their children showed signs of readiness.

The weaning process seemed to be individual and gradual, based on children's changing needs for nursing, and took place over several years. Mothers in the study followed child cues for weaning, much the same way they initiated nursing and interacted with their children during and in between nursing sessions. Respect for children's individual rhythms and needs for nursing and the understanding that nursing is an encompassing behavior with physiological and emotional elements, helped these mothers make decisions about weaning. Several salient styles were apparent; naturally all were affected by individuality. Children's needs and views were always taken into account when weaning was considered, regardless of the specific pattern.

Mother-Led Weaning

Mother-led weaning was the least common form of weaning in this population and the most common form of weaning in children who weaned prior to age three. Reasons included maternal breast discomfort resulting from an existing pregnancy or a desire for another pregnancy, alongside fears that nursing might interfere with the ability to conceive in mothers with previous infertility issues. Mothers contemplating taking fertility medications worried about the possible harmful effects of the medication on the nursing child, and weaned for that reason.

Mothers also contributed to weaning in tandem nursing relationships. They might precipitate weaning for the older child in the relationship when they perceived that tandem nursing was detrimental for the younger child, who seemed to need nursing more than the older one. For example, a mother of two adopted children was concerned that her milk supply was not sufficient for both children and thus helped the older child wean at around age two for the benefit of his younger sibling.

Most mothers, who initiated weaning, felt ambivalent about their role in this process. This was especially pronounced in mothers of children younger than age three. Maternal narratives were often complicated by themes of guilt and emphasized that nursing took place in a child-led manner prior to precipitous weaning. Mothers' statements demonstrated their empathy towards their children, and they talked about their children's perspectives of the apparently enforced weaning process. They also mentioned their concern about the possible harm they might have caused their children. They made special efforts to compensate their children. One mother, who terminated the nursing relationship in order to take fertility medication, explained to her preschooler that they had to stop nursing because mommy had to take medication that would make her milk taste bad. She compensated her child in various ways, including by fulfilling her daughter's requests to sit together in the kitchen in the middle of the night while the mother prepared special scrambled eggs for her daughter. According to the mother, both were apparently quite pleased and weaning went smoothly. Like this mother, other mothers also made extensive efforts to compensate their children by giving them extra attention and providing other forms of physical comfort, including increased cuddling. Maternal ambivalence, emphasis on child centrality prior to and during the weaning process, and the efforts the mothers made to ease the weaning process and to compensate their children suggests that mothers retained a child-focused approach even though they seemed to act in a contrasting manner.

Child-Led Weaning with Maternal Contributions

Children's contribution to leading was more apparent in the weaning processes of children over three years of age in the study, suggesting that weaning over this age was more in line with children's natural processes than prior to this time. The mothers continued to respond to their children's cues in a flexible manner and accepted older children's periodic increased needs for nursing. Between age three to five years, children progressively reduced the frequency of nursing in a fluctuating manner, reminiscent of the way toddlers boomeranged back and forth from the nursing mother. As weaning progressed, many children displayed a more predictable pattern in comparison to the ongoing nature of nursing prevalent prior to this point. For example, a few three-year-olds in the observational group changed their all day nursing patterns to once a day, usually in the evening. Individuality within this age group was demonstrated by another four-year-old little girl, who nursed more frequently than many of her younger counterparts, albeit in a set pattern. This little girl nursed in the morning, at a few set times during the day, at bedtime, and sometimes during the night as she slept by her mother's side.

Key informants and lay literature (La Leche League, 2004) often referred to the weaning style demonstrated by children at approximately age three to five years of age as child-led. However, a careful analysis of the observations and descriptions of apparent child-led weaning processes in this study indicated that mothers contributed to this process, albeit in a minimal fashion. Maternal contribution was especially apparent when the weaning style of children under five was compared to the process of weaning in subsystems who weaned between five and eight years of age. The data suggest that mothers of children younger than age five, in comparison to mothers of children who wean later, encouraged them to wean, usually subtly. Naturally, one might wonder what causes mothers and key informants to disregard maternal contributions. One might venture that maternal contributions were discounted because the main determinant of weaning at this age was the child. This implies that participants and mothers felt that since children's needs were the central factor, this was the main ingredient considered. The centrality of the child in this style of parenting caused a mother to discard or even hide her contribution in her narrative. Nevertheless, mothers did expedite weaning, suggesting that normal weaning processes in children from ages three to five were mainly based on children's cues, but they were also minimally influenced by maternal intervention.

Maternal contribution to weaning included intermittently providing children with other means of comfort, distraction, or by limiting the frequency of nursing. The last option seemed especially prominent in the mothers with children over the age of three who intermittently lost their patience with nursing. Mothers who set limits often discussed their plans with their children. Mothers made statements such as, "we just nursed a few minutes ago, let's do something else now, and then you can nurse later on again." A mother recalled how she told her children that her breasts hurt when she nursed too much and asked her children to help her by reducing the frequency and length of their nursing sessions.

Other mothers reduced nursing in order to ensure that the needs of all children were met. One mother limited the number of times that she nursed in the afternoon in order to pick up her older children from school and deliver them to their after school activities. Most older children coped well when mothers intermittently withheld nursing. Furthermore, their behaviors and older children's narratives about past nursing experiences suggest that the children in the study felt comfortable with their weaning processes.

Child-Led Weaning

Child-led weaning implies that children's cues are the only impetus to weaning and that maternal prompting is minimal or absent. Fully child-led weaning usually occurred in the early stages of mid-childhood, from approximately ages five to seven, implying that this might be the normal time for children to wean when they are allowed to develop in tune with their natural processes. It seemed that only a small portion of nursing subsystems continued to nurse into early mid-childhood. The apparently small number indicates that perhaps despite their child-led philosophies, some mothers were uncomfortable with a nursing relationship after a certain age. Their discomfort might have reflected the influence of the non-nursing culture on families. The salient non-nursing culture might also lead some families to hide breastfeeding after a certain age, even in apparently accepting contexts, suggesting that nursing at this age was more prominent that it seemed. The closeting of nursing behaviors was exemplified by a mother who hid her school-aged daughter's nursing from the father, implying that some mothers might not have felt comfortable nursing in their own families after a certain point. Yet, children who nursed into early childhood seemed to feel quite comfortable with their weaning processes. One ten-year-old boy who had nursed until the age of six proudly proclaimed that he had nursed until this age and exemplified the positive attitudes children who nursed for many years had of their nursing experiences.

Feelings for Nursing after Weaning

The views expressed by the young boy in the example also demonstrates the strong connection between children and nursing that continued following weaning. Young children talked about nursing and continued to pay attention to their mothers' breasts after they were fully weaned. Similar to the twins who were referred to earlier and who continued to play with their mothers' breasts after weaning, other children also liked to touch, kiss, look at, and refer to their mothers' breasts after they ceased nursing. This behavior seemed most prominent in newly weaned children. Furthermore, the finding that some children, especially younger children, continued to touch and play with the breast after apparent full weaning suggests that perhaps children needed to nurse longer and were weaned before they were truly developmentally ready. This idea fortifies the earlier proposal that mothers contributed to the weaning process prior to age five. Older children usually focused more on the internal feelings or the mother as a whole following weaning. The centrality of breastfeeding in older children's narratives suggests that they retained feelings for the breast long past weaning. Usually, children transferred their feelings for the breast to the mother and other relationships. However, for some the actual breast object might actually still have been considered a tangible symbol of comfort. This was suggested by a twenty-one-year-old independent adult, former nursing child, who touched her mother's clothed breast lightly during a physical and emotional crisis.

Responsive Cue-Based Interventions Outside of Nursing

Behaviors associated with nursing affected the interactions between nursing mothers and their children in areas outside of nursing. The practical experience that mothers had reading cues during and in between nursing seemed to set the tone for parenting interventions that followed children's leads. Mothers allowed their children to determine their rate of development, especially in regards to their relational needs.

Similar to how mothers acknowledged their children's needs for closeness, they also recognized, accepted, and facilitated their children's increasing needs for distance. The process of separating from mothers resembled weaning from the breast. This was similar to nursing children boomeranging back and forth from their mothers as they ventured out to explore their environment. Younger children often nursed when they rejoined their mothers. Older children increasingly replaced nursing with other forms of warm contact with their mothers. In most cases, children determined their rate of separation from mother and home. Eventually, these children slept on their own, engaged in lively social interactions with others, and attended programs away from their mothers and homes.

Interactions in the Nursing Subsystem and Child Development

Our description of the cue-based interactions through nursing has important implications for child development. First of all, nursing provided infants with the opportunity to interact with a good enough and giving object. The likelihood that nursing was seen as positive was suggested by infants and children in the study, and the young children's demonstrations of affection for the breast. Infants turned to their mother's breasts frequently including, but not only, when they were in need. When in need, nursing immediately appeased their distress and the infants stopped crying. Nursing infants and children often exuded an air of calmness and positive regard. The relaxed behaviors and signs of positive affect exhibited by most nurslings suggest they felt their needs were well taken care of. The internalized feelings facilitated the development of a positive sense of self in relation to others.

That good enough feelings are retained was suggested by older nursing children who talked about nursing and how much they loved it. One three-year-old nursing boy saw that his mother's breasts were exposed as he got dressed for the day. He ran over, touched her breasts, and said "I love tzi tzi!" Young and newly weaned children under five spoke about the physical attributes of nursing, often with a smile on their faces. They made statements exemplified by, "I have fun sucking." A six-year-old little girl mentioned that it was "nice to be close to mom." The narratives and descriptions of children who had weaned demonstrated the long lasting positive regard that children had for their first relationship, the nursing relationship.

Along with good enough and contained feelings, these children were provided with opportunities to engage in intricate cue-based interactions. From infancy onwards, they were able to learn how to communicate their needs, and they experienced good enough feelings when these needs were met. They were provided with opportunities to refine cueing. Through intricate interactions during cue-based nursing, children were provided with a means of developing a repertoire of interactional tools.

Experiences through nursing likely facilitated these children's ability to feel good about themselves in relation to others and enhanced their tools for interaction. It seems that nursing served as an important interactional template that children carried with them as they interacted with others. As these children grew, they increasingly mirrored the warm interactions that they had during nursing in their interchanges with others. Although these children continued to prefer their mothers as their central comfort figures for the first few years of life, they increasingly looked to others for comfort and play.

Summary of Interactions in the Nursing Subsystem

The nursing relationship was a central aspect of mother-child interactions during the first few years of life that contributed to the development of reciprocal interactions between the mothers and children in the study. Through nursing interactions, mothers internalized that children had naturally occurring needs that they expressed through cues. Mothers watched, interpreted, and responded to their children's cues that changed to reflect naturally paced needs and growing developmental capacities. Children initiated and nursed frequently, exclusively for approximately the first six months of life, and they continued to nurse into early childhood and weaned from the breast gradually, mainly at their own rate. Child-paced practices were also evident in between nursing, with children remaining close to their mothers until they showed signs of readiness to change existing behaviors.

Interactions in the Nursing Subsystem and Maternal Development

Patient and Attuned Mothering

Nursing seemed to help the mothers develop sensitivity to their children's signals. Mothers' ability to see, read, interpret, and respond to their children's cues was facilitated by the frequency, closeness, intensity, and intimacy of nursing. Their capacity to read and respond to children's cues was indicated by the fluctuating frequency and length of nursing sessions that corresponded to their children's changing needs. As nursing progressed, mothers increasingly demonstrated more patience and understanding towards their children. For example, mothers were noted speaking to their children in patient tones and allowing the offspring to approach them as needed. In a circular manner, mothers' contributions enabled the children to continue to signal their needs in a way that promoted the frequent nature of nursing and also allowed them to decrease their cues for nursing when they no longer needed it as much. The same sensitive qualities allowed mothers to integrate special nursing conditions, such as tandem nursing. From a very early stage of parenting, mothers internalized that infants had needs that they were able to express through signals and that it was important to answer these needs accordingly. The tools internalized during nursing were generalized to additional aspects of parenting.

Mothers' Personal Growth and Emotions

Observations and descriptions of mothers indicated that their ability to interact with their children in a sensitive manner was also affected by the impact of nursing on their personal needs and growth and their perceptions of these events. Nursing affected mothers' feelings about themselves and their relation to their child. By the same token, the nursing relationship was influenced by the mother's interpretations of this experience and her subsequent function as a nursing mother.

Self-Confidence

It seemed that the nursing relationship contributed to the mothers' sense of efficacy as mothers and this contributed to their self-confidence. The case study sample demonstrated that mothers felt pride and self-confidence when they spoke about their apparent successes at meeting their infants' needs through nursing. The good enough feelings that mothers internalized about themselves facilitated continued sensitive interactions. Mothers who progressively displayed increasing self-assured behaviors as they demonstrated increased skills in reading their children's cues through nursing illustrated this. The significance of self-confidence for responsive parenting was exemplified by a new mother who demonstrated an increasing capacity to withstand her infants' needs as she became more confident in her capacity to mother him.

A mother of two children, who felt insecure about her capacity to read her children's cues, further demonstrated the significance of feelings of self-confidence for maternal sensitivity. She periodically stated, "I don't think that I understand my children." She appeared to miss some of her infant's cues for nursing, despite trying so hard not to do this. In addition, she periodically made demands of her older child that did not match his developmental aptitudes. In circular fashion, the infant continued to cue for attention and the older child acted out, fortifying the mother's sense of inadequacy. The frequent nature of nursing compensated for some of the missed opportunities for interaction. When nursing calmed the baby or the baby expressed positive affect during nursing, the mother responded with positive affect and patience, implying that positive reinforcement seemed to help her keep on trying to meet the baby's cues.

Exclusivity and Intimacy

Mothers seemed to cherish exclusive interactions with their infants. The compassionate feelings that mothers felt about exclusivity were exemplified by the steps mothers took to ensure exclusivity in the postpartum period. Many mothers withstood family and cultural pressure, and nursed exclusively for approximately six months. After that, mothers continued to ensure that they had intimate nursing sessions with their children in between their offspring's growing repertoire of interests outside of nursing. Exclusivity seemed to provide mothers with a sense of uniqueness in relation to their children. For example, an adopted mother claimed that her ability to provide her children with something special endeared them to her. She said emphatically, "I am the only one who can do this for them (nurse, calm them this way)."

Another implication of exclusivity was that it provided mothers with the sense that their interactions with their children were intimate. Mothers repeated that the feelings of closeness and intimacy were important to them and very enjoyable. Like many other mothers, the adoptive mother noted above stated that she relished the intimacy of nursing above all else. This mother claimed that nursing helped her connect emotionally to infants who were not biologically related to her.

In another case, a mother forced to relinquish nursing for apparent medical reasons relactated, despite the obstacles, in order to engage in an intimate relationship with her baby. She claimed that the intimacy she experienced in her previous nursing relationships facilitated her attachment to her older children. This feeling was missing in her relationship with her non-nursing infant, from whom she had felt estranged.

While mothers for the most part revered the sense of intimacy, occasionally they found it overwhelming or confusing. This was illustrated by a first time mother who tried to overcome her desire for intimacy with her infant in order to fulfill cultural expectations that she retain distance from her infant. Many other mothers reported that they initially felt ambivalent about their strong feelings toward their infant and their desire to remain close to them. They gradually accepted their feelings of being stirred up by their babies and allowed themselves to fully respond to their babies' needs.

The intense and ongoing nature of nursing challenged some mothers intermittently. A mother with four children, two of whom were nursing twins, generally demonstrated a great deal of patience towards all of her children. Yet, she readily admitted that she periodically felt exhausted by the intensity of the relationship. She claimed that she overcame her periodic impatience with ongoing nursing by reminding herself of her personal goal of "meeting children's needs above all else." In addition, she acknowledged that the intense feelings of love and the genuine enjoyment that came with the intimacy enabled her to withstand the intermittent periods of ambivalence.

Reparative Functions

Mothers seemed to feel that nursing had reparative functions. Maternal narratives implied that nursing helped restore a sense of wholeness and well being to mothers who had undergone trauma that they perceived had impeded normal female development. This was especially relevant to this population due to the significance of normal processes to their worldview. One mother recounted how nursing returned her sense of normalcy following "botched" breast surgery and a horrifying birth experience. Several other women, who had suffered from infertility and traumatic birthing experiences, designated nursing as the healing element that restored their capacity to feel normal and more open to their children. The mothers named different aspects of nursing that helped them repair their apparently damaged parts. It is important to remember, for example, that the adopted mother also mentioned intimacy as important for her. Nursing also helped mothers regain a sense of competency and normalcy that was hindered following the birth of children with health issues. As was noted above, mothers' feelings about themselves increased their patience for their children.

Key informant interviewees repeated a most interesting claim that nursing made mothers feel relaxed. Several attributed this to the hormonal effects of nursing. It seems that the relaxed feeling enhanced mothers' abilities to interact with their children in a patient and calm manner.

Mothers expressed pride that they were nursing mothers and that they met their children's needs above all else. Some mothers made significant lifestyle changes that allowed them to be more available to their children at all times. For one mother, this included giving up a high powered and satisfying position at work to be home with her children. Like many other mothers described and observed, she felt proud of this decision. The centrality of nursing for maternal sense of self was suggested by the large number of mothers who remained active in organizations and academic and professional work affiliated with breastfeeding after their children were no longer nursing.

Summary of Interactions in the Nursing Subsystem and Mother–Child Development

Through their experiences with nursing, mothers internalized tools that helped them respond in a sensitive manner to their children. In addition, mothers enriched their personal needs through nursing, and this further advanced their capacity to interact with their children in a patient and responsive manner. Children appeared calm and displayed a positive attitude about interaction with others that contributed to their relationships with their mothers and others. Nursing appeared to set the template for a child-paced and responsive parenting style that was transmitted to the family.

Clinical Implications

The description of the development of the nursing subsystem following the early stages of initiation and establishment indicates that nursing is an optimal context for the growth of sensitive mothering styles. This implication indicates that clinical support of nursing is more than simply enabling latching on. The tasks here are to provide support to mothers as they internalize cue-based interactions through nursing. In some cases, this might mean education and encouragement.

Educating mothers and helping them develop attuned mothering styles includes teaching them about cues and helping them identify their infant's specific signals. Nursing is a wonderful context for teaching about cues that can be extended to other areas. The facilitative clinician will explain and point out cues indicating an infant is ready to nurse. These might include explaining infant sleep cycles, signs of REM (rapid eye movement) sleep, and signs of wakefulness that indicate a young infant is getting ready to nurse. Following the explanation, the professional or lay support person might point out these signs in the mother's infant. This makes the information tangible and available to the mother. Next the clinician can continue to explain and point to other actual infant cues, including those associated with latching, optimal suckling, satisfaction and dissatisfaction, reduced milk let down, desire to terminate nursing, and all other apparent communicative signals.

Teaching includes helping mothers learn about proximity behaviors and nursing beyond infancy. Mothers, like clinicians, are also members of a culture that values distance over connection, so these concepts might be new for some mothers. One might teach, for example, about the value of proximity, child-led distancing, and the implications of these behaviors for child development. In addition, mothers value the names of other resources, such as mothering groups supportive of nursing.

Encouragement should always accompany teaching. Remember the impact of maternal sense of efficacy on mothering and consistently provide mothers with positive reinforcement. Mothers should be lauded every time they read a cue appropriately, even the easiest cue. Naturally, the last clinical intervention should reflect the mother's stage of mothering development and should not be condescending.

Optimally, use language conducive to physiological nursing teaching and supportive interactions with clients. Remember that language has important implications for nursing mothers and infants and can alter the meaning of their behaviors. Hence, it is imperative that counselors use language carefully and in a way that reflects the dynamics of the nursing couple. For example, one might refer to the encompassing acts associated with nursing while refraining from using terms associated with food.

Providing mothers with opportunities to talk about their feelings about nursing and mothering has important therapeutic value. Some clients may indicate that they need help with nursing when they are actually looking for a warm ear and supportive exchange. Empathetic discussions between mothers and practitioners often positively affect the quality of the nursing relationship, including technical aspects. The empathetic practitioner is a good listener, validating maternal expressions as mothers create their unique mothering narratives. The meaning that mothers ascribe to their experiences is always central. Practitioners might remind themselves that mothers' individual scripts influence their views and capacity to mother. Individuality is respected during counseling, and it is important to remember that there is no right or wrong way to feel. In some cases, a good enough listener will notice and take advantage of opportunities to help mothers reframe difficult experiences and turn them into tolerable events that promote growth.

In some cases, clinicians might be called upon to provide intense support, for example, in cases where mothers are trying to cope with ambivalence. Clinicians might enhance their capacity to support mothers in this case when they recall the source of ambivalence for many mothers in this population, while at the same time always remembering that internal meaning is individual. This book indicates that for some mothers ambivalence stems from discomfort with a newfound and, most certainly, overwhelming desire to be with her baby. A conflict arises when the sense of being stirred up negates former self-concepts and cultural norms. At the same time, mothers rarely state the problem clearly and often talk instead about a need to get away from the baby and feelings of intense longing, unhappiness, or guilt during separation. Others mothers are unable to leave their babies and feel guilty for not acting in accordance with cultural, family, or their own apparent values. It is easy for clinicians to get caught up in the dilemma and to try to relieve the mother by dismissing her needs for contact. When this happens, clinicians mirror the existing pressure on mothers and encourage mothers to leave their infants, even for short periods of time. This non-validating experience might distance the mother from the clinician, losing an opportunity for helpful support. Clinical work may be advanced when one tries to help mothers explore their true feelings. This work might be enriched by discourse with colleagues and by recalling that clinicians are also humans impacted by their experiences and culture.

In many cases, clinicians may feel unprepared and unable to tolerate a client's immense emotional complexities. For example, clinicians trained primarily in lactation consulting might feel challenged by mothers presenting with signs of depression. Referring clients to other practitioners is an important aspect of clinical interaction. One might continue to engage with the client as part of a team of consultants, with the mother's permission, of course. In situations of team interaction, clinicians should remember that they are obligated to the client above all else.

Mental health professionals unacquainted with maternal and child development through nursing might benefit from ongoing consultations with lactation specialists. It is important to remember the positive impact of nursing on mothers' emotional function. For example, physiological aspects of nursing decrease the risk of depression and facilitate the return to health in mothers with depression. When medications are necessary, it is important to choose interventions that are compatible with nursing.

Acknowledging the contribution of nursing to maternal function implies that one important role of the therapist is to help mothers retain nursing relationships in difficult situations. Reframing is an integral part of saving a threatened nursing relationship. Helping mothers break up difficult situations into small parts is one means of reframing apparently overwhelming nursing relationships. The therapist might help the client climb through the emotional clutter and gain a sense of control and well being by locating positive aspects of the nursing relationship. This process is gradual and small steps are celebrated. Some psychotherapists might have difficulty supporting mothers' needs for closeness if they are unfamiliar with the specific closeness and gradual separation processes associated with nursing. In these cases, the therapist might have difficulty deciphering pathological processes from physiologically based goals. Ascertaining underlying and real issues and differentiating between the client's agenda and the clinician's issues are always central to psychotherapeutic interactions.

The task of respecting the clients' agenda might be extremely difficult. Some clinicians might feel uncomfortable with the concepts and behaviors that facilitate sensitive nursing patterns. Remember the importance of self-awareness, accepting one's difficulties, and the need to assess whether one can engage in genuine interactions that advance growth with nursing dyads. It might be helpful for clinicians to review themes that distance them from nursing and associated behaviors and to assess their personal view of these themes. The task of working with nursing families might also be facilitated by remembering the developmental implications of this seemingly different style of interaction. Clinicians might discuss the impact of working with mothers who engage in ongoing apparently caring relationships on their own parenting. These concepts might trigger a sense of deficiency for some clinicians. Peer or individual support may be useful in these cases. At other times, it is also valuable for clinicians to recognize their limitations and to refer clients to more suitable practitioners when they feel unable to provide adequate support. And just like for clients, it is important for clinicians to also celebrate small steps and rejoice in novel conceptualizations and practice.

Chapter 7
Interactions with the Nursing Subsystem and the Development of Sensitive Fathering

In this chapter, fathers' contributions to the nursing subsystem will be reviewed. Key informant interviewees and fathers in the case study indicated that responsive and child-based interactions in the nursing subsystem were facilitated by the fathers. At the same time, fathers internalized themes and emulated behaviors and patterns associated with nursing. Fathers mirrored their partners' sensitive interactional styles in their interactions with their nursing children. However, their paths to sensitivity were different from the mothers' developmental trajectory. Fathers internalized responsive parenting themes by supporting and, at times, facilitating their partners' efforts to match their infants' cues through nursing, watching the nursing dyad, discussing issues related to nursing with their partners, and increasingly responding to their infants' cues directly.

Internalizing Sensitive Fathering

Matching Support to Needs

Much like the way mothers read and matched their children's cues, fathers observed and supported the nursing subsystem accordingly. Fathers' actions mirrored the needs of the nursing unit and the phase of nursing development in the family. The support that fathers provided in the initial postpartum period was intense and included caring for the mothers' physical needs. In the early postpartum period, fathers engaged in a high degree of involvement in direct child care while mothers focused mainly on nursing. Following the intense early postpartum period as mothers regained strength, no longer needing intense nurturing as nursing became an established behavior, fathers decreased their direct supportive actions and child care, although most remained highly involved. They reduced the direct care and protection they provided for their spouses. Intermittently, they increased their degree of involvement when they believed that more help was needed. Fathers seemed especially aware of their protective duties when they perceived that others were denigrating the nursing relationship.

Observing and Emulating Cue-Based Nursing Behaviors

Fathers seemed to learn how to interact with the nursing unit and children by observing interactions associated with nursing. It seemed that much like the way that the frequency of nursing sessions enabled mothers to watch, interpret, and respond to infants' cues, recurrent nursing sessions also provided fathers with ample opportunities to view sensitive interactions associated with nursing. Fathers watched and replicated behaviors intrinsic to nursing, including distinguishing between cues for nursing and other needs. For example, fathers frequently stopped playing with their babies when they seemed to perceive that their infants wanted to nurse. Usually, infants validated their fathers' actions by latching on to their mothers' breasts.

The impact of observing nursing on fathers was also evident in the fathers' abilities to assess the quality of nursing, including suckling patterns and positioning. At times, fathers made suggestions or provided hands on help with nursing that further advanced the ability of mothers to answer their infants' needs appropriately. One father of formerly and actively nursing children proclaimed with great pride, "I helped with latching!"

Fathers also mirrored mothers' responses to cues for nursing. They used cue names for nursing with ease and warmly validated their children's needs for nursing. This was demonstrated by a father of a twenty-four-month-old boy, who joined his spouse and responded to his son's cues for nursing with, "Do you want "Pa?" He then watched as the little boy latched on and nursed. His body tone was relaxed and matched the calm demeanor of the interactions that took place between the mother and nursing toddler beside him.

Along with noting, responding to, and emulating the cues associated with nursing, fathers also acknowledged the unique features of the nursing relationship. Fathers' actions and words indicated that they recognized and respected the emotional closeness between nursing mothers and children. Fathers talked about the closeness in a very positive way and took steps to ensure that nursing children and mothers remained close. For example, they accepted and encouraged ongoing mother-child proximity behaviors, including co-sleeping. The supportive attitude displayed by most fathers was exemplified in father's comments. One father said, "If you are a nursing mother and you are raising your children in that particular mode of breastfeeding ... that we do ..., then there are things that we prescribe to. You are sleeping with the baby and the baby is with the mother constantly. So that is obviously going to build a strong bond."

Tactile and Proximity Behaviors

Fathers also demonstrated reverence for the physical intimacy of nursing by incorporating the tactile aspects and the physical proximity between nursing units into their interactions with their nursing children. Fathers observed how mothers used touch and engaged in similar strategies. A father explained, "She (the mother) would get as much skin-to-skin contact as possible. I remember trying that myself as well. I would take his (the baby's) little shirt off and put him down on my chest. I might have gotten that idea from my wife. I used the sling a lot and I guess that that came out of the nursing. Also the general mode that you are always with your kids, that spills over on to how you father."

Like this father, others fathers mirrored closeness in their interactions with their children. They remained at home with their children outside of their hours at work. They also held, carried, and hugged their children frequently. Fathers often wore their children in slings when the babies were young and immobile.

Fathers also mimicked the comforting aspects of the nursing relationship. For example, one father put his newborn son on his bare chest at night in order to calm him. Yet, along with mirroring nursing, fathers' actions also showed that they recognized that nursing has unique features that cannot be replicated. One father stated, "I could actually cope with the babies pretty well with their comfort, but the ultimate comfort could come from Amy (his wife). Which was fine. There was more pressure on Amy, but that was also more wonderful (meaning that the father enjoyed that his son loved his wife so much). Some little part of me was jealous of that, and would like to know what that would be like, but that would certainly not lead me to do what is apparently not possible medically which would be to develop breasts. It's not that important to me! (He laughed). ... But I never felt deprived; I felt that that was a good thing." Like this father, most fathers read their infants' cues, recognized their limitations as comfort objects, and relinquished this role to their spouses when necessary.

Mothers Tutor Fathers Follow

Along with watching and imitating aspects of nursing, fathers were also provided with opportunities to internalize the parenting associated with nursing through their interactions with their partners. Although mothers stated they cherished their time alone with their infants, they also said they relished their partners' direct involvement with the children and took an active role in facilitating this. Most mothers encouraged their children to build relationships with their fathers, who welcomed their offspring's advances. Some mothers indicated that they truly appreciated the intermittent breaks they had when the children were with their fathers and seemed genuinely pleased that the children had relationships with their fathers. Their pleasure was suggested, for example, by the happy facial expressions that some mothers displayed as they watched their children interact with their fathers and the positive regard they expressed while speaking about this issue in their narratives.

Similar to the prenatal period when mothers initiated ideas, mothers introduced their partners to novel parenting concepts and often guided them. For example, maternal direction of paternal behavior was illustrated by the way that one mother told her partner what to do as he held the baby. Mothers also supported their partners' behaviors through discussion. Like in the prenatal period, mothers researched novel parenting issues which they later discussed with their spouses. One couple proudly presented the mother as the "researcher." The mother said, "I tell my partner about things that I read and research concerning parenting. Then we discuss the issues and decide what we want to do." The discussions that couples had about parenting were an extension of open communications patterns that were prevalent in this population.

Feedback from Nursing Children

Children also contributed to their fathers' growth. It seemed that children's feedback helped fathers internalize ways of responding to their children. Even young infants showed an interest in their fathers, and it is this interest that sometimes drew fathers into interchanges with them. This might occur during or in between nursing. For example, a four month infant made loud sounds and smiled directly at his father while holding his mother's breasts in his mouth. The father reciprocated by smiling, briefly talking to, and gently touching the baby. Some older toddlers also initiated physical contact while they nursed. For example, an eighteen-month-old toddler touched her father with gentle little motions with her foot as she nursed happily. Child-initiated interactions increased as children grew, providing fathers with opportunities to practice responding to their children.

Shared Connection to Nursing

Fathers shared connection to nursing helped them support and internalize fathering that mirrored interactions associated with breastfeeding. Proof of fathers' sense of connection to nursing was suggested by the passion they displayed as they discussed nursing and their own narratives. For example, a father genuinely thanked me for giving him and his family the opportunity to discuss the present nursing relationship and to reminisce about past nursing experiences during the research process. He said, "We never have this opportunity to talk about these things and we appreciate it." This enthusiasm was repeated by others fathers. One grandfather cried during the entire interview, and like his younger counterpart, he emphasized that the interview was important to him and that he enjoyed having an opportunity to talk about his feelings.

Fathers' appreciation and joint ownership of nursing, as well as associated behaviors, was also noted in the way fathers continued to protect nursing under all circumstances. Their protective duties included guarding the exclusivity and closeness of nursing beyond the early postnatal period. Appreciation of nursing was also evident when fathers proclaimed that it was wrong for dads to interfere with nursing by bottle feeding or any other means. One father, for example, who had fed a nursing infant under duress, emphasized that he felt ambivalent about interfering with nursing exclusivity, and that from his perspective, interactions during bottle feeding were not like those that take place during nursing and did not mimic the feelings of closeness.

Protection in later stages of nursing moved from ensuring exclusivity to protecting the dyad from external pressures to wean or to decrease the degree of closeness between the nursing pair. Fathers and mothers frequently talked about coping with the ongoing pressure that others, including family, friends, medical practitioners, and mental health professionals placed on families to wean and use distancing strategies in their parenting. It is noteworthy that fathers played an important role in filtering insensitive external interventions. Very often, it was the fathers who strongly refuted negative comments. Most significantly, it was interesting that some fathers, who disputed aspects of nursing with their wives, defended breastfeeding when others made comments. By protecting and relating to the nursing relationship as their own, fathers contributed to the proliferation of a family style that reflected concepts stemming from the nursing relationship.

Applying Lessons Learned Through Nursing to Fathering

Fathers applied the cue reading skills that they learned by watching and emulating nursing when they interacted and cared for their children. It seemed that many fathers had a positive attitude towards their tasks that included giving baths and changing diapers. This positive regard was evident in the comments of a father of three children, all of whom had nursed. He said, "She (the lactation consultant) showed us that this was a part of parenting (meaning changing diapers) and a part of the body that was also important...as a joyous thing in itself. It showed us that it was something special. We saw that it was something to be appreciated. At least I did and I guess that (my wife) felt that even more. Changing a diaper is part of life and it does bring you closer to the baby. It is one of the natural functions of the child. I guess that our society frowns on anything from that end. We like to talk about eating food, whatever, but we don't talk about that. But it is part of it. There is something so innocent, so totally dependent. You know they lift up their legs and they spread them for whatever you need to do and it is just trust!" This father's comments also pointed to his reverence for nature, an important theme in these families.

The fathers' growing capacity to respond to their children's cues was illustrated when they played and engaged in child-centered activities with their infants and older children. Fathers matched their activities to their children's needs, speaking gently to their offspring as they explained things to them and calming them when appropriate. One father emphasized proudly, "I could get the baby to laugh in a way that no one else, even my wife, could."

Fathers' caregiving, playful, and social interchanges with their children complemented maternal parenting. A father of a school-aged son and an older toddler who nursed during the study exemplified the complementary actions between parents in nursing families after the initial early postpartum period. He said, "I would be doing things that Wendy (his wife) couldn't do if she was busy with the baby. Whatever needed to be done.... Just have to go with the flow. I have always been a very involved person with people around me. I have always cooked. I have always cleaned. I have done things like that... I might be sitting on the computer, but when it is time to get things done, I get things done."

In most families, mothers stayed at home as full time parents, at least until the nursing infant was one year old. Even though fathers worked at outside employment and spent less time parenting than mothers did, most continued to complement their partners' parenting. They were highly involved in childcare and household activities when they returned home from work. One father in the case study group, who worked long hours away from home, downplayed his involvement and said that his wife did the majority of childcare. Yet, upon observation, the father engaged in all aspects of childcare from the moment he walked in the door and throughout the night. Like this father, other dads remained active in childcare, and this facilitated additional interactions with their children.

Fathers increased their caregiving responsibilities as children grew. Like mothers, fathers' growing repertoire of tasks reflected their children's changing needs, natural processes, and individual rhythms. In addition, fathers took into account the needs of the system and their partners' changing capacities as they altered their tasks to suit the situation. For example, fathers often took over the exclusive care of older siblings in the early postpartum period after younger siblings were born and mothers were intensely involved in new nursing relationships. It also seemed that fathers' capacity to comfort and patiently support children increased as children grew.

The fathers' capacity to respond to their children in a cue-based manner that reflected respect for individuality was illustrated when they tolerated and responded to children's varying degrees of interest in them. The degree of children's focus on the father and the rate of development of the father-child relationship varied over time and differed between children. The two sets of twins in the case study group illustrated how fathers responded to their children's diverse displays of affection. In both of these families, one twin fell in love with the father much more quickly than the other sibling did. Reasons for the discrepancies in the twins' behavior and attitudes were not apparent in the parents' narratives or in the observations of family interaction. Both fathers seemed to initiate contact with their twin sons in an equal manner. They also referred to the twin siblings with like affect and demonstrated similar levels of interest in and affection towards both twins. Observations of one of these families over a four year period indicated that the apparently unequal interest in the father remained a stable component of the father-twin interchanges, and the father remained more important for one twin than for his brother over time. The father suited his interactions to each son's needs in a different way, while remaining equally absorbed in, and accepting of, his sons' differences.

Fathers Facilitate Weaning

Fathers patiently supported their children and facilitated weaning. Their role was usually passive, and some did not even seem to be aware that they were part of the process. However, when fathers supported nursing and proximity behaviors, and calmly read their children's cues for closeness much like mothers did, they seemed to facilitate the transfer of their children's attention from the breast to them. In some cases, fathers took a more active role in weaning by purposely diverting the child's attention to the father instead of nursing. This information implies that the quality of the father-child relationship also seemed to play a role in children's capacity to wean when it was developmentally appropriate.

Children's Focus on Fathers

An interesting aspect of the weaning process was that children demonstrated an increasing interest in their fathers instead of their mothers. Sometimes the change of interest included preferring the father more than the mother. Many children did this in a very obvious manner, even when they were still nursing. In one family, a young girl initially demonstrated her intermittent preference for her father in her second year of life. She repeatedly asked the mother to leave her alone with her father.

Children's obvious preference for their fathers was also very apparent in two families with little boys. One was four years old and the other was three years old. These little boys verbally declared that they preferred to be with their fathers when they were home. As claimed by both sets of parents, the love that these boys displayed towards their fathers was reminiscent of the intense love that had been shown to their mothers when they were younger. It is interesting that the three-year-old boy was still involved in a tandem nursing relationship at the same time that he developed a passion for his dad.

Both of the little boys spoke about their fathers incessantly and often with passion in their voices. They followed their fathers around closely, looked up to them with love in their eyes, and sought out tactile interactions with them. The three-year-old engaged in frequent wrestling matches with his dad that seemed to excite the youngster to no end. The four-year-old little boy refused to accompany his mother and sister on a short family trip in order to be alone with his dad, much to the parents' surprise. He stayed with his father and had a wonderful time, according to his and his parents' narrative. These cases show the transfer of children's focus on the mother, established in the exclusive mother-child relationship, to the father-child relationship, an act facilitated by paternal sensitivity.

Challenges to the Trajectory of Sensitive Fathering

Paternal Envy

Despite the circular processes that facilitate the transfer of sensitivity to paternal scripts, some fathers seemed to be intermittently challenged and unable to internalize ideas associated with nursing. Although most fathers seemed to appreciate the unique characteristics of the nursing relationship, some also appeared to find these same attributes disturbing. Their ambivalence disabled them from consistently supporting the nursing subsystem and internalizing parenting themes and behaviors associated with nursing. Interestingly, fathers' respect for the closeness between nursing mothers and their children also triggered ambivalence for some dads.

Envy of Mothers and their Closeness to Children

Paternal envy was a normal part of the nursing process for some fathers. In some cases, fathers talked about things that they missed openly, then continued to support nursing and all of the associated behaviors with great commitment. The issue that seemed to trigger envy was the same closeness associated with nursing that they revered and supported. One father quite openly admitted that he envied the intimate relationship between his wife and their nursing children. He had actually tried to feel the closeness that nursing mothers and infants experienced by trying unsuccessfully to nurse his older children. As he recounted his feelings, his family smiled, indicating that this was a well known family story and that it was viewed in a positive way. He explained, "It is not fair...I mean that there are a lot of not fair things. I am not saying that women have all of the luck or anything. But it is something (nursing) that is so special that kind of, you know. They talk about penis envy, this is the opposite! I think that fathers would like to be able to do it (nurse). I don't think that it is envy in a negative way, like in a jealousy sort of way. It is more like wow that is such a great feeling to have that closeness and to give from your own body. If you just try and imagine it, you want it." This father also indicated that he relished his role as a father and his parenting tasks, he was highly active, and his actions were important and affected the quality of the nursing relationship.

In contrast, in the words of a key informant interviewee, some fathers felt "excluded, like second wheels, and insignificant." A father of a child who had nursed in the past and a toddler who nursed during the study exemplified the frustration that some fathers felt. This father claimed that he felt excluded as soon as his daughter was born and started nursing. His tone was angry as he blamed nursing for interfering with his relationship with his children. He said, "I didn't bond to her (his daughter) until after she weaned." He felt especially angry and displaced by his inability to comfort his children as long as they nursed. As was noted earlier, most fathers acknowledged and accepted that their children were comforted best by nursing. However, this father, like a few others, found it intolerable to not be able to comfort his children. He stated that being unable to resolve his children's distress made him feel helpless, and this caused him anxiety. He claimed that, if his children had bottles or pacifiers, he, too, would have been able to soothe them. The father's suggestions that his children receive artificial feeding contrasted with his enthusiasm for natural processes and his view that nursing was important because it was natural.

This father also remarked angrily, "I have been told that if I were to change a diaper more often or burp a kid more often that that would have helped. (Meaning helped him emotionally attach to his daughter). That is crap! ... I would never tell him (meaning another father) that the way you can bond more is if you change the diapers more often. That doesn't help you love the kid. How could that (changing diapers) possibly help. No child likes to have his diaper changed! You are intruding on that. He sees you as something that is intruding on his space. They don't enjoy that. Burping him. What's that, tapping him on the back?" This father, it is interesting to note, admitted that he had never actually engaged in most of the parenting tasks that he described with his older child and that he was only beginning to look after a few of his younger child's needs.

Although this father claimed that nursing was devoid of emotional significance, he simultaneously blamed the emotional closeness between his wife and nursing children for the distance between him and his children when they nursed. His negative expressions decreased when he began to enjoy closer relationships with his children, especially when it seemed that he was able to do special things with them that no one else could do. This suggested that he wanted to experience the same emotional closeness – that he simultaneously was denied – with his children that his nursing spouse experienced. Furthermore, when he became more involved with the younger nursing child, he also increased his support for the nursing relationship.

Envy of Children and their Closeness to Mothers

While some fathers longed to replace the mother, others wanted to switch places with their infants and experience the closeness associated with nursing with their spouses. One father exemplified this type of envy when he frequently took his daughter away from the breast before she finished nursing. Initially, he replaced the breast with his finger, then a pacifier, and eventually he added a baby swing. Furthermore, he interpreted his daughter's apparently robust nursing pattern as excessive, and seemingly lovingly, called her a "monster." He said, "Well she was eating my finger. She wasn't settling. We didn't create this monster; she (meaning the baby) did it herself." He denied that nursing had emotional characteristics and stated that it was merely a means of feeding. However, dissimilar from the former father who felt that nursing was taking the children from him, this father's attention was on his wife, who routinely ignored his advances. His efforts at distancing the young infant from his wife resembled his ongoing attempts to ensure increased separation between his older child and the mother. In the case of the older child, the father claimed that he did this to enhance his child's development.

Another father was less aggressive in his efforts to separate his wife and son, and was more accepting of his nursing toddler's needs for his mother. This first time father openly, and quite proudly, disclosed that his son had a pacifier and slept solitary, suggesting that he attempted to place limitations on the mother-son relationship. It was interesting that this contrasted with the pride that he expressed regarding the nursing relationship, the efficient way that he read his sons cues for nursing and facilitated nursing sessions, and the way that he enjoyed watching his wife and son as they interacted at the breast and otherwise. Furthermore, this dad was absolutely enthralled by his son with whom he interacted with in sensitive interactions. Nevertheless, it seemed that there were limits to the amount of special closeness that he was able to withstand between his wife and child.

Desire to Protect Mother

The desire to protect was another interesting challenge to paternal sensitive parenting that also stemmed from a behavior usually associated with promoting the development of sensitivity through nursing. However, in this case, fathers wanted to protect their spouses from the closeness associated with nursing or a nursing child who apparently took too much from the mother. In a way, this challenge was similar to the apparently protective feelings, but more likely a sense of being overwhelmed or guilty feelings, that fathers felt when they perceived that their partners had endured too much pain.

A father of four children, all of whom had nursed or were nursing, wanted to limit mother-child closeness out of a concern for his wife's welfare. He stated that he did not like how his children constantly used his wife as a comfort tool. In this case, the father's personal script seemed to play a role in his ambivalence. On one hand, he cherished the closeness and comfort that his wife provided to the nursing children. He worked hard at emulating the same components in his interaction with his children and had successfully developed warm and child-led interactions with his children. Yet, at the same time, he felt that his wife was overextended, and this interfered with her right for privacy and time alone – issues that were central to the father's personal script. It appeared that he had displaced his own needs for privacy onto his wife, and this reduced his capacity to fully see or respond to needs that he otherwise valued.

Fears of Overdependence

Others fathers attempted to reduce mother-infant or child closeness due to their fear that these children might otherwise never become independent.

It was most interesting that in the research study, some of the fathers who worried about independence also seemed to experience envy towards members of the nursing dyad. The fathers' focus on apparent independence impaired the fathers' capacity to read and consistently respond to their infants' needs for closeness. In addition, their concerns sometimes clouded their ability to see the actual signs of autonomy in their growing children. In addition, paternal concerns about independence may have caused friction between parents. The discord was likely due to the apparent lack of relevance of this issue for mothers who seemed content with their children's development.

Resolving Ambivalence

It seems that paternal knowledge, maturity, and experience helped fathers accept aspects of the nursing relationship over time. Fathers seemed more open to the ongoing nature of the nursing system as children grew. Fathers, especially those with several former nursing children, became more vocal in their defense of the nursing relationship. In addition, fathers seemed to be less concerned about their children being too dependent after they had a few children. Although some fathers with older children in the study continued to imply that their older children had been overly dependent when they were younger.

Fathers also seemed to overcome some of their ambivalence when they recalled their reverence for natural processes. For example, the father who blamed nursing for the apparent distance between him and his children said, "There is nothing wrong with it (meaning nursing). It is natural." Other fathers also expressed relief when they remembered the health enhancing factors associated with nursing.

Like the way that fathers learned to read their children's cues by observing interactions between nursing mothers and children, their ambivalent feelings seemed to be relieved when they watched their children. For example, fathers' acknowledged that the closeness associated with nursing was valuable when they observed how their children were quickly relieved at the breast. Fathers who expressed anxiety regarding their children's apparent overdependence on their mothers were relieved when they noted these children's emerging signs of independence.

Most significantly, children's direct feedback appeased fathers. This feedback was a direct result of the interactions between nursing subsystems, and the father-child relationship. Interactions between fathers and children during caregiving and play interludes provided dads with opportunities to experience the emotionality that they associated with nursing and relieved some of their envy. The prominent tactile aspects associated with nursing that fathers integrated into their interchanges with the children seemed especially important for relieving anxiety. The happy facial expressions and relaxed body language that fathers displayed during tactile interchanges suggested that they experienced extreme enjoyment during those moments. Father-child interaction seemed to reinforce the father-child system and in a circular fashion encouraged fathers to continue with their supportive and fathering tasks. A father who displayed more satisfaction with nursing when his level of involvement with his children increased illustrated the impact of direct interaction between fathers and their children on paternal ambivalence and nursing.

Interactions between the parental couple also helped fathers cope with their ambivalence. The processes were similar to those that helped mothers transfer and fathers internalize parenting themes and patterns associated with nursing. For example, parents discussed issues, and this helped fathers alter their views. Open communication and the ability to discuss feelings and receive feedback appeared to contribute significantly to the development of paternal sensitivity.

Summary of the Interactions in the Nursing Subsystem and Paternal Development

Fathers demonstrated a sense of ownership of the nursing relationship and took steps to ensure that the nursing unit developed accordingly. By altering their behaviors to suit the needs of the nursing system, they practiced cue reading and responding. They internalized themes of responsiveness associated with nursing by supporting the nursing relationship, observing nursing sessions, and replicating attuned behavioral patterns; through tutoring by and discussions with mothers; and when children reinforced their efforts with interaction. By complementing their partners' mothering tasks and mirroring the mothers' interactional style, fathers strengthened the nursing relationship and provided children with a sense of consistency. In circular fashion, when fathers' reinforced the nursing system, they also enhanced children's capacity to interact with them. Infants increased relational capacities reverberated back to the father, enriching further paternal interaction. Although fathers internalized, appreciated, and emulated the salient issues associated with nursing, at times they were challenged by their role and the dominant issues related to nursing. Paternal envy, concerns that offspring hurt the mother, and concerns about independence were issues that challenged paternal support and their trajectory to sensitive fathering. Fathers were able to resolve conflicts, increase their supportive and responsive tasks, and enhance their trajectory to sensitivity through validating interactions with children and their spouses.

Clinical Implications

At this stage of family development, clinicians should continue their efforts to support fathers' distinct trajectory to parenthood. There are several elements that match paternal development in the early stages of family development. Clinicians should continue to help fathers realize, experience, and celebrate their unique traits. This intervention enriches paternal ability to internalize sensitivity through nursing.

A father's continued need for tangible feedback implies that clinicians provide fathers with practical information about ways they can support their partners and participate in the care of their newborn infants. Information should be specific and include applicable tools. Clinicians might turn specifically to fathers and point out infant cues associated with nursing. They might discuss ways that fathers can respond to these cues and enhance nursing. These steps will provide fathers with a sense of inclusion and a means of experiencing positive feedback when they read cues successfully.

Clinicians might point out paternal successes and help fathers see their tasks as unique and meaningful. The enhancing impact of feedback on paternal function indicates that practitioners may use this as a means of helping fathers support their nursing systems and internalize sensitivity. Much like the way that this tool is used in the initiation stage, clinicians might help fathers see their success. An empathetic clinician might comment on how well a father carries, bathes, or looks after an infant in between nursing. One might also advance nursing by commenting on how the father enhances the nursing relationship in his family. Giving fathers specific examples, such as how the father accurately assessed that the baby was ready to nurse, is encouraging. The finding that paternal efforts are advanced by child feedback indicates that pointing out children's positive regard for their fathers is a potent means of enriching function.

In addition, clinicians might help fathers see that relevant issues, including health, growth and independence, are actualized in their children. This task is of greater importance for fathers with less experience than those with older children. The value of experience indicates that paternal knowledge and confidence might be enhanced through the creation of father support groups led by experienced dads. However, this is said with caution due to the salient finding that fathers learn best through their partners' guidance and not through reading or group meetings.

The established pattern of maternal leading remains significant over time. It is helpful for clinicians to see this pattern as a facilitating tool readily available within the family context. For example, one might strengthen the apparently existing maternal tutor –father learner paradigm if this is working for the parents. Educators might provide information for mothers and help them find ways of disseminating the information to fathers. In addition, clinicians might help parents enhance or create open communication systems that not only help paternal learning, but are also a valuable means of resolving feelings, such as distress over a perceived traumatic birth or envy, should they appear.

Anticipatory guidance about potential paternal feelings is an important measure easily incorporated into prenatal teaching. Along with teaching fathers about possible future feelings, educators should also promote discussion between dads in group contexts. These tactics will normalize difficult feelings.

An important issue that should be included in discussions at the prenatal and early postnatal stages is the impact of birth on fathers and their ability to support perceived difficult nursing relationships. Clinicians might follow up by providing fathers with a means of talking about their feelings, including negative feelings about the birth, and their concerns about the mothers' associated physical state.

Many practitioners are likely familiar with lactation consulting situations where mothers seem to be able to handle difficult nursing situations, while their partners simultaneously disrupt nursing under the apparent pretext of protecting the mother or baby. This situation is often very difficult for clinicians and impedes our ability to repair or enhance nursing. Discussions with the parental couple during lactation consulting in these cases might include a focus on the mothers' desire to nurse. One should point out existing strengths in the nursing relationship and celebrate small changes. Focusing on what is working and how mothers are happy is helpful for fathers who fear that they are causing more harm to partners whom they perceive they have already hurt. The most powerful means of conveying maternal well being to fathers is through direct discussion between the couple. A skillful clinician might find a way of helping fathers listen and mothers talk about the good feelings they get from nursing.

Paternal envy is another issue with clinical implications. It is extremely important for clinicians to be aware of the significance of paternal envy and to normalize it, not only for families, but also for themselves. This is another issue that should be discussed at the prenatal stage. Implying that many healthy fathers experience envy normalizes feelings. Reframing this feeling as a normal part of a development trajectory makes it easier to break down and learn about the meaning behind the feeling for the client at hand. This intervention opens up the paths of communication, the door to resolution, and enhances paternal function. The tools for resolution point to a systemic component, and clinicians will benefit by continuing to look at the impact of this feeling on the parental couple.

Some fathers might require more in-depth opportunities to process feelings. Referring fathers to clinicians more specialized in this type of discussion will advance paternal ability to internalize sensitive fathering styles though nursing. Again, counselors should use nursing as the term of reference as they try to help fathers understand and process their emotions.

Counseling fathers with complex emotions can feel overwhelming for clinicians providing different services. For example, a lactation counselor might feel overly burdened by a father's apparent anger when attempting to help a crying mother nurse a lethargic or screaming baby. A natural response for some might be to agree with the father who wants to put an end or reduce an apparently harmful nursing relationship and give the baby an artificial feeding apparatus. Another counselor might overly identify with a father's perceived sense of exclusion and support a father's efforts to separate the mother from her nursing child. It is very natural to feel overwhelmed and to look for apparent immediate solutions. This conflict might be resolved by reviewing information about emotional process in nursing families and recalling the negative impact that short term solutions might have on the family in the long run. In addition, one might remember the impact of countertransference on our interactions with clients, accept our feelings, and seek support from empathetic colleagues.

Hence, supporting nursing families includes containing fathers as they sustain the nursing dyad or triad and internalize sensitive fathering. Counseling should include practical information and emotional support. Working with fathers as they go through the transition to parenting a nursing child can be emotionally trying for clinicians when extraneous issues impede paternal function. It is important to remember the significance of our personal scripts on clinical work, the importance of retaining support from our colleagues, and the necessity of referring clients when needed to clinicians who counsel using nursing as the term of reference.

Chapter 8
Interactions with the Nursing Subsystem, Couple Development, and Parental Sensitivity

In this chapter, interactions between the parental couples in the study group are reviewed. Like in earlier chapters, this section also includes examples provided by key informant interviewees and case study families. Knowledge about maternal and paternal development is described and how parents' distinct developmental trajectories affect and are influenced by their relationship as a couple are discussed. Insights about couple interaction are combined with knowledge of the impact of nursing on infants and children. This cumulative view provides increased understanding of systemic interactions and the transfer of themes in the family, and enriches clinical interactions.

Complementary Interactions

Parents' capacity to internalize themes and display behaviors associated with nursing was influenced by their interactions with one another. As they went through the process of internalizing novel concepts, they also had to integrate their differences stemming from their diverse developmental trajectories. This task was facilitated when each parent was able to engage in distinct tasks and complement their partner. The complementary structure remained stable over time, even after children grew and parents shared similar tasks.

Most mothers spent a proportionally increased amount of time at home in comparison to fathers who were employed outside of the home. Mothers continued to function as the primary innovators of parenting ideas in cases where they returned to work following maternity leaves or when their children were older. Even though children eventually related to their parents in a more equal manner, fathers and mothers continued to interact in distinct ways with them and complemented one another's actions.

Another task that the parental subsystem coped with was integrating parents' diverse perspectives of issues related to parenting. Diverse views of independence exemplified this aspect of couple interactions. The section on fathers demonstrated that some fathers had concerns about their children's future capacity for independence, an issue that was not apparent in maternal narratives. It seemed that this issue was more prevalent with less experienced parents of younger children versus more experienced families with older children. In all families, mothers and fathers seemed to understand independence differently, even when their children were very young. Mothers seemed to recognize their children's developing signs of independence before fathers did, perhaps due to the salient pattern of maternal leading and the increased amount of time that mothers spent with their children in comparison to fathers.

Observations of two families with toddlers demonstrate these parents' diverse trajectories. The mothers remained calm when their infants wandered off and explored the house, including when they were momentarily out of sight. In contrast, both fathers became uneasy when they were unable to observe the actions of their children, and they eventually chased after their children. The mothers acknowledged the fathers' behaviors and warmly explained why their partners acted this way. One mother said, "I understand the baby better (than the father). I am with him (the toddler) more than his father is." The more time that mothers spent with their children in comparison to fathers seemed to enable mothers to see signs of autonomy in their children that were not apparent to fathers. The diversity between the parents regarding this issue was ongoing and was temporarily resolved through discussions, maternal tutoring, paternal observations, mothers' capacity and desire to understand their partners, and fathers' capacity to revise their perceptions of age appropriate independence.

Open Communication

The capacity of parents to integrate differences suggests that couples engaged in facilitative processes that advanced their development as a couple. Growth was enhanced most when couples engaged in open communication patterns, inclusive of validation and mutuality. The study findings indicate that most couples in families that nurse in tune with physiology displayed open communication styles. This style of communication pattern helped them discuss and establish joint themes. Mutuality between the parents was evident in paternal supportive actions, maternal tutoring, discussions, and complementary parenting actions. Couples were in accord about their parenting style and shared the goals of meeting children's needs as they engaged in open discourse. This style of communication also allowed couples to validate one another's feelings, a tool especially important for resolving differences.

A family with four children exemplified how parents used open communication to resolve a disagreement related to nursing. The father in this family was described earlier and was concerned about his wife, whom he believed overextended herself as a mother. Following the birth of twins, this father convinced his wife to give the twins pacifiers. Although the mother strongly detested pacifiers, she said that she understood her partner's position and made this compromise for him, despite that she enjoyed being with her infants in an ongoing manner and that she was not bothered by what her husband perceived as persistent demands from the twins. Her distaste for pacifiers was demonstrated by the joy that she expressed when one of the twins outright refused it. She rarely used a pacifier with the other twin who did not reject it, and she successfully stopped giving it to him a few months later. Throughout this period, the couple openly discussed their feelings. In addition, the father observed his wife and her interactions with the babies and listened carefully to her perspective in the same way she listened to him. Like the way the mother compromised her views for her husband at an earlier stage, the father accepted his wife's decision to discard the pacifier after the short trial. He supported her and accepted the outcome. This case demonstrated the process of open communication, mutual understanding, and compromise in parental couples that also led to increased sensitivity to children's needs.

The impact of open communication patterns was evident in couples' shared visions of family life. It seemed that when parents shared common beliefs and goals about issues related to nursing, it was easier for them to internalize themes associated with nursing. Most couples shared many of the themes related to nursing and complemented one another's efforts as they engaged in associated behaviors. The nursing relationship seemed to contribute to the interactions between the couple subsystem by allowing the couple to work on joint ventures, such as parenting, together. The complementary parenting interactions of tutoring and discussions exemplified the joined nature of this subsystem in many families.

An adoptive father exemplified the view of nursing as a shared behavior. He said, "I don't know if breastfeeding helps me bond. Most importantly, it helps establish that most important critical connection with the mother... There is definitely something like a magical connection there. The breastfeeding in an adoptive connection really helps solidify that…. But as much as Amy and I are a unit, parental unit, it helps the parental unit bond to the baby."

Closed Communication, Ambivalence, and Decreased Parental Sensitivity

The proportionally less visible group of parents with closed communication styles in this population indicates that closed systems might not be not conducive to physiologically based nursing patterns and associated sensitive parenting styles. Closed communication means that one hides one's feelings and does not receive validation or a means of resolution of issues. Observations of couples with closed systems helps one understand how closed communication patterns at the couple level impair the establishment of responsive parenting styles associated with nursing.

The fathers in two separate families with closed systems were ambivalent about nursing, yet they did not discuss their feelings honestly. One father, described earlier, expressed his unresolved discomfort with the frequency of mother-infant contact by interfering with nursing. He insisted that nursing was merely a means of feeding, and he refuted his wife's claims that nursing was also comforting. The mother in this case was also described in the section on mothers. She admitted that she was not confident in her ability to understand her children, and she was ambivalent about the comforting aspects of nursing. Observations indicate that the ongoing tension between the couple weakened the mother's stance, contributing to her husbands' efforts to separate her and the baby. His efforts reinforced the mothers' lack of confidence, and she forfeited her ideals, likely also to appease her husband. The mother mirrored her husband's insincerity and withheld her angry feelings when her husband grabbed the infant from the breast before the infant cued that she had finished nursing. The mother also reluctantly ignored her baby's cues for nursing when the father gave the baby a pacifier or finger instead of allowing the child to meet most of her needs at the breast. The parents' silence exacerbated the tension between them and impaired their ability to respond sensitively to their infant's cues.

In another family, the mother acknowledged that, "We never spoke openly about things even before the kids were born." The father in this family was described earlier and implied that he felt distant from his children when they nursed. He retained an angry position towards the nursing relationship and anyone from the nursing community. He often compared his children to other children in his extended family, implying that his offspring were too close to their mother and not as close to him as his nieces and nephews were to their fathers. The mother despised these comparisons and insinuated that her in-laws tried to interfere with her parenting style. She did not disclose her anger to her husband, and this contributed to the tension between the couple. In addition, the mother claimed that she had concealed that her older daughter had nursed in early childhood from her partner. Interestingly, the father later disclosed that he knew how long his daughter had nursed, reinforcing the closed nature of interactions between the couple. Although this couple engaged in some complementary parenting task allocation, this was less apparent than in most families in the study. Yet, despite the closed communication pattern and compared to the family discussed in the previous paragraph, this mother was extremely responsive to her children and refused to give her nursing children pacifiers, fingers, or bottles.

Compensatory Measures

Both of the families discussed above never discussed their issues at length, and contentious issues, such as the closeness inherent to nursing, remained unresolved. In addition, in both of these cases, the mothers attempted, often successfully, to tutor their partners and discuss parenting issues with them. In both couples, the fathers intermittently engaged in complementary parenting tasks and were sometimes attuned to their children. The difference between these two couples was that the second mother, who managed to retain ongoing sensitive interactions with her children, also made an effort to appease her partner. She said, "With everything else (meaning conflict over parenting interventions), I made sure that that was still working (meaning sexual intimacy)." In contrast, in the first family described, the couple did not engage in interactions, sexual or otherwise, that might have compensated for the dissension between them.

The comparison of these families suggests that when couples do not have the capacity to resolve issues through open communication, they require other means of compensating for the deficit. Sexual relations enabled one couple to temporarily dissipate the accompanying tension and allowed normal nursing interactions to occur. While compensatory measures did not fully resolve the tension between the couple, the mother seemed to have a stronger hold on her convictions than the mother who did not have other ways of appeasing her partner.

These two family systems provide additional insight into mechanisms that help families remain attuned to the needs of their nursing children despite their unresolved issues. These families show that although couple dissension interferes with some parents' ability to internalize and apply all of the themes and behaviors associated with nursing, they nevertheless were able to fulfill parts of this task. The processes, including maternal tutoring and discussion, facilitated the task of responding to the nursing child's needs. However, the most influential factor was that both fathers continued to share family themes associated with nursing. Reverence for natural processes and the view that nursing contributes to children's health seemed to be especially reinforcing for the parents who had trouble resolving issues related to nursing and some of the associated behaviors. For example, the father who perceived that nursing distanced him from his children was the father noted in the section on fathers who claimed that nursing was important, "because it is (was) natural and normal." Similarly, the father who felt that the nursing children displaced him proclaimed that he supported the nursing relationship and accepted some of the associated parenting interventions because it was healthy for his children.

Retaining and Reinstating Homeostasis

The couples with unresolved issues demonstrate the importance of reinstating homeostasis for couple interaction. The same processes that boosted parental sensitivity, including open communication and complementary interactions, were used as means of helping the couples improve their relationship with one another. Couples also enhanced their relationship and retained a sense of balance as a couple by engaging in unique and separate interactions outside of parenting.

Couple Time

One consequence of ongoing proximity behaviors between members of the nursing subsystem was that the marital couple had very minimal private time. Parents indicated, however, that they were not disturbed by this and felt that they were actualizing their joint themes of parenting by being close to the nursing child. One of the ways that parents managed to meet their children's needs and their needs as a couple was to engage in shared activities together. These activities often included children, especially when they were very young. Special time for one couple, for example, meant talking together while they shared a pot of tea and a special snack after the oldest child was in bed. These parents were pleased that the younger child, a toddler, played nearby.

When children reached early childhood and began to attend programs, there was more time for parents to be alone. Yet, like with younger babies, some couples continued the tradition of special time at home. One mother explained how this worked in her family. She said, "For many years, Tom has been working out of the home. So we have time in the middle of the morning...We don't have time in the night because children are here. So we will be talking. He will be working and I will walk in and tell him things. We are always talking. We are always telling each other things - communication times." Similar to this mother's narrative, many families indicated that discussion was a central element of couple interaction.

Sexual Intimacy

Other than in early infancy, many couples engaged in satisfying sexual intimacy, despite the ongoing presence of nursing children, including at night in the parental bed. Many parents implied that parent-child co-sleeping had little effect on couple relations and did not impede physical closeness between the couple. Interestingly, most of the aforementioned fathers in the case study group, who demonstrated diverse levels of ambivalence regarding the intensity of nursing, also stated that they were pleased that their children slept with them or with their wives. Some implied that they liked co-sleeping since it provided them with a means of remaining close to their children or wife.

It seems that many parents found places other the bed to be intimate with one another. In fact, some participants were perplexed that one might associate parent-child co-sleeping with parental intimacy. A remark made by one mother exemplified parents' views. She stated, "You don't have to have a bed to have sex!" One key informant interviewee said that some families believed that co-sleeping actually "put some spice in their lives." A common and repeated view was that the need to find special places and times for physical intimacy made sexual interludes more exciting, creative, and interesting. There were also some parents who engaged in sexual relations in the parental bed, including when babies were close by. One father explained, "You take care to not rock the boat so much."

It seems that some couples found that intensive parenting, not necessarily parent-child co-sleeping, complicated couple intimacy. In some cases, sexual intimacy was impeded due to parents' diverse levels of sexual desire, rather than the presence of infants or children in the bed. In most families with young infants, fathers seemed to desire sexual intimacy to a greater degree than their spouses. The term "all touched out" was frequently used to describe the maternal rationale for low libido.

One mother described how she felt when her children were young infants. "You don't realize you're not doing it (having sexual relations) because you are so ...so completely touched constantly and those constant cuddles twenty-four hours a day, and you don't realize that he's (the father) getting nothing." Her husband, in turn, described his sense of exclusion that came with feeling that he was no longer important. The couple claimed that this was resolved when the wife confirmed that her husband was still worthy to her, and that her lack of desire was not related to their relationship, but rather to the intensity of the nursing relationship. The father added that they compensated for the lack of sexual intimacy by meeting their couple needs in other ways. The dad said, "The lack of that (sexual intimacy) had to still be met in other ways of couples communicating about how they feel about each other. I needed her to tell me that this was not because of anything other than just her hormonal picture right now.... Even little things like hugs and kisses...became much more important."

In contrast, there were cases where mothers were more interested in sexual contact than their partners were. Some women attributed these feelings to a heightened sense of femininity. A breastfeeding professional and former nursing mother said, "Nursing makes you feel all womanly." Differences between couples when mothers desired sexual intimacy more than their partners did were resolved through mutual discussions and empathy.

Social Pressure

Nursing parental couples reiterated that family, friends, and professionals urged them to periodically separate from their children, apparently for the good of the couple relationship. Parents found this advice was non-validating and intrusive. This dilemma was particularly trying for couples with minimal parenting experience. They indicated that they struggled with the desire to remain with their child and their need to fulfill cultural expectations of them. More experienced parents were more likely to ignore the advice of outsiders and remain with their children most of the time.

Summary of Couple Processes Facilitated and Influenced by Interactions in the Nursing Subsystem

Although mothers and fathers traveled diverse trajectories in the nursing families, they supported and influenced one another as they facilitated the development of nursing and associated behaviors and themes. When mothers were supported, they concentrated on the nursing relationship that enabled them to develop sensitive mothering styles. Mothers' sensitive styles were reinforced by the children's responses to their care, their consequential positive affect, and their ability to interact with others. Children and mothers contributed to the transfer of a parenting style by providing fathers with cues for observation and interpretation. This system was facilitated further when children cued directly to their fathers. Fathers in turn reinforced the sensitive nursing system by responding to children' cues in an attuned manner like their partners and by engaging in complementary parenting tasks. Complementary interactions remained a central aspect of the couples' relationships as they responded to the changing needs of the nursing subsystem.

Parents were challenged along the way by personal and couple issues. Functional communication patterns and couple processes helped couples return to a state of homeostasis and respond to their children in a sensitive manner. Open communication and the capacity for mutual caring was an important means of resolving issues for these couples. The overall sharing between the couple subsystem was an important factor that sustained the parents, facilitated nursing, and upheld associated sensitive parenting.

Couples' relations in busy, child-centered nursing families were impacted by the quality of interaction between the parents, rather than the quantity of alone time. This aspect of family life was influenced by couples' abilities to find special activities that had meaning for them and that they enjoyed together. Couples also engaged in satisfying intimate interactions.

Parents in nursing families engaged in mutual parenting and couple ventures. These processes were influenced by and facilitated the transfer of themes of sensitivity and patterns of responsive parenting associated with nursing to parents' scripts of parenting. Interactions between the parents facilitated the transfer of these themes and patterns to the whole system.

Clinical Implications

Clinicians support parents as they make the transition to parenthood or to parenting another child, and integrate nursing into their system. Educators and healthcare professionals may use an educational model to promote concepts associated with nursing. Mental health professionals might use a systems models, psychotherapeutic tools, and verbal discussions to help couples come to the conclusion that makes the most sense for them.

Our review of counseling mothers and fathers clearly demonstrates the important impact of couple interaction on individual function and vice versa. Acknowledging that individual behavior is the function of systemic interaction has different applications depending on one's profession and clinical role. Practitioners primarily focused on advancing the nursing technique may use a systemic approach to decipher apparently inexplicable nursing problems. For example, one might recall that paternal distress might interfere with maternal function and impede one's ability to help a mother learn how to latch an infant to her breast properly. Clinicians focused on advancing interaction will use the same information as they help couples work out the emotional aspects of the transition to parenting.

Work with couples focusing on role transition is an extension of practice with mothers and fathers at the individual level. At this level, one helps parents undergo the role and task changes and integrate individual themes into the couple relationship. The clinician may scaffold parents' processes as the partners learn more about the other's gender specific roles and tasks. This task might be facilitated by first providing parents with a means of discovering and celebrating their unique qualities. Next one might help the partners explain the emotional meaning and challenges of their roles to one another. Supporting parents' transition includes reinforcing existing helpful processes, including patterns of paternal support and maternal tutoring.

In some cases, the transition to differentiated parenting tasks might be challenged when parents' views reflect the salient cultural perspective that self-worth and equality is based on sameness. Validating parents' feelings, including their sense of loss of their former non-parent selves, provides mothers and fathers with a sense that the clinician is joining them in their efforts to incorporate novel concepts. This sense of being heard will increase their capacity to examine existing perspectives and decide whether they are still valid in the novel of context of parenting. This task might also be facilitated when parents become more aware of the source of their negative views of gender differences. Providing parents with knowledge about the multiple influences on human behavior and attitudes, including cultural views, will increase their awareness. This task will be even more meaningful when parents are also asked to recount their narrative and the possible source of their discomfort with the change. Supporting parents as they incorporate novel roles and tasks will enrich their capacity to develop or reinforce differentiated and complementary task allocation systems.

These tasks are facilitated by helping parents reinforce or create open communication patterns. Open communication will help couples form joint meaning, a task that facilitates sensitive parenting and couple interactions. Working with couples with closed communication styles can be challenging for clinicians. Their pattern of hiding real feelings might make it difficult for the clinician to decipher their reasons for seeking help. In addition, one or both partners might be feeling extremely upset and not heard. An important role here is to contain the parent who does not feel heard and find ways of correcting the situation. One step is to validate disclosure, however small, and to model open communication until a proper resource can be found. In cases where it seems overly difficult to facilitate better communication, one might help couples create compensatory measures that have meaning for them. It is imperative to listen carefully to the couples and hear examples of what they think can help make themselves feel better.

In some cases, the clinician might be the first person the couple has met who talks to them about the impact of couple interactions on nursing and vice versa. Couples might be exhausted by non-validating experiences where nursing is blamed for couple problems and the real issue is neglected. In those cases, one must spend time listening and validating their sense of being unheard. Clinical understanding of processes associated with nursing also means that one will be able to help couples initiate and develop models of interaction that facilitate sensitive nursing interactions, enrich maternal sense of competency and self-worth, and define and give positive feedback to supportive and active fathers.

Listening carefully to couples can be very difficult when one recalls the impact of cultural themes on our views of interaction and family life. Couples attempting to integrate physiologically based nursing associated with responsive parenting into their lifestyles clearly have a different view of couple precedence and distancing than what is regarded as the salient perspective in this culture. The clinician should develop a clear awareness of their own views on this topic, as well as on sexual intimacy, in order to help the couple find a way that suits their lifestyle.

 It is also important to note that underlying couple functions, not nursing, are what usually plague couples. For example, closed communication styles plague the resolution of issues, such as paternal envy. Bearing this in mind will help the clinician focus on the actual couple issue, rather than blaming nursing. It is important to remember that the goal of helping couples is to understand and enhance underlying function. Couples may present with nursing problems when in reality functional issues are the reasons they are seeking help.

Thus supporting the parental couple in the nursing family enhances nursing at all levels. Work at this level is an extension of work at the individual level. This information has significance for those primarily focused on advancing nursing technique and for those who help couples with emotional issues. Clinical focus should include a systemic approach using nursing as the term of reference.

Chapter 9
Interactions with the Nursing Subsystem, Parents, and Siblings: Children Reverberate Sensitive Behaviors

In this section, the impact of nursing on individuals and subsystems in the nursing family will be reviewed. Earlier chapters looked at the impact of nursing on infants, young nurslings, and newly weaned children. Also discussed were the impact of nurslings' interactions with parents, and the mutual influence was noted. In this section, the trajectory of sensitivity in older children and siblings will be discussed. This data will provide further insights into the systemic transfer of themes and clinical interactions in nursing families.

Trajectory of Sensitive Interaction

In this study, key informant interviewees and case study families demonstrated that children echoed the sensitive behaviors that they had experienced since infancy. Children's behaviors suggested that their experiences also facilitated the development of several other characteristics that enhanced their interactions with others, and advanced their capacity to function in and outside the family context. All of these factors affected the system and reinforced processes that originated in the nursing subsystem.

Experiencing, Observing, Learning and Practicing Interactions with Siblings

The most apparent example of family processes on children was their interactions with their siblings. Siblings were sensitive to one another's needs and remained this way over time. Observations of children confirmed that siblings were attuned to the needs of their brothers and sisters.

Children initially experienced sensitivity through their own cue-based nursing interactions as nurslings, the maternal interactions that accompanied nursing, and their similar experiences with their fathers. As was noted earlier, children reinforced sensitive systems when they gave feedback to their parents. Children with nursing siblings were provided with additional ways of internalizing responsive conceptualizations when, like their fathers, they watched nursing from the side.

The almost constant nature of nursing in most families provided older children with ample opportunities to experience, discuss, watch, and internalize optimal responsive communication styles. In one family, for example, twin babies were almost constantly in their mother's arms and, for most of the time, at least one of the twins also nursed. Nursing took place as the mother engaged in diverse activities with her daughters inclusive of symbolic play. At times, the little boys were rarely referred to while the mother and her older children went about their activities. Yet, at the same time, the mother gently touched, positioned, looked at, and softly spoke to her babies as she concentrated on her older daughters.

In another family, a six-year-old girl watched as her brother, the toddler, intermittently crawled on top of his mother to nurse. She observed her mother's soft-spoken style and her warmth. She also noticed how her father also allowed the little boy to crawl over him and watched as her father hugged her brother frequently. This little girl's behavior suggested that she incorporated her parents' patience in her own serene and loving interactions with her brother. Her capacity for empathy towards her brother was exemplified by the way that she confidently explained why her brother liked nursing, uttering that, "...maybe he also enjoyed being close to mommy." Also, like her parents, she often laughed at her brother's antics and withstood his occasional rough play and periodic demands for assistance.

In addition to modeling sensitive behavior, mothers and fathers also simultaneously tutored their children in the art of empathetic interaction through verbal directions and lively discussions. A mother and father, who responded to their three-year-old after he kicked his infant sister, apparently by mistake, illustrate the way that discussions accompanied modeling. The older child watched how his father immediately picked up the baby in a warm and reassuring manner and gave the baby to her mother to nurse. The little boy also saw how his mother pulled the baby close to her breast and spoke softly to her. Signs of a developing capacity for empathy in this three-year-old were suggested by his apparent uneasiness over his sister's distress. His erratic movements and the nervous laughter that he displayed as he tried to busy himself suggested his sense of discomfort with the apparent harm that he had done. After the infant had calmed down at the breast, the mother called her older child over, provided her son with insight into the baby's perspective, and gently asked him to apologize to his sister. At the same time, she responded to some of his needs by validating his grief and confirming that she understood that he had not meant to hurt his sister. These actions provided the little boy with an outlet for repair of the emotional damage. They also tutored him in empathetic and responsible interactions.

Parents continued to simultaneously model and tutor attuned interactions as their children grew. This was illustrated in the way that parents enhanced their ten-year-old son's interactions with his three-year-old sister. These two children demonstrated a great deal of interest in one another and engaged in frequent mutual interchanges. Like his parents, the ten-year-old answered his sister's cues regularly and helped her when needed. For example, he retrieved and cut an apple for her when she was hungry. He also patiently engaged with her in activities that suited her level of development, inclusive of play. Often the parents witnessed these interactions and sometimes they intervened. This occurred, for example, when they felt that their son's play was too instructional and contradicted their child-led position. At that time, they gently tutored him and reminded him, for example, to allow his sister to make her own decisions. The older child was able to accept the tutoring as was illustrated by his continued interest in and engagement with his sister and his ability to implement different strategies in his play with her.

Parents provided positive feedback and demonstrated immense pride when their children were responsive to one another. This was illustrated in the way that a mother of three children proudly claimed that everyone in her family was very responsive to one another and knew how to meet one another's needs. She said that if the baby fell and she was temporarily unavailable, then someone else would immediately go to the baby. She explained that the children had learned since infancy that their needs had been met, so they had learned that other's needs were also important. The behavior of the oldest child verified this learning. This eight-year-old was able to recall his sister's nursing cues and other behaviors. Most importantly, he was very comfortable and happy in realizing his capacity for empathy. With pride in his voice, he said, "I am a very responsive person!" This suggests that not only was he able to interact sensitively, but also that he had internalized that responsiveness was an important value.

Along with obvious signs of responsiveness and empathy, many children intermittently teased and argued with one another. This was more prevalent in certain subsystems than in others. Siblings seemed to be most empathetic to the youngest children in their families, and often the older children bickered or teased one another. The same young and responsive eight-year-old boy who had exclaimed that he was very responsive also periodically teased his siblings, especially the sister who was closest to him in age. In a similar fashion, both of the daughters in the family of four children with twins were very patient, understanding, and loving towards their twin brothers. However, these two sisters quarrelled frequently which caused immense distress to their mother. Diverse subsystemic activity was also apparent in another family with three children. In this family, the oldest daughter, who was eleven years old, often took on a parenting role and helped both of her siblings when they required assistance. She was almost consistently kinder to the three-year-old than she was to her seven-year-old brother, about whom she complained from time to time.

Like the older siblings, younger children also intermittently displayed ambivalence. This, too, was mixed with overall responsive interactions. For example, a four-year-old boy displayed anger towards his nineteen-month-old sister when she bothered him while he tried to play with his trains. The toddler responded with minimal signs of frustration to her brother's animosity and consoled herself at her mother's breast. Outside of consoling the younger child through nursing, this mother allowed her children to resolve the issue without intervening. While the younger child nursed, her brother brought her little offerings that she accepted nonchalantly. This conflict was quickly resolved and, for the most part, these two siblings were quite pleasant towards one another.

Children appeared to be mostly very empathetic towards their siblings. Despite that the aforementioned eight-year-old boy periodically teased his middle sister; he chose to share a bed with her at night. In addition, these two children were quite aware of the others' needs, and on occasion, the brother helped his middle sister when needed, proving that his responsive nature prevailed after all. Similarly, in the family with twins, the sisters who bickered occasionally also chose to be close to one another and often ended up sleeping together at night, even though each child had her own bed. The older daughter, in particular, looked after her younger sister and ferociously defended her when needed. This was exemplified by the way that the older sister empathetically explained her younger sister's behavior when the little girl made a mess. Moreover, the ten-year-old tended to minimize the arguments with her sister when she discussed this issue during the study. She said, "The fighting is not really that bad."

When parents' modeled behavior, talked to children about sensitivity, and provided them with opportunities to repair their actions, children developed genuine positive regard for their siblings that was sustained over time. A participant who had married into a nursing family described the interactions between her husband and his siblings. She said, "They all really seem to like one another." A five-year-old boy exemplified the manner that this was manifested in the case study group. Along with momentary displays of frustration with his younger two-year-old sister, this little boy was also very enthusiastic about everything that his sister did. He spoke about his sister in a genuine and warm tone, seeming to demonstrate a true love in his eyes as he watched her. This was also evident in the soft way that he touched her and welcomed her when she joined him in bed at story time with their dad. Most remarkably, he used an adult tone when he said, "Look how cute she is. Do you see how cute she is? Get her on the videotape."

Extending Themes and Patterns to Contexts outside the Family

Nurturing Behaviors

The overwhelming capacity of children to engage in nurturing and responsive behaviors with their siblings was extended to relationships outside the family. Older children spoke about satisfying relationships with relatives and peers alike. The kindness that a nine-year-old girl showered on children who were maltreated by others at school was an example of how these children expressed caring for others, even when it was not popular with their peers.

It seems that these children continued to develop and display empathy to others. Former nursing children from families displaying sensitive patterns were overwhelmingly described as "extremely nurturing." This applied to their relationships with their family members, peers, partners, and others. They thrived in social settings and enjoyed interaction with others, even those who were shy. It was also significant that many adult children of former nursing families were social activists who carried the notion of nurturing to the macro level where they tried to create empathetic settings for all individuals. The fortitude of nurturing as a value was also illustrated by the way that adults from nursing families carried on the responsive behaviors in their interactions with their children.

Optimistic, Confident, Responsible, and Independent

A common trait observed in older children was optimism. They seemed to be very enthusiastic about the full lives they led away from their parents. They exuded confidence, initiated and attended a variety of extracurricular activities, enjoyed social interactions with peers, and demonstrated an overall very positive worldview that seemed to sustain them as they coped with insensitive teachers, periodic social struggles, and the tension associated with academia and sports.

These children demonstrated flexibility and most coped well with diverse settings, including those that differed from their child-centered homes. Older children in the study attended schools and participated in a wide range of activities that were very distinct from their home environments. Parents continued to support their children, and this likely contributed to the children's capacity to deal with diversity.

Many key informant interviewees, especially those with decades of experience, provided important insights into the issue of separation and individuation, and the development of autonomy in nursing families. They admitted that the continued closeness between mothers and children often gave the impression that young nursing offspring were less independent than their non-nursing peers. However, as older children, they not only caught up to the other children, but they apparently also surpassed their age appropriate behaviors. This was illustrated in the case study group whereby all of the older children were extremely responsible students and independently fulfilled their homework assignments and other projects.

A central characteristic of older or adult children of nursing families was that they exuded independent behaviors. Several key informants actually used a common statement, "They go by the beat of their own drum," to describe their behaviors. The connotation was positive. Apparently, their independent ways of thinking usually enabled them to make wise decisions. This was most poignantly exemplified by the repeated descriptions of how as adolescents these children were not likely to sheepishly follow their peers. These offspring were also described as creative, responsible, and moral. These characteristics likely contributed to adult children's involvement as social activists. Most interestingly, adult children from nursing families were cognizant of their independence. An adult who had grown up in a nursing family very nonchalantly stated, "I am very independent."

Reverence for Nursing

Key informant interviewees suggested that reverence for nursing was also passed onto children. As nurslings, they expressed their love and adoration by turning to the breast in great frequency. The few examples, provided earlier in this summary, of older and weaned children who continued to touch, kiss, or talk about their mothers' breasts, imply that older children remembered what their mothers' breasts had meant to them when they were younger. The likelihood that older and weaned siblings empathized with their younger siblings' persistent cues for nursing was suggested by their ability to withstand persistent nursing needs of their younger siblings. At times, this meant that their needs were temporarily put in second place, or in other cases, that they rarely had time alone with their mothers. For example, a five-year-old boy acknowledged that his sister needed to nurse in order to go to sleep. He happily let his father put him to bed so that his mother could nurse his younger sibling. In all families, children seemed to patiently accept the constant presence of their nursing siblings at the breast.

While it is likely that the children's patience was merely an expression of their sensitivity to their siblings' needs, the ways that children referred to nursing suggests that they were attuned to their siblings' nursing behaviors. Children often reminded their mothers to nurse when it seemed to them that their siblings needed comfort. A poignant example of the way that children participated in nursing was illustrated by a family where the mother had to relactate after coming out of a coma. According to the family history, the children understood the critical nature and significance of the relactation process and patiently allowed their father and mother to work together to help the mother establish nursing with the youngest sibling.

Other examples of children's reverence specifically for nursing are demonstrated by the positive regard and pride that children expressed about the nursing relationships in their families. A seven-year-old brother proudly told me that his sister nursed. He happily urged his little sister to tell me how much she loved "booby" (family name for nursing). Some, such as a six-year-old girl and her nine-year-old sister, enjoyed showing their friends how their mother nursed their twin brothers. They also proudly exclaimed that they, too, had nursed in this manner.

Nursing is Normal

In addition to feeling proud of being part of a nursing family, children seemed to internalize the normalcy of nursing and considered it a natural part not only of their lives, but also of life in general. Nursing was part of children's play, and children nursed their dolls and spoke about nursing in their symbolic play. The normalcy and essentiality of nursing in their lives was also evident in the way that children described their nursing experiences, and most portrayed it in a very functional way. A six-year-old who had weaned the year before said, "nursing is like drinking, sucking ... like this with a straw." She pretended to use a straw as she spoke. However, it also seemed that she retained some of the emotional memories of nursing, as was indicated by the way she explained that her younger brother nursed because he "liked to be close to mom."

School-aged children were affected by the reactions of others to nursing and the associated family patterns. Yet, overwhelmingly, these children saw nursing as normal and were perplexed when others didn't nurse or engage in interactions they were used to in their families. One ten-year-old boy was very aware of the existence of a non-nursing culture and often discussed this issue with his mother. He was aghast at the appearance of bottles and cribs in children's books. He made comments such as, "It makes sense (to nurse) otherwise G-d wouldn't make have made us like that...That reminds me when I am picking a wife I will not marry her if she does not promise to breastfeed the baby... Breastfeeding is healthier than, what do you call that other thing (meaning artificial baby milk)?" It was also interesting that he, like the other children in the study, felt comfortable about his former nursing relationship. This little boy said, "I am fine with it (nursing into early childhood). I don't care. I think that the kid should nurse as long as the kid wants to. I nursed for six years...Oh yes, I do remember nursing. I remember going to sleep nursing... I remember lying in your bed (looked at his father and meant his parents' bed) with mom beside me and nursing. ...That is a good memory..."

The adolescent years challenged these children's capacity to retain views of nursing as normal as they coped with age appropriate tasks of reverence for peers. The discomfort that some teenagers felt discussing nursing, breasts, and related issues during adolescence was temporary. In addition, teenagers' comfort around nursing mothers implied that they accepted the motherly components of the female breast. This was true even though it appeared that children also knew the breast had other meanings.

Carrying Traditions of Nursing and Sensitive Interactions to the Next Generation

Like children, adult members of nursing families passionately defended their family's stance and retained their sense of pride and ownership of nursing. A few stated that they had been embarrassed as teenagers; however, their perspective changed as they reach adulthood. Then, they reverted back to notions of pride. Many of these children became social activists and one attributed this to her early realization of her mothers' efforts to nurse in "a culture that frowns on nursing."

Like their parents, adult children tended to simultaneously admire nursing and natural processes. Statements that many former nursling adults made about the importance of engaging in natural acts referred to natural birth and nursing in tune with nature. Many carried on the tradition and nursed their own children. One nursing mother in the case study group who had grown up in a nursing family exemplified this finding. She said, "My mother nursed the rest of the children. Two of my siblings were nursed for four years and my youngest sister was nursed for two years. I grew up watching this. Breastfeeding was an example in our family, my mother breastfed and I remember it."

Summary

Living in a sensitive nursing family impacted children and their relationships beyond their nursing experience. Children enjoyed sensitive interactions at the breast and eventually echoed associated themes and behaviors. Their parents' sensitive style was reflected in the nurturing way they treated first their siblings and then others. The process of child-focused weaning facilitated the development of independent, responsible, moral, and creative older children and then adults. Offspring of nursing families internalized a view of nursing as a normal and natural behavior. Adult children carried and transferred the responsive themes and behaviors associated with nursing to the next generation of nursing children.

Clinical Applications

The information in this section demonstrates that children are affected by and may influence the nursing relationship. In these families, older children remain an important part of family function. Parents continue to read and attend to their cues carefully. By the same token, the children's early and continued experiences with nursing contribute to the sensitive system by providing children with a means of internalizing attuned interaction. Their ability to mirror their parents' attuned style in their interactions with one another, their parents, and eventually others outside of the family points to the contribution of ongoing interaction with the nursing system to positive child outcome. From a clinical perspective, this implies that one should encourage these behaviors in families.

Encouraging existing family patterns implies that one should acknowledge the impact of the older children on the nursing unit. This principle indicates that along with assessing the quality of latching, for example, one might assess how the mother's interactions with the older child influence the presenting nursing issue. An associated task is helping the family find ways to facilitate the older child's transition to the new family composition and his/her new role.

One might suggest that parents use existing skills as they help older children incorporate novel tasks into their repertoire. Parents might learn how to help their children use their existing scripts of sensitivity in their interactions with the nursing unit. This task includes teaching children tangible means of deciphering and responding to siblings' cues for nursing. This intervention is similar to the techniques used to encourage fathers and provides them with a sense of inclusion. These feelings might be reinforced further by positive feedback displayed by their siblings or by pleased parents.

Reinforcing children's existing scripts of cues reading not only facilitates role transition, but also seems to enhance parents' capacity to remain attuned to older children. Clinicians may play an important role in increasing parents' sense of efficacy and associated sensitivity by pointing out the older children's advanced capacity to respond to their sibling. In addition, parental patience might be increased when clinicians discuss the long term implications of sensitive parenting through nursing on child outcome.

This same information might encourage clinicians. The data pointing to enhanced development might also be especially reassuring for practitioners previously unfamiliar with the family interactions associated with physiological breastfeeding patterns and those holding cultural views of distancing in their scripts of healthy growth. The contribution of nursing and associated sensitive patterns to positive child outcome reinforces the need to support nursing and parents in these systems.

While it seems easy to support families with pre-school children, school nurses and counselors in high school, for example, might have to offer additional support to youngsters, realizing that their family themes and behaviors differ from those of their peers. In addition, the evidence that some adolescent members of nursing families temporarily feel uncomfortable with otherwise salient themes has important implications for practitioners supporting teen parents. This information indicates that they might also experience a heightened sense of cultural pressure regarding the multiple meanings of breasts and require additional support.

Taking older children's development into account has diverse clinical implications depending on the practitioner's role and the stage of family and child development. Clinicians working with mothers with newborns might help parents include and remain attuned to older children by providing tangible tools for signal reading and by pointing out children's capacity for sensitivity to parents. The positive impact of nursing on child outcome might help clinicians continue to support families over time. This perspective will also help clinicians contain older children as they become aware of prevailing cultural themes that differ from their family patterns.

Chapter 10
Interaction Between All Individuals and Subsystems: The Extension of Themes Associated with Nursing to the Family System

The interaction between individuals and subsystems in the nursing family has been covered in earlier chapters. In this chapter, the circular impact of all of these interactions on one another and the transfer of themes associated with nursing to the family context and vice versa will be reviewed.

Family Interaction

The impact of interactions in the nursing subsystem on individual family members and the parental couple, and the interactions between these components of the system, set the tone for family themes that were exhibited by the whole family beyond nursing. Nursing families exhibited specific and perpetuating behavioral patterns. The themes, including attitudes, specific behaviors, and recurring behavioral patterns, resembled those in the nursing relationship, were reflected in overall family interactions, and reverberated back to the nursing subsystem.

Proximity in the Midst of Family Activity

Key informants' descriptions and observations of case study families demonstrated that children's cues for nursing were answered at all times, including during active periods of family interchanges. Nursing was an ongoing behavior. At times, it seemed that fathers and siblings were oblivious to the nursing dyad as they went on with their activities. Mothers focused their attention on additional family interchanges during many of their nursing sessions. Some mothers played with their children while they nursed a younger sibling. For example, one mother nursed her five-month-old son and played house with her four-year-old daughter at the same time.

It appears that nursing sessions had a calming effect on the family. Observations indicate that mothers and the nursing children appeared relaxed when they nursed. The calm interactions in the nursing subsystems were mirrored in the interchanges of other family members in the same room.

The centrality of physical closeness in the nursing subsystem and the parents' positive attitudes towards this was apparent during family interchanges. Mothers and nursing children engaged in tactile interactions and remained close to one another during busy family interchanges. Mothers and fathers held and carried nursing children while their older siblings were nearby. In many families, both parents wore their children in slings at home and on outings. Older children calmly watched as active toddlers and younger siblings periodically returned to their mothers and fathers for physical reassurance. All family members emulated the physical closeness in the nursing subsystem by holding and carrying the youngest family member in between nursing sessions. Siblings sat close to one another and hugged, held, and carried younger brothers and sisters. Parents touched and hugged older children, although touch was not as prominent in interactions between parents and older children as it was with preschoolers and babies.

The common theme of reverence for parent-child closeness in these families was also indicated by the commonality of joint family activities. Until children were approximately school-aged, families spent most of their time together and engaged in child-centered activities in and outside of the home environment. All family members enjoyed going out together. Parents rarely went out without their children when they were young and seldom left their children with babysitters.

Co-Sleeping

Families demonstrated that mother-child closeness was important to them at all hours. Reverence for continuous mother-child closeness explained why parent-child co-sleeping was the most common sleeping arrangement in nursing families. Apparently, most nursing children woke up several times a night to nurse for the first few years of life, and thus co-sleeping was also practical. A mother of twins explained, "They nurse through the night ... I just roll over from side to side. They nurse whenever they get up." A father of two children also justified co-sleeping as a means of meeting all family members' needs. He said, "I think people without children don't realize that once you have children no one is getting much sleep. Now if you can manage to get more sleep with everyone sleeping in the same bed, then that's better. Sleep is critical for Jody (his wife), and if she doesn't get enough sleep, then she doesn't feel well and she can't function.... And if that means that our child has to be in our bed for her health (Jody's health), then that is how we are going to do it."

Different families carried out co-sleeping patterns in varied ways. In the majority of families, children slept with their mothers for a few years. In other families, co-sleeping was considered a temporary solution in infancy. Most commonly, children slept in the parental bed for the entire night, and both parents were in the bed. A family of four, for example, had only one bedroom and one large bed where everyone, including the parents and two children, slept. Other forms of co-sleeping included arrangements where children slept alone for part of the night and with their parents for the rest of the night. In some cases, mothers and fathers joined the children in their beds. A few fathers left the bed, while the nursing child slept with the mother in the parental bed. Some fathers who slept on their own claimed that they were comfortable with the arrangement because it gave them more physical space, was in the best interest of the child, and moreover, both parents were aware that these arrangements were temporary.

Changing sleeping routines was common in these families and reflected the flexible patterns associated with nursing and the theme of following children's leads. Families allowed children to co-sleep until they showed signs that they were ready to sleep alone. This was similar to and often accompanied the process of weaning from the breast and from the mother. Most children initiated the move away from the parental bed between the ages of four to six years. The transition was smooth, resembling the process of gradual weaning from the breast, and was viewed positively by the child and the family alike. Many children continued to visit the family bed from time to time.

It was very common for children to move from the parental bed to a sibling bed. Older and younger siblings seemed to enjoy this arrangement. For example, an eight-year-old brother and four-year-old sister in a family of three children shared a double bed in the young girl's bedroom. Their younger nursing sister sometimes joined them prior to going to sleep with her parents.

Solitary Sleeping Arrangements

Although it was apparently uncommon, some nursing families engaged in separate sleeping arrangements. Two young families exemplified this pattern. Both couples were first time parents. The babies had slept in a cradle by their mothers' side until they were a few months old and were moved to another room when the parents perceived that the babies were ready. The parents emphasized that they continued to answer the babies' cues during the night. In one family, the father instigated separate sleeping, and in the other family, the new mother stated that she was too nervous to sleep with her baby. Most importantly, these cases demonstrate the association between separate sleeping and potential distancing of mothers from their infants and from the breast. In one case, the baby was given a pacifier at night and slept through the night – a behavior that was rare for most nursing children. In the other case, the baby also began to sleep through the night at an early age and, according to his mother, this, together with his growing interest in roaming his environment, led to a precipitous weaning prior to the age of one year. It is important to note that both of these families were new to parenthood, and one might wonder whether the pattern of single sleeping would remain a permanent pattern in these families in the future.

Extending Interactions from Mothers to Family Members

Most families seemed to accept that mothers remained the children's central love object for most of early childhood. The section on fathers highlighted that this issue can be complicated by paternal ambivalence in some families. However, most families acknowledged the mothers' special role, and at the same time, also provided nursing children with opportunities to interact and form loving relationships with all family members at their own rate.

Parents' reverence for natural processes of child development and their desire to consistently meet their children's needs helped them facilitate their children's growing interest in interacting with other family members. The exclusive interchanges between mothers and children decreased over time, although children continued to turn to mothers more than to other family members for comfort during early childhood. Children increasingly asked their fathers to do things for them, went to them for physical comfort, and as they got older, also confided in them. Fathers demonstrated a capacity to patiently support their children.

As was documented in the section on fathers, young children increasingly turned to their fathers, even when mothers remained the central comfort figures. Many of the interactions between older children and their fathers suggest that the children internalized them as trusting objects. The secure nature of the father-child relationship was exemplified by the way a four-year-old former nursling told her father that she was very angry with him. The tone in her voice and the clear way she expressed her feelings suggested that she felt her father would accept her despite her apparently negative feelings. Her father, in turn, validated her feelings and accepted the artwork she offered him in an apparent reparative gesture.

The apparent trust children have in their fathers was also suggested by the way a ten-year-old was able to withstand inconsistencies in his fathers' behaviors and to disregard momentary outbursts of parental frustration. This boy approached his father with ease despite the father's infrequent, but existent bouts of impatience. The capacity of children to withstand momentary pain in their relationships with their fathers was also observed in a six-year-old who reacted to her father's claim that he had not bonded to her until after she had weaned. Initially, she seemed distressed by her father's outburst and hid under a blanket as she said, "That is not very nice what daddy is saying." Yet, the parents joined together to reassure her, and as she emerged from underneath the blanket, her body language and facial expressions suggested that she felt relieved. The daughter's ability to accept her father's ambivalence was suggested by the way she sought him out in a confident manner and initiated warm tactile interactions with him. He returned her touch by remaining physically and emotionally engaged with her on several occasions. This seemed to advance their relationship further.

Interviews with adult members of nursing families and with key informant interviewees with decades of experience indicated that fathers and mothers were viewed eventually as equal comforting objects. Many of the interactions between older children and their fathers suggest the children had internalized them as trusting objects much in the way they had earlier turned to the breast. Young children's interests also included older siblings, to whom they turned for support and assistance, although to a lesser degree than they did to their fathers.

Mothers promoted child-led interest in interactions with others outside the nursing system. However, it seems that some mothers experienced ambivalence about the changes that took place in their relationships with their children. One mother, for example, seemed to have a hard time accepting her three-year-old nursing son's obvious and growing preference for his father. She looked anxious and continued to try to interact with her son even after he repeated, "I don't want to read with you. I want Daddy to read to me." This mom's temporary insensitive reaction suggested that perhaps she had difficulty letting go of her central role. One might wonder if other mothers also felt ambivalent about changes in their relationship with a growing nursing child.

Retaining a Child-Paced Focus as Children Grow and Develop Beyond Nursing

Parents' interactions with children over time remained as intense and validating as they had been in infancy. Interactions remained focused on children's cues. As their offspring grew, parents altered the interactional components they used in their interchanges with their children to suit their changing needs. This included accepting children's reduced needs for tactile interaction and physical proximity to their parents as they grew. Although families continued to hug, touch, and intermittently co-sleep with one another, touch did not remain the central feature of the interactions between parents and children. Instead, families engaged in deep and genuine discourse that mirrored the validating nursing relationship and open communication style established in nursing that was prominent in earlier parent-child relationships and in parental couple interactions.

A young adult key informant who had nursed until six years of age exemplified the combination of physical and emotional aspects of adult relationships in nursing families. She recalled how she still enjoyed sleeping beside her mother when she came to visit. However, her descriptions of warm discussions with her mother and her sense of being validated and accepted constituted a far more prominent aspect of her narrative. Like this young woman's story, it seemed that families in the study with older and adult children continued to touch one another and enjoyed being physically close to one another. Yet, deep and genuine discussions replaced tactile interactions and physical proximity as the central means of communication.

Along with noting children's needs for closeness, parents also demonstrated an awareness of their children's growing needs to venture out and build relationships with others outside the family. The concept of child-led weaning from the breast was extended to child-paced separation from mother, family, and home. However, it is most significant that separation was not the goal of the families. Rather, their goal was to boost the individual needs and traits of each child. Separation was rarely forced on these children and parents responded to their cues for distancing in the same way they answered their signals for closeness at the breast. They promoted separation in response to their children's signs that they were interested in gradually exploring the world outside the family. At the same time, parents accepted children's needs for renewed closeness when it was expressed.

Child-paced weaning beyond the breast, mother, family, and home was illustrated by the way that children determined their readiness for school and other programs. Parents seemed to understand that their young children's needs for closeness preceded cultural expectations that they attend preschool programs. Some of these children remained at home until they started elementary school.

A mother of a three-year-old boy used a child-centered approach to determine and explain her sense of her child's readiness for preschool. She said, "We (the parents) made the decision not to send him. ...No one cares about his development more than us. So I don't want to send him to school so early when he is not able to make those decisions that he knows are right, but he is just not mature enough to fulfill them. So we are very flexible when we send him to school, we are just going to really take our time."

Similarly, parents also responded to children who cued that they wanted to intermittently separate and have experiences outside the home, even if the parents felt that this was earlier than expected. For example, a mother in the case study group sent her two and a half-year-old nursing child to preschool at a much younger age than she had sent her older child. She explained, "I didn't intend on sending her to school until she was three, but when she was two and a half, she said that she was going to go to school and that, (mother quoted her daughter) 'I would drop her off and then when she was done, I could pick her up'. Just like that. What was amazing was that she didn't ask me, she told me that she was going to school! So I had to find a school."

Parents continued to support their children as they entered school and other activities far from home. Many parents remained active participants in their children's lives, including in specific school activities. Yet, it was also significant that parental participation also diminished as children's capacity for independence or desire to be away from home increased.

Just as parents assessed their children's state of readiness for closeness and separation, they also took note of their children's individual qualities. It was commonplace for parents to take steps to nourish their children's talents, much in the way that parents had nurtured children's early development at the breast. Individuality was respected, and the children were provided with resources that suited their special needs. In one case, parents acknowledged their son's unique talents and provided him with many opportunities to reach his individual scholastic and athletic potential. The parents' efforts resembled the way they had responded to their son's cues for nursing and closeness when he was a young child.

Like these parents, most parents made extensive efforts to find educational settings that promoted their individualistic philosophies and allowed each child to actualize their uniqueness. Some parents got discouraged when they were unable to find settings that fit this perspective. Despite how hard this was for them, parents compromised their ideals and sent their children to schools and activities that differed from the home philosophy. Some families resolved their frustration with existing schools by home schooling their children.

Parents continued to respond to their children's needs, signals, and rhythms. The responsive parenting style was apparent in interchanges between parents and adult children. Evidence that parents supported their older children's unique rhythms was apparent in a comment reiterated by several key informant interviewees. They said, "Sometimes parents were challenged by choices that their children made, yet they continued to support them." Similarly, an adult child of a former nursing family claimed, "I did some things that they (my parents) might not have liked, but I always knew that they were there for me and that I could talk to them and depend on them to support me."

Summary

Nursing in the case study group took place in the midst of an active family environment. All family members experienced the interactions between the nursing subsystem. By the same token, family members engaged in behaviors that enhanced the function of the nursing subsystem. The mutuality of this process was demonstrated by circulation of a sensitive and child-paced parenting style established through nursing that reverberated throughout the system and affected behaviors unrelated to nursing. The same family behaviors boomeranged back and reinforced the nursing subsystem. Sensitive family interactions established through nursing enabled children to nurse at will and to wean from the breast, mother, and home. This style of interaction was sustained as parents altered interactional components to reflect their children's changing needs and as they supported them through other significant developmental milestones. Most significantly, the validating communicative style that was established through nursing was retained by parents and valued by children over time.

Clinical Implications

Clinicians may meet families as a whole. It is always important to remember the clinical implications and applications at the individual level and to see their contribution to the entire family. By the same token, a practitioner might support development at individual levels by facilitating behaviors at the family level. Our insights about family interchanges demonstrate the circularity of themes in the family system.

The clinical role at this level is to support and encourage families to uphold behaviors generated by the nursing subsystem, while acknowledging the effect that these behaviors have on the family as a whole. It is easy to see how many of the behaviors might be difficult for families to tolerate. For example, a review of interaction at the family level indicates that families must be able to tolerate ongoing nursing and proximity behaviors. Yet, the contribution of these ongoing behaviors to the development of sensitive family interaction is apparent. It is important to help families see what is meaningful for them and to assist them in fulfilling their own agenda.

One might understand the challenges that the family feels as a whole by understanding the impact of nursing at all levels. For example, a clinician might support a father as he protects the nursing dyad or a mother as she reluctantly lets go of her central role by helping the system compensate her for the loss in others ways. The clinician might help family members talk about what these tasks mean to them as a means of enriching family function. This role points to the significance of open communication in these systems and implies that clinicians might want to facilitate optimal communication when possible.

Educators might teach families about child-led processes, proximity behaviors, and altering interactional components to suit the levels of development. Again, it is important to help families implement these concepts in a way that has meaning for them.

As in clinical interactions at other levels of interaction, some clinicians might find it difficult to support behaviors, such as co-sleeping, that contrast with personal scripts of parenting and family life. The use of self-awareness, enriched understanding, and validating support from peers is one means of enriching clinical practice. And, as always, practitioners have the right to let go of tasks that are unbearable.

Thus supporting individual nursing functions includes acknowledging systemic processes. Family-focused practitioners reflect this acknowledgement in their assessment of nursing issues. This assessment includes looking at salient family themes and helping families establish themes that augment the development of physiologically based nursing and sensitive interaction. An acknowledgernent of the impact of the family system can also be integrated into interventions that advance nursing and educational interactions. While one may use a general view of family system interaction to guide clinical interaction, it is also important to verify individual meaning and the unique way that families integrate nursing into their specific family system.

Chapter 11
The New Breed of Breastfeeding Families: Adult-Focused Nursing

In this chapter, data that was gathered about another kind of nursing family that differs from those included in the study will be described. These families did not nurse in accordance with physiologically based nursing patterns. Instead their themes concur with the prevailing patterns in western culture that were described in chapter three. The likelihood that many clinicians will encounter families displaying these patterns suggests a brief review is in order.

Adult-Focused Nursing

Earlier in this book, we reviewed how breastfeeding is portrayed as a supreme substance in the present context. This notion was apparent in the narratives of parents in this group who strived to provide their infants with the perfect substance. According to the data used to prepare this book, these families see nursing as a feeding choice that is fashionable and healthier than other choices. Their narratives indicate that they see nursing as "in," "the right thing to do," and "the healthiest way to feed babies."

The view that nursing is primarily a feeding choice concurs with parents' attempts to remain in control. Many become parents after years of organized living. A salient theme in this group is retaining former pre-parenting selves and control over their lives. This is actualized by the efforts they make to fit their infants into their schedules rather than following their infants' signals. Their desire for organized schedules is reflected in nursing behaviors based on parent-focused timing rather than infant signals.

Missed cues for nursing are suggested by observed nursing patterns. In these families, nursing sessions were proportionally infrequent in comparison to the constant pattern described earlier in this book. Other signs of missed cues for nursing were the use of oral pacifiers, early supplementation with artificial substances, the use of artificial feeding apparatus, and the use of breast pumps. Many of these young parents invested emotional energy, time, and sums of money learning about the best pumps prior to even holding their infants. For some, this act enabled mothers to distance themselves from their infants, retaining their former selves, while simultaneously providing their infants with the supreme substance. In addition, pumping allowed them to fulfill the cultural myth that fathers must feed their infants.

Distal strategies (Valsiner, 2000) were also evident in these families, aside from distancing from maternal nursing. Mothers retained emotional distance from their babies and upheld strict boundaries that hindered them from becoming overly physical with their infants. Although some parents started off with babies in cribs or bassinettes close to their own beds immediately after birth, many quickly moved their offspring to their own rooms. Solitary sleeping was common in this group. Rather than parental holding and carrying, these infants were often placed in multipurpose infant seats that enabled mothers to move their babies from place to place without ever touching them. Additional distancing objects observed in these homes included infant swings and similar apparatus.

The distancing behaviors at the breast and beyond were both a symptom of the parents' philosophy and, in circular fashion, also contributed to this style of parenting and nursing. In some cases, parents initiated distancing steps, and in other cases, they did it to comply with directives from medical personnel, family members, and, of course, the domineering non-nursing culture. All of these steps pulled parents away from the developmental task of answering children's cues through nursing and were missed opportunities for the development of sensitive parenting.

Precipitous weaning was an unfortunate consequence of adult-focused and distance nursing and strategies. Early supplementation, including with pumped breastmilk, were the first steps in the process to full weaning. Many children in this group were only nursed for short periods of time, fully weaned after only a few months of nursing.

Clinical Implications

No doubt that many readers are familiar with the family style of nursing described in this chapter. Clinicians holding western concepts of nursing and family will likely feel comfortable working with these families. On the other hand, once one has internalized concepts conducive to physiologically based nursing patterns, one may find it challenging to work with these families. This seems to be especially likely when one notes the contribution of nursing to optimal family function and positive child outcome.

At this point, we can apply our understanding of the development of sensitivity through nursing to the context of distance and adult-focused nursing. First we note that perceptions of nursing as a supreme feeding choice rather than views of nursing as part of a physiological process interfere with the establishment of physiological nursing patterns. Next we note the impact of distancing on cue reading through nursing and how this style of parenting interferes with the important process of internalizing sensitive parenting. In addition, we note that parental sharing of feeding through expressed milk or intermittent artificial feeding, for example, interferes with the development of gender-based trajectories to the fullest. It is important to remember the important role that gender-based development through nursing plays in the advancement of self-esteem for parents and how this seems to facilitate further their capacity for sensitivity. One might concur that in these families opportunities for missed cue reading and subsequent sensitive parenting are missed on several levels, directly through nursing and also through paths of individual script enhancement.

It is difficult and not recommended to confront these families, or any clients for that matter, considering that respect for clients is basic to ethical practice. However, at the same time, it is also ethically appropriate to provide parents with optimal information that might change the quality of family interaction and child outcome. It is important to remember that families nursing in this style are reflecting salient western concepts of parenting and nursing. They will likely not hear any different views, other than from a clinician aware of the information presented in this book.

On one hand, clinicians should always respect clients and see them as adults responsible for their welfare. On the other hand, that exact same view implies that our clients are adults and have the ability to internalize or ignore information. Moreover, we are ethically obligated to provide clients with accurate and evidence-based information in a manner reflecting the client's learning style. This principle applies to all clinical work, yet interestingly, many clinicians might feel uncomfortable fulfilling this task with these families. Some adhere to the guilt myth that was reviewed earlier in this book. One might offer that self-awareness discussed at the beginning of the book might facilitate practice in this area.

Based on principles of ethical practice, one would therefore respect family decisions and listen carefully to the family agenda, while providing educational material. Interested families may receive additional support through referrals to peer support groups. Of course, clinicians should always remain open to questions and supportive of ambivalence. All clinicians, including healthcare providers, social workers, and psychotherapists, might gently contain clients as they internalize novel concepts and embark on a path to enhanced parenting.

Chapter 12
Themes Promoting Physiologically Based Nursing Patterns and the Development of Sensitivity

The previous chapters described the development of sensitive interaction at individual, sub-systemic, and systemic levels. This chapter will augment the understanding of nursing families by describing the interconnected themes that facilitate the development and reverberation of sensitive interactions in the family system. Several of these themes are established prior to nursing, others stem from experiences associated with nursing, and all themes are refined as they circulate throughout the system and reflect the needs of the evolving family.

Reverence for Physiology

Respect for Physiological Processes

Family narratives and behaviors suggest that reverence for physiological processes was a salient family theme. Reverence for physiology was evident in families' language. However, the word physiology was rarely used and instead terms such as healthy, natural, and normal were used to describe physiological processes, such as birth, nursing, and child development. Physiologically based events were described as normal points on a continuum of naturally occurring development. For these families, birth and nursing were just as normal as other physiologically based processes, such as breathing and digestion. Families also repeated that they had never considered anything other than nursing - it was not a decision, it was a fact. This viewpoint contrasts with the common cultural perception of nursing as a feeding choice discussed earlier in this book.

Prevalent patterns of natural birthing processes, allowing babies to nurse exclusively for approximately the first six months after birth and to continue nursing for at least the first few years of life, exemplify family behaviors suggesting respect for physiology. Themes of admiration for physiological processes were evident in the specific way that families nursed. Mothers, with the support and encouragement of fathers, nursed immediately after birth. Joint efforts were made to ensure that nursing units nursed exclusively for approximately the first six months of life, and that they continued nursing for a few years. The significance of nursing in tune with natural processes for families explains data showing that parents suffered emotionally when physiologically based nursing was interrupted, for example, when supplements were provided to their infants. This view also clarifies the efforts families made to repair damaged nursing experiences, nurse in difficult situations, and nurse naturally despite cultural and sometimes systemic opposition. These behaviors reinforced the existence of respect for physiology and indicated that families felt that it was not good enough for them to merely nurse, they must nurse in a specific manner, namely physiologically.

Respect for natural processes seemed to contribute to families' understanding that nursing had multiple physiological functions and could be used to meet a variety of needs. This attitude reflects the physiologically based interdependence between mothers and infants discussed in the first chapter in this book, and explains why families used nursing as the most common way of meeting infants' needs. This perspective also contributed to the exclusivity and duration of nursing patterns. Accordingly, respect for the physiological development continuum prompted families to nurse exclusively from birth until approximately six months of age. In circular fashion, exclusivity facilitated mothers and infants to actualize their physiologically based interdependence. From a practical point of view exclusivity for these families meant that there were tasks associated with nursing that could not be replicated, namely nutritional and comfort needs until a physiologically defined age. All tasks contributed to the relationship between the mother and child. Some tasks were physiologically based and included oral nutrition in the early months. Infants received all of their oral nutrition and liquids, and most of their comforting through nursing until they were approximately six months of age. Fathers actualized themes of respect for physiologically based task specificity by refraining from feeding their infants, and in most cases, babies did not have any form of oral comfort other than the breast. Respect for physiological continuums and the associated understanding about change over time enabled families to modify specific tasks to suit the growing nursing child and changing nursing relationship. When complementary nutrition was added at approximately six months of age, it was done in a gradual manner matching the infants' slowly maturing system. Nursing remained the main source of comfort for children until they weaned, usually several years later.

Regard for physiologically based interdependence between mothers and infants, and the associated understanding that nursing meets most infants' needs, provides insight into the finding that mothers and children nursed frequently. One might venture that it must have been hard for mothers and their fellow family members to withstand ongoing nursing, especially since it took place in the middle of ongoing family activity. Yet the study discussed in this book shows that both mothers and their families demonstrated immense patience and tolerance for nursing. Repeated references to the normalcy of this situation implied that reverence for the perceived natural flow and functions of nursing likely enabled families to withstand nursing behaviors. This perception contributed to parents' capacity to tolerate the fluctuating and often ongoing nature of the nursing sessions and to engage in nursing patterns that were consistent with physiologically based recommendations. Similarly, respect for natural processes also contributed to families' capacity to sustain nursing into at least early childhood and to welcome continued exclusive emotional interchanges between nursing mothers and children.

Respect for physiology remained salient as children grew reinforcing the salience of this theme in families demonstrating physiologically based nursing patterns. For some this theme stemmed from their life experiences prior to parenthood and was exemplified by the prevalence of this theme in some families' stories of their first birthing experience. The likelihood that many families had at least a minimal investment in physiological processes prior to nursing was suggested by family regard for nursing as the only next step after birth, an attitude that facilitated the initiation of nursing. Some families internalized themes of reverence for natural processes only after giving birth and nursing, suggesting that engaging in physiological processes also contributed to families' respect for nature. An important process enhancing the circulation of this theme was the pattern of maternal leading. Mothers seemed to have more information on the normalcy of nursing than fathers did, and led the process. Findings show reverence for physiology continued as families supported nursing over time. Moreover, the centrality of this theme to the narratives of families with older children, including those who did not have this attitude at the onset of parenting, suggested that this theme became more relevant as children grew. This change seems to suggest that the experience of nursing contributed to the development of respect for natural processes, and by the same token, this theme enabled families to continue nursing. The salience of similar views in older children's narratives indicates that this theme was transferred to all family members, reinforcing behaviors between nursing mothers and children.

Thus an analysis of family interaction points to the existence of themes of reverence for physiology, usually termed as respect for nature and natural processes. This concept is actualized through nursing and additional behaviors. The viewpoint that nursing is a step on a natural continuum facilitates physiologically based nursing processes and evolves over time.

Nursing is Normal

A component of respect for nature that appeared to affect family behavior is that nursing is normal. Families rarely used superlatives when referring to nursing, and instead referred to nursing a normal life cycle event that they expected to experience without interference. Interference for this population included medical intervention during birth, artificial feeding or pacifiers during nursing, and lack of regard for child, female, and male biologically based development. The circulation of this theme in the family system was evident in the actions and words of older children who portrayed nursing as normal in their narratives. They were proud to tell others about their nursing siblings and that they too had nursed. Views of nursing as normal were also indicated in the comfort they displayed when mothers or other women nursed. Moreover, they were perplexed when it became evident to them that others didn't nurse, something abnormal in their view. It seems that views of nursing as normal and the "other" as abnormal might have enabled families to remain strong in the face of controversy associated with salient cultural perspectives of family, children, and nursing.

It seems that families' perception of nursing as normal fostered an environment enabling them to accept behaviors associated with nursing, and enhanced their responsiveness to nursing. On a daily basis, this outlook seemed to help families allow ongoing nursing and to accept that they were surrounded by nurslings nursing frequently and remaining close to their mothers. Respect for the natural continuity of nursing also clarifies why families included nursing children in all activities, including outings. By the same token, when families allowed mothers to nurse in tune with nature, in all locations, mothers were close to the rest of the family and could tend everyone's needs, fulfilling another interconnected family theme. This behavior likely contributed to the cycle of reverence for natural processes and sensitivity towards nursing. Furthermore, the responsive tools that children internalized through nursing enabled them to reinforce the cycle by providing others with positive feedback for their efforts.

The likelihood that family members, and most remarkably young siblings, accepted physiologically based nursing patterns as a normal and regular part of family life was suggested by their tolerance of the nursing unit. Older children's internal models of relationships, the good enough feelings that they internalized through their own nursing experiences, parents' well defined role and task allocation, and parents ongoing responsiveness, likely reinforced older siblings' patience. It also seems that children's views of nursing as normal were strengthened by watching ongoing nursing. This experience likely fortified the notion that nursing is an essential part of normal development and "normal in our family."

Respect for Gender-Based Processes

Families' reverence for natural processes and the view that nursing is a normal part of nature was also indicated by the gender-based parenting task allocations that were salient in these families. This style of organization likely eased the transition to parenting by providing parents with shared definitions of their novel tasks, reducing conflicts regarding the creation of novel tasks. Couple function was likely enhanced by parents' clear expectations of one another. Parents' comfort with each one partners' physiologically based and gender specific capacities ensured that infants were nursed by their mothers without interference.

Complementary, Mutual Respect, and Support

Themes of reverence for natural and complementary processes also enriched couple interactions by helping parents actualize personal agendas and biologically based developmental needs. Discussions on maternal development implied that female biologically based processes were admired by mothers and perceived as essential to their development. Similarly, gender-based task allocation in these families enabled fathers to actualize their scripts of support and protection. Each parent was afforded a means of actualizing individual scripts, a task that enhanced self-satisfaction and patience for one's partner and children.

Self realization was accompanied by mutual admiration and respect for the other's unique biological traits associated with parenting. For example, fathers appreciated mothers' exclusive biological capacity to nurse, and mothers lauded paternal support and caregiving behaviors. Parents' sense of fulfilment, mutual respect, and clear definitions of their parenting tasks facilitated the development of a complementary style of interaction. Complementary interchanges enabled both parents to be highly involved in parenting while they engaged in different tasks.

The tutor and learner relationship between parents was another expression of the complementary nature of parents' processes. It is interesting that descriptions of maternal leading are congruent with the sociocultural model of learning (Kruger & Tomasello, 1996; Wertsch, 1985). Mothers modeled their behaviors, and instructed and scaffolded their partners' learning processes in line with the role of tutor in this paradigm. As worthy tutors, mothers transferred their novel conceptualizations about sensitive mothering learned through nursing to their partners, a task facilitated by paternal practices and observations. The pattern of maternal leading facilitated the growth of sensitive parenting styles. One might venture that mothers' apparently enhanced understandings about nursing and similar issues stemmed from the increased time they spent as parents compared to fathers, and the centrality of nursing to female development. In addition, it seemed that mothers' behaviors seemed to correspond to fathers' needs for information. This pattern seems especially relevant considering that fathers refrained from reading material related to nursing and parenting, regardless of their educational background. It is possible that fathers avoided reading due to the prevalence of female voice in the lay literature. However, the resilience of this pattern established prior to birth and the positive way that it was presented, especially by fathers, suggests that families were not interested in altering the present pattern and were comfortable with their roles in this process.

Maternal tutoring resembled fathers' supportive actions and thus might have played another important role in the parents system of mutuality. Just as fathers protected, and emotionally and physically supported nursing when needed, mothers supported fathers' learning processes through tutoring, supportive discussions, and by setting examples of parenting. Thus parents mutually contained one another by incorporating differences, respecting one another's unique talents, and by taking turns facilitating one another's efforts in these families.

The functional nature of complementary interactions between parents was also suggested by the way parents altered their task allocations to fit the changing family constellation. According to the findings, most mothers readily accepted their children's gradual interest in others outside of the nursing unit, and fathers mirrored this by meeting their children's incrementing interest in them as comfort objects. At the same time, parents accepted that mothers remained the central comfort object even after children lovingly engaged with others. Thus the complementary interactions and flexible nature of couple interchanges were conducive to the family theme of meeting children's needs in a child-paced manner. The important implication of this analysis is that parents in nursing families integrated difference into their relationship and used it to meet their common goal of meeting children's needs in a sensitive manner. Thus reverence for physiologically based difference, a concept stemming from parents' respect for natural processes, helped mothers and fathers follow trajectories enhancing their unique qualities, facilitating nursing and the development of sensitivity.

Views of Breasts as Multifaceted Organs

Another important factor associated with families' comfort with natural processes and the unique physiological functions that seemed to help parents facilitate nursing was their regard for the maternal breast as a multifunctional organ. Perspectives of breasts as motherly were exemplified by the practice of nursing freely in different environments and by repeated references to the significance of motherly breasts for females' natural development. Families also referred to the sensual components of nursing and implied that this was normal. Yet despite families' comfort with breasts as sensual mothering objects, most mothers covered their breasts in public settings, suggesting that families also perceived breasts as sexual. Conceptualizations of breasts as sexual was demonstrated further by participant and family narratives that showed that fathers and mothers regarded the female breast as sexual and relevant to their intimate relations, although the exact role that breasts played in the sexual interactions between parents was not clear. Parents' capacity to hold onto views of breasts as multifaceted organs was suggested by data implying that parents' views of the breasts did not interfere with the quality of a couple's sexual life or with their ability to nurse in all contexts.

The duality of breasts from the mothers' perspectives was also suggested by mothers' nursing actions. Although mothers covered their breasts, they did not conceal that they were nursing. These actions suggest that mothers hid the breast partly in compliance with the sexual connotation, but not the breast action associated with sensuality and mothering. The emphasis that many key informants, including mothers, placed on discreet nursing, while at the same time advocating for nursing in all locations also point to the likelihood that mothers accepted that breasts were sexual and mothering at the same time.

Mothers' ability to differentiate between varied roles and to simultaneously hold onto various perspectives of the female breast facilitated a style of nursing that allowed mothers to nurse in tune with natural processes. There appear to be several factors that enabled mothers to feel this way. The finding that mothers of older children were more comfortable with nursing in public than were mothers of infants suggests that maternal conceptualizations of the female breast were influenced by experience. It is interesting that participants spoke about family themes of reverence for natural processes and children's needs when they explained this phenomenon, suggesting that themes were connected and became more salient as mothers gained more experience. Accordingly, mothers became more comfortable with the notion of breast duality and nursing in all locations as they increasingly saw their children's needs as central. Their focus on the child, a central theme in these families, overshadowed other issues, including cultural disdain and individual discomfort. One of the few mothers in the study group who did not conceal her breasts in public illustrates this point. Despite that she came from a religious background emphasizing modesty, she explained that she nursed openly due to her view that her children's needs were her priority, and they were uncomfortable when she concealed her breasts.

Thus reverence for physiology establishes gender-based parenting tasks that ensured that mothers nursed. Similarly, respect for the physiological functions of the breast helped families see breasts as multifaceted organs. This last step helped families feel comfortable that mothers used their breasts for nursing in all contexts, despite culturally based views of breasts as sexual objects.

Reverence for Children's Natural Needs and Cues

Needs are Naturally Occurring Processes

Themes of reverence for natural processes and nursing seemed to predispose parents to accept that infants have naturally occurring needs. Like other naturally occurring processes, children's needs are viewed as valid and respected. This belief explains the finding that parents focused on their children's needs from the onset of parenthood. This emphasis remained a salient facet of parent–child interaction over time. Since nursing was perceived as the natural means of meeting children's needs, it was matched to their needs.

Some parents' experiences in their families of origin affected their focus on children's needs in their present nuclear families. For some, meeting needs fulfilled salient family themes from the past. Other parents came from families of origin with contrasting themes and strived to meet their children's needs in order to repair their own experiences. These behaviors suggest that meeting children's needs is one salient theme with deep psychological meaning extending beyond the here and now. It seems that future research on the intergenerational transmission of themes related to parenting and nursing is warranted and might provide interesting insights into this issue.

Respect for Children's Needs and Cues

A concept that is associated with parents' growing understanding of and respect for children's needs is the idea that young children are able to convey information about their needs to others. This conceptualization commenced with the onset of nursing. The evidence suggests that parents based their interventions on infant cues right from birth. They demonstrated recurring patterns of watching and responding to cues, indicating that parents acknowledged that infants can convey information about their states, and that the information was valid enough to receive a response.

Parents responded to a range of cues from subtle changes in infant movements to more obvious signals, such as signs of distress. The act of responding to cues for nursing provided parents with repeated opportunities to read, interpret, and respond to their children's signals. Repeated cue-based interaction fortified their understanding, strengthened the theme, and enhanced the associated behavioral pattern. Infants and children contributed to this process by validating their parents' efforts through positive feedback when their needs were met. The behaviors infants displayed included signs of calmness or excitement when they were brought to the breast. Infants rarely cried. The lack of crying indicates further that parents were attentive to infants' needs, matched their interventions to the needs appropriately, and infants appreciated their efforts. All of these behaviors contributed to a feedback cycle that seemed to help parents continue using nursing as the means of responding to cues, contributing to the development of sensitive parenting and a responsive family style.

Respect for Frequent Cue-Based Nursing Sessions

The emphasis on nursing in tune with children's needs and the cues signifying these needs explains the frequent nature of nursing observed in the study and also clarifies the tolerance that family members demonstrated towards the ongoing nature of nursing. Furthermore, the frequent nature of nursing perpetuated and perfected behaviors associated with nursing. Frequent nursing sessions provided families with many opportunities to practice and develop the child-based interactional style established through and associated with nursing. Parents of older children were more confident about their capacity to interpret children's needs and were more skilled at answering children's cues. This suggests that practice at cue reading improved the skill. In circular fashion, cue-based nursing contributed to frequent nursing sessions and further enhanced parents' capacity to interact with and understand their children in an attuned manner.

Nursing is an Encompassing Experience

The interconnected nature of family themes is demonstrated further by the emergence of the salient family view that nursing is an encompassing experience. This acknowledgement stemmed from the reverence for physiological processes and respect for the naturally occurring cues associated with nursing. The frequent cue-based nursing sessions took place in response to diverse cues and in different situations, implying that nursing was viewed as a means of meeting a variety of children's needs. Nursing was regulated by children's signals, and children appeared content when their cues were answered. This behavior suggests that infants and children likely regarded nursing as a multifaceted experience. Similarly, parents responded to most children's cues with nursing, indicating that they accepted and shared their children's perspective of nursing as an encompassing behavior. Thus the theme of nursing as encompassing contributed to parents and children's relationships by providing them with opportunities to develop a sense of shared meaning. Joint ownership of nursing as encompassing sustained the system further by enhancing parents' capacity to accept nursing without regard for time, frequency, or amount of breastmilk, and perpetuated the nursing cycle. Views of nursing as encompassing further verified families' tolerance for ongoing nursing sessions.

Views of nursing as encompassing were also demonstrated by the pattern of responding with nursing to a wide range of cues, often without always defining the exact need. On one hand, this behavior suggests that parents seemed more concerned with answering signals than understanding the actual meaning of each signal and the underlying need, possibly pointing to insensitivity on the part of the parents. On the other hand, this behavior indicates that parents trusted the physiologically based behavior of nursing to fulfil their ultimate goal of meeting children's needs.

Nursing is an Emotional Experience

The theme of nursing as an encompassing behavior concurred with and also facilitated the development of the theme that nursing is an emotional experience. The theme of nursing as an emotional experience had meaning on two planes. On one level, families noticed and spoke about the emotional aspects of nursing. On another level, the emotionality was something experienced, affecting behavior that was not necessarily expressed by families, but was obvious to an observer. The complex emotions associated with nursing and the implications of the emotional impact of nursing on development reinforced other themes that veered from the prominent cultural view that nursing is mainly a means of feeding. Thus this theme implied that nursing was a behavior that evoked emotions and was also affected by feelings. The quality of the emotionality of nursing affected the developmental trajectory of other associated behaviors, especially sensitivity.

Themes Develop over Time

The intense feelings that accompanied parents' descriptions of early nursing sessions imply that nursing induced an emotional reaction immediately. Body language and interaction during early nursing sessions confirm that a deep emotional relationship was established early on in the nursing relationship. The emotional component of nursing increased over time and was exemplified by changes in parental narratives. For example, even though parents, especially first time parents, referred to the emotionality of nursing in their narratives, they also frequently referred to latching (the physical attachment to the breast), hunger, and their children's physical status. While some of these issues appeared in the narratives of parents with older children, they were far less central than parents' references to the emotional aspects of the nursing experience. The change in the centrality of emotions in parental narratives and their increased capacity to understand the role of nursing as a comforting behavior suggest that the experience of nursing contributed to the attitude that nursing is an emotional experience and also a function of the impact of nursing on parents' emotions. This increased understanding suggests this theme also contributed to parents' tolerance for ongoing nursing sessions and nursing into early childhood.

Shared Meaning

The shared efforts family members made to fix and reinstate nursing, and the loss that they felt when this was not successful, was testament to the shared ownership of nursing as an emotional experience. Point in case are the efforts that adoptive families made to induce and sustain nursing, even when mothers did not apparently have sufficient breastmilk to sustain infants. Although family members often implied that they maintained nursing for physiological reasons, in-depth analysis of their narratives showed that they repeatedly referred to feelings. Family members' emotional experiences varied and reflected personal experiences with nursing. These varied emotional experiences contributed to the shared meaning of nursing as an emotional experience.

Nursing as an Emotional Experience for Children

Comfort and Love

The emotional relevance of nursing for children was suggested by the way that they were comforted through nursing. Infants turned to the breast frequently without apparent regard for their state of satiety. The likelihood that infants felt warm feelings towards the breast was also suggested by the way they touched, played, smiled at the breast, and displayed overall feelings of positive regard and relaxation when they nursed. Older nurslings who ate full diets and nursed frequently, spoke lovingly about nursing and created names for the breast that often had relational connotations that reinforced the view that children loved the nursing breast and saw it as far more than a feeding object. The likelihood that children felt deep emotional feelings for the breast and nursing, clarify further the frequent nature of nursing noted repeatedly. It was also quite compelling that some children continued to touch their mothers' breasts and to talk about nursing after weaning. The remnants of nursing in children's interactions with their mothers and others also point to the emotionality of nursing.

Emotionality of Nursing for Siblings

Recognize Siblings Needs for Comfort through Nursing

Further evidence attesting to the existence of the theme of nursing as an emotional experience in these families was suggested by children's recognition and acceptance of the emotional bond between their mothers and nursing siblings. This acknowledgement associated their view of nursing as an encompassing behavior was apparent in their descriptions of nursing and their behaviors towards the nursing mother and child. Descriptions of older siblings prompting mothers to nurse when they perceived that siblings required calming, illustrated their views of nursing as a comforting experience. The capacity of older children to withstand temporary exclusion from deep sensual and sensitive exchanges between nursing units points to their understanding of the meaning of nursing for their siblings. This understanding was likely enhanced by their own sense of being emotionally filled up from their own previous nursing relationships and from the attention that they continued to receive in between nursing. These feelings in combination with their growing experience of observing, and discussing sensitive interactions, helped them assist the family take steps to ensure the continuation of the nursing relationship. The experience of nursing contributed to their understanding of and tolerance for nursing as an experience encompassing many facets including emotional comfort.

Adoration over Time

Another indication of the emotional implications of nursing for children is the fervor that they displayed when they talked about nursing. This quality is apparent even in young children and in their narratives of love for the nursing breast and nursing. It is as if they had a love affair with the nursing object. The emotions that nursing evoked for older children were apparent in their narrative of admiration for breastfeeding and pride that their younger siblings were nursing. The way that older and former nursing children defended nursing and replicated this behavior with their children also attests to the strong emotional impact of nursing on children over time.

Nursing as an Emotional Experience for Mothers

The theme of nursing as an emotional experience was also evident for mothers. They acknowledged the emotionality of nursing for their infants and responded with nursing frequently. Nursing was also an emotional experience for them, affecting their development and feelings about themselves as women and as mothers.

Self-Efficacy and Sensitivity

The impact of emotions associated with nursing on mothers was suggested by the contribution of feelings of efficacy through nursing and sensitivity to infant cues. Mothers internalized a sense of efficacy and confidence through their cue-based interactions with nursing infants, and this prompted a cycle of continued cue reading, positive feedback, positive self-regard, and increased sensitivity. The impact of emotions internalized through and associated with nursing on maternal sensitivity is suggested further by comparing these mothers with their counterparts who felt deficient in their ability to understand their infants' cues through nursing and intermittently ignored cues and missed opportunities to nurse, perpetuating the negative cycle. Accordingly, when mothers internalized good enough feelings about themselves through the experience of nursing, they were able to partake in additional experiences that increased good enough feelings further.

Experience Female Processes

Maternal positive self-regard was also increased through nursing due to mothers' perception that nursing provided them with the opportunity to actualize celebrated and essential aspects of female development, a concept consistent with themes of reverence for natural processes. Mothers who forfeited promising careers outside of the home to become fully immersed in their nursing children exemplified the efforts that mothers made to experience nursing and mothering to the fullest. The finding that many women altered their career plans only after becoming nursing mothers shows the emotional impact of nursing on mothers' development. For some women, nursing remained a central component of their sense of self over time. This phenomenon was illustrated by women who continued their involvement with nursing beyond mothering through academia, volunteer work, and social activism, and as professionals in fields related to lactation. Thus it appears that mothers perceived that nursing enriched their sense of self by allowing them to partake in an essential and revered growth-enhancing experience, and the positive feelings that arose from this augmented their capacity to mother.

Repair and Healing

Similarly, nursing contributed to mothers' good enough feelings about themselves due to perceptions that nursing was a healing experience compensating for processes that decreased their sense of self as women. Nursing seemed to play a special role in correcting mothers' feelings of deficiency when their sense of self as a female had been disturbed by infertility, disfiguring surgery, disappointing birthing experiences, the birth of unhealthy children, and prior negative nursing experiences. Nursing seemed to provide mothers with the sense that they were "back on track" and "in tune with" the natural rhythm that was an integral aspect of their personal scripts and family reverence for normal physiological processes. Thus it seems that the feeling of normalcy associated with nursing enriched mothers' positive feelings about themselves, contributing to their capacity to understand and respond patiently to their children.

Frequent Nursing Sessions and Sensitivity

There are specific aspects of the nursing relationship that helped mothers internalize positive self-regard and affect. The frequency of nursing enabled mothers to experience good enough feelings in a recurring fashion. Mothers' sense of competence was also enhanced by the ample opportunities to refine their skills and also to receive affirmation from their infants, perpetuating the cycle of competence and sensitive cue-reading.

Exclusivity

The exclusivity of early physiologically based nursing and of later nursing sessions also contributed to mothers' perceptions of nursing as a positive emotional experience. The intense emotional meaning of exclusivity explains why mothers cherished this aspect of nursing and suffered immensely when it was interrupted. The emotional component of exclusive nursing clarifies the anger and disappointment that mothers demonstrated when their efforts to nurse exclusively in early infancy were disturbed. The emotionality of exclusivity also clarifies maternal disdain for artificial feeding, their refusal to bottle feed, and in most cases, their rejection of artificial soothing objects. One might propose that mothers felt disappointed, since interrupting nursing was perceived as a deviation from the natural physiological processes that they adored and that were central to their personal scripts. This perspective implies that when exclusive nursing was obstructed mothers felt robbed of the biological connection, the sense of physiological interdependence, and the opportunity to establish and maintain physiologically based nursing patterns. While these factors were likely important to mothers, it also appears that mothers cherished exclusivity due to their perception that this allowed them to engage in unique and close emotional interactions with their offspring. Mothers who attempted to sustain exclusive functions, even when low milk supplies or other physiological deficits challenged their capacity to nurse in an exclusive manner, reinforced the importance of aspects besides physiology for mothers.

Special and Irreplaceable

The emotional aspects of exclusivity were also apparent in maternal perceptions that nursing provided them with a sense that they were special and irreplaceable, and this advanced their capacity to mother. The significance of feeling special was most poignantly demonstrated by the efforts adoptive mothers made to nurse, even when they were unable to physically produce enough breastmilk. Mothers felt that nursing, especially the emotional interchanges associated with nursing, was something that only they could give to their children, and this increased their attachment to the infant. Mothers' desire to feel special in relation to their children clarifies why some mothers had difficulty letting go of their central role as comfort figures when their children grew older.

The sense of being special acted as a form of compensation, reinforcing the proposal that nursing was perceived as a reparative experience by some mothers. This point was relative for mothers with perceived negative birthing experiences, infertility, and in cases of adoption. In cases of adoption, feeling special helped mothers make up for their perceived loss of a symbiotic state inherent to pregnancy and increased their attachment to their infants. Thus exclusivity through nursing helped mothers feel special and functional, making up for perceived dysfunction in other areas.

Additional aspects of exclusivity cherished by mothers included the intense and physical nature of nursing. Maternal passion that was evident in their narratives demonstrated that they were passionate about the intimacy and sensuality of nursing. Mothers seemed to be able to tolerate sensuality since they associated it with the intimacy of nursing, a perceived positive aspect of the nursing relationship. Intimacy also seemed to advance maternal affinity towards their infants, maintaining the cycle of frequent nursing, cue-based mothering, and the cluster of emotions that advanced the interchanges further.

Frustration, Deviation, Reduced Sensitivity

Since maternal appreciation of exclusivity appeared to be central to nursing mothers' scripts, findings that some mothers periodically deviated from this behavior were perplexing. The use of artificial soothing, including fingers, pacifiers, or infant swings exemplified the deviation in this group. Firstly, the rarity of the use of these objects strengthened the notion that nursing exclusivity was important for this population. The anger, frustration, or embarrassment expressed by a few mothers who had periodically used in the past or who continued to use artificial means of soothing their infants reinforced the irregularity of these acts and the ambivalence that it caused for mothers.

It seems that some mothers were most likely to veer from normal nursing behaviors when they were pressured to do so by the father. The impact of paternal pressure on nursing was most evident when couples experienced dissension, illustrating the influence of systemic function on mother–infant exclusivity. Yet some mothers remained fully committed to exclusive nursing and other physiological process, including nursing into early childhood, despite immense pressure from partners. The second group of mothers appeased their partners through compensatory measures, such as sexual intimacy, showing the impact of interactions at the couple level on maternal nursing behaviors. The most salient factor that seemed to enable mothers to withstand paternal pressure was their commitment to the prevalent family themes of reverence for physiology, meeting infants' needs before all others, and a view that nursing was a multifaceted behavior that was central to optimal child development.

Ambivalence

The emotionality of nursing was also evident in the ambivalent feelings that arose for some mothers due to the intensity of the nursing relationship, including the impact this had on their lifestyle. The evidence suggests ambivalence about lifestyle changes was resolved easily when mothers focused on the welfare of the child and the positive feelings that arose from meeting the offspring's needs. Most mothers seemed to feel comfortable with and proud of the lifestyle associated with nursing, reinforcing that meeting children's needs was a significant theme for these mothers.

A more salient and complex form of ambiguity in this population indicates that some mothers had difficulties coping with feelings of being "stirred up" (Weininger, 1999) by their infants. New mothers in particular felt confused by their overwhelming desire to be close to their infants and to meet their babies' needs at all times. At the same time, mothers felt pressured to periodically separate from their children, a feeling reflecting the influence of culturally predominant concepts of distancing. The capacity of mothers with extensive nursing experience to ignore cultural messages better than their less experienced counterparts reinforced the circularity of the mothering experience through nursing. Like in other areas of mothering, it seems that the experience of nursing caused mothers to change their priorities and focus on the child above all else in an increasing fashion, decreasing maternal ambivalence. This evidence reinforces again the importance of meeting children's needs from the mothers' perspective and their capacity to develop attuned mothering styles. It seems that the good enough feelings mothers internalized about themselves when they believed that they had fulfilled that goal enabled them to overcome most obstacles.

Thus it seems that the theme of nursing as an emotional experience was very relevant for maternal development through nursing. Many of the emotions triggered by and associated with nursing affected maternal function beyond breastfeeding. In this regard, mothers shared their children's meaning of nursing, contributing to the interchanges between mothers and children.

Nursing as an Emotional Experience for Fathers

There are many indications that fathers not only understood that nursing was an emotional relationship for mothers and nursing children, but that they were also affected by the emotionality of nursing. While reverence for physiology likely contributed to their supportive and protective actions, the efforts they made to ensure nursing exclusivity during infancy, and unique and intimate exchanges in later nursing exchanges, and their references to the relational aspects of nursing, suggested that they sensed the same emotionality experienced by mothers and children. The feelings that arose in them regarding nursing affected their capacity to fulfil their unique tasks and, by the same token, their interactions with nursing evoked deep emotions for them.

Shared Ownership of Exclusivity

The intense emotional involvement of fathers in nursing was demonstrated by their fervent opposition to feeding their young infants. The tone and words that fathers used to describe paternal feeding, including pathological and a break in physiology, demonstrated their ownership of and investment in a physiologically based nursing pattern. The emotionality of nursing for fathers was suggested further by the sorrow displayed by fathers who had intermittently fed their infants as a last resort to sustain infants during perceived periods of severe infant, maternal, or nursing deficiencies. The distress that fathers felt when they were forced to feed their children due to the aforementioned conditions matched their partners' frustration. Paternal narratives indicating that feeding during crisis periods did not endear fathers and children to one another contrasted with the feelings attached to preserving physiological nursing, protecting their nurslings and their partners, the mothers. The association between positive emotions and fulfilling tasks ensuring physiology and negative feelings under contrasting conditions was demonstrated further by the finding that paternal feeding was associated with couple tension. One might suggest that this tension stemmed from shared distress over the situation or that paternal feeding signified existing pathology in the system.

Tolerance of Maternal Centrality, Intimate and Sensual Nursing Interactions

Fathers' understanding and sharing of the emotional meaning of the nursing relationship was suggested by their tolerance of maternal centrality. Emotional investment in nursing was suggested by their ability to tolerate that their infants initially saw them as secondary comfort objects, while at the same time they longed for closeness with their infants. Their capacity to withstand the intimate and sensual interludes in a culture where sensual maternal-infant interactions are not the norm was remarkable. Granted reverence for natural processes and children's naturally occurring needs and views of nursing as encompassing likely helped them prioritize meeting infants' needs over other concerns. Yet the analysis of paternal narrative implies that their support stemmed from deep emotions symbolized by their statements pointing to an underlying belief that children required intimacy just as much as they needed food. This shared understanding of the meaning of nursing was clearly an emotional one that matched children's and mothers' perspectives.

Validation and Sensitivity

Fathers' behaviors were not only guided by benevolence, but also by the contribution of nursing to their emotional agendas. Like mothers, paternal capacity for attuned parenting was increased when they felt fulfilled emotionally, and several of the tasks associated with nursing enabled them to have this experience. Paternal need for validation was demonstrated by their jubilant reactions to mothers' stories about their accomplishment and their increased sensitivity after receiving positive feedback from their children. It seems that the good feelings that fathers internalized when they were lauded contributed to their capacity to support nursing in a sensitive manner and to withstand a temporary secondary stance in relation to their children. In others words, protecting the physiologically based nursing relationship made fathers feel good about themselves.

Protection and Sense of Efficacy

Specific issues affected fathers' sense of self and their capacity to support nursing. It is important to remember the centrality of protection in paternal scripts. Interactions with the nursing sub-system enabled fathers to actualize themes of protection. Fathers' need to protect their families contributed to their capacity to uphold themes of reverence for nature that they shared with mothers. Fathers' associated natural processes with health and felt fulfilled when they perceived that they contributed to children's health by protecting nursing. Paternal need to feel efficient at protecting health was actualized when they initiated and established nursing, repaired perceived damaged nursing relationships, and supported nursing exclusivity. Again one notes that the emotional impact of nursing was associated with additional themes, and in this regard, specifically reverence for nature.

The likelihood that a sense of efficiency affected fathering and that fathers internalized confident feelings through nursing was also evident in findings that fathers saw their tasks as highly significant. This perception contributed to fathers' capacity to accept their apparent exclusion from the special nursing relationship. It seems that fathers' perceptions of themselves as important guardians of the nursing relationship and as significant caregivers served as compensation for their apparent exclusion. Fathers' sense of importance was also suggested by the way that fathers, including those who worked full time, increased their involvement in parenting over time. As fathers remained involved, they were provided with additional opportunities to internalize good feelings about themselves as supporters and protectors of the nursing sub-system.

Ambivalence

The strong influence of interactions associated with nursing on fathers' emotional well-being was also suggested by the ambivalence that some fathers felt. Evidence showing that otherwise supportive fathers sometimes interfered with nursing illustrates this. Feelings of ambiguity were not consistent for all fathers, or even for the same fathers with different children. Nevertheless, several similar and relevant themes seemed to trigger ambiguity for fathers. Paternal ambivalence was most prevalent during moments of heightened family stress when fathers lost sight momentarily of their cognitive-based notions and family themes. At these times, fathers' personal issues were triggered, including reverence for sole time, preoccupation with apparent independence, and regard for couple precedence over child centrality. The similarity between these themes and salient cultural views negating nursing implies that some fathers were most vulnerable to cultural perceptions when they perceived that excessive demands were being made of them or their partners. The fathers most influenced by cultural themes were those who were ambivalent about the encompassing nature of nursing, pointing to the importance of this theme for sustaining physiologically based nursing patterns. Accordingly, fathers who were genuinely invested in protecting emotional and physiological processes were most likely to be safeguarded from the influence of cultural themes during crisis periods.

Guilt, Helplessness, and Reduced Sensitivity

Descriptions of the anxious and demanding behaviors displayed by fathers who perceived that their partners had suffered excessively during birth exemplified how fathers' stressful feelings impacted their capacity to support nursing. While interactions associated with nursing generated strong feelings of efficiency, strength, and the ability to guard and protect, they could also evoke feelings of helplessness that paralyzed fathers emotionally, reducing their self-esteem and capacity to support nursing. This situation is poignantly suggested by the behaviors displayed by fathers who perceived that their partners had suffered excessively during birth and who were unable to tolerate nursing difficulties. It is important to remember that during this early transition period after birth, these fathers seemed to focus more on their partner's welfare than on their infants or anything else, including the nursing relationship. Their desire to alleviate maternal pain came before anything else and interfered with nursing. Their excessive demands for immediate pain relief for their partners, suggested that they felt a strong need to fix their partners' condition. The association between the desire to repair and guilt (Klein, 1998) implies that some fathers likely experienced guilt. The urgency of their demands and other anxious behaviors suggests that perhaps they felt responsible for the pain their partners endured and needed to make amends. One might wonder if fathers felt bad about the role they played in conception, the creation of the pregnancy, and the consequential apparently difficult birth. The resulting guilt was exacerbated when mothers experienced difficulties or frustrations associated with nursing. One might offer that nursing was at this point perceived as a bad and hurtful object, something to avoid. Thus they demanded immediate solutions for perceived nursing problems, often without regard for the harmful effects of their actions. It seems that fathers demanded supplemental bottles and other forms of interference in order to temporarily relieve their own anxiety.

The association between paternal anxiety and a sense of helplessness explains why fathers reduced their support and ignored cues for nursing when they perceived that they were unable to resolve maternal distress. Again helplessness is the opposite of feelings of protection and efficiency that were central to fathers' scripts. The fortitude of these themes for fathers was also suggested by the extreme frustration some fathers experienced when they were unable to comfort their children. Fathers' apparent grief in the absence of tangible solutions explains why some fathers impelled their partners to discard nursing and replace it with apparently practical artificial feeding practices during times of crisis. These examples suggest that some of the erratic behaviors that fathers displayed were attempts at reinstating their protective roles and feelings of competence, ridding themselves of emotional turmoil. These behaviors reinforce that the experience of nursing was an emotional affair for fathers.

Envy, Unresolved Envy, and Reduced Sensitivity

The complex nature of paternal emotionality, anxiety, and nursing is poignantly suggested by the existence of paternal envy. The finding that father's longing to experience the same closeness that mothers had with their infants was more common than the desire to experience the same closeness with their spouses that infants felt, points to fathers' deep understanding of the emotionality of nursing. This feeling, in combination with the general disdain for methods of artificial feeding and the negative connotation of paternal feeding, implied that fathers recognized their inability to replace mothers and experience the desired emotions.

It is also important to remember that fathers' subsequent capacity to support nursing was contingent on the way envy was resolved in the family. This important conclusion reinforces that envy was not the emotional culprit interfering with nursing, rather the factor determining paternal function was the capacity of fathers to find a means of resolving envy. The inability to resolve envious feelings culminates in contemptuous actions (Klein, 1997b). In keeping with this theory, incidences of paternal insistence on pacifiers, supplemental bottles, adult rather than child-led processes of independence, pressure for early weaning, and other distancing processes may be explained as contemptuous expressions signifying unresolved envy of the closeness inherent in nursing. This seems especially true when one recalls that some fathers displayed harmful actions despite apparently well-founded cognitive bases for nursing.

The negative impact of unresolved envy on paternal function in nursing systems points to the importance of outlets for fathers' envious feelings as a means of enriching both paternal support and the nursing relationship. This suggestion explains that beyond paternal understanding of children's needs, fathers treasured tactile interactions. By engaging in tactile interchanges and proximity behaviors, fathers were able to replicate the physical closeness of nursing. The idea of imitating maternal tasks associated with maternal-child interaction concurs with the underlying premise of theories that promote paternal feeding. However, the emphasis on tactile interactions, rather than on actual feeding, takes into account the physiology of nursing and the unique tasks of the nursing unit, again pointing to the significance of interdependent themes. In addition, using touch as the compensatory interactional element rather than feeding differs from the cultural perspective of nursing as feeding and reflects the reality of nursing to a far greater degree. An analysis of paternal narratives where fathers emphasized tactile interchanges with their infants reinforces that fathers enriched their sense of self and resolved frustration when they emulated the tactile and proximity aspects of nursing in their interchanges with their infants. Through touch and closeness, fathers not only acknowledged and accepted the sensuality of nursing that they longed to experience, but by doing so, they repaired some of their damaged feelings.

Along with experiencing the physical closeness of nursing, the reverberating effects of paternal support and caregiving tasks also seemed to help fathers integrate their envious feelings constructively. The compensatory and reparative features of these behaviors seemed to mitigate envious feelings and reframe them. This relates to the earlier discussion on the way nursing increased paternal self-regard and suggests that when fathers felt good enough about their roles, they were able to cope with envious feelings.

The process of resolving envy was also advanced when fathers openly discussed their feelings and came to accept them as normal. Yet paternal disclosure was associated with the type of envy that fathers experienced. It seemed that fathers talked openly about their desire for closeness to their infant and were less open about envious feelings towards their infants and longing for sole interactions with their spouses. The finding that fathers were less likely to disclose that they longed to replace their infants is interesting, considering that couple precedence is valued in western culture. This difference implies that concepts other than couple precedence had more credence in these families. This is likely considering the significance of child-centered themes for this group. Thus the desire to replace the infant might have been perceived as shameful, and it is plausible that fathers hid this feeling. This implies that, in this population, the resolution of fathers' envy of the infants' position was more difficult to resolve than paternal envy of mothers' close relationship with the infant.

The significance of open discourse for the resolution of envy indicates that the process was also contingent on the quality of systemic interaction. This was pointed out by examples of fathers who were not fortunate enough to be part of open communication systems and who continued to obstruct physiologically based nursing relationships. One might venture that the finding that some mothers forfeited exclusivity, as was described earlier in the section on mothers, was a manifestation of this unresolved process and that some mothers gave up nursing-friendly behaviors in an apparent effort to appease their partners' unspoken envious feelings. In contrast, mothers' acceptance of fathers' feelings, open discourse, and compensatory measures in the couple sub-unit, played an important role in facilitating the integration, as well as the reframing of otherwise difficult feelings.

Thus envy was not a threatening force in nursing families. Instead, the culprit was unresolved envy. Moreover, paternal yearning for closeness might have also played an important role in augmenting paternal understanding of the unique nursing experience and provided fathers with further impetus to support nursing. Paternal comprehension of mothers' and babies' needs for closeness, albeit from a different point of entry, facilitated the shared ownership of nursing and mutual desire for successful physiologically based nursing relationships. From this perspective, the strong desire to be close to an infant was not negative and instead contributed to fathers' participation in nursing as a shared family experience.

The Emotionality of Nursing for Siblings

Further evidence attesting to the existence of the theme of nursing as an emotional experience in these families was suggested by children's recognition and acceptance of the emotional bond between their mothers and nursing siblings. This acknowledgement associated with their view of nursing as an encompassing behavior was apparent in their descriptions of nursing and their behaviors towards the nursing mother and child. Descriptions of older siblings prompting mothers to nurse when they perceived that siblings required calming illustrated their views of nursing as a comforting experience. The capacity of older children to withstand temporary exclusion from deep sensual and sensitive exchanges between nursing units points to their understanding of the meaning of nursing for their siblings. This understanding was likely enhanced by their own sense of being emotionally filled up enough from their own previous nursing relationships and from the attention that they continued to receive in between nursing. These feelings, in combination with their growing experience of observing and discussing sensitive interactions, helped them assist the family take steps to ensure the continuation of the nursing relationship. The experience of nursing contributed to their understanding of and tolerance for nursing as an experience encompassing many facets, including emotional comfort.

Another indication of the emotional implications of nursing for children is the fervor they displayed when they talked about nursing. This quality was apparent even in young children and in their narratives of love for the nursing breast and nursing. It is as if they had a love affair with the nursing object. The emotions that nursing evoked for older children were apparent in their narrative of admiration for breastfeeding and pride that their younger siblings were nursing. The way that older and former nursing children defended nursing and replicated this behavior with their children also attests to the strong emotional impact of nursing on children over time.

Summary of Nursing as an Emotional Experience

A strong theme in families displaying physiologically based nursing patterns is that nursing is an emotional event. This theme is actualized in demonstrated understanding of the significance of nursing for the breastfeeding sub-unit. In addition, the prevalence of the theme of nursing as emotional was suggested by the impact of nursing on all family members' scripts. Parents and children's emotional scripts affected nursing and, by the same token, the nursing relationships influenced their feelings.

Themes Interfering with Physiologically Based Nursing and Sensitivity

The significance of themes facilitating physiologically based nursing and associated sensitivity were demonstrated further by the impact of contradicting themes. These attitudes and behavior negated the meaning that nursing had for parents and interfered with the implementation of cue-based nursing. Not only did negating themes interfere with nursing, they also reduced parents sensitivity to cues, reinforcing the contribution of interactions associated with physiological nursing patterns to the development of parental and family sensitivity.

Views of Nursing as Feeding

Feeding, Missed Cues, Broken Continuum, Decreased Sensitivity

It appears that veering, even occasionally, from the perspective that nursing is an encompassing relationship impeded parents' cue reading capacities and children's experiences of being heard. The view that nursing is feeding was a common view negating the concept of nursing as encompassing. Even periodic disregard for nursing as an encompassing behavior impacted the everyday interactions associated with nursing. Misnaming nursing as feeding was associated with missed cues for nursing. Even though some parents revered physiological processes like other parents in the population, the act of naming nursing as feeding seemed to impair their view of physiology. They focused on digestive functions and implied that they saw the central role of nursing as a way to relinquish hunger. According to this perception, once this task was completed, babies' cues for additional nursing were ignored under the premise that the infant must be satisfied as he/she had already "been fed." This view was especially relevant for parents who also disregarded the emotionality of nursing. Parents' misconstrued images of nursing as a means of feeding explains the periodic use of pacifiers, baby swings, and cribs that were otherwise extremely rare in this sample population.

Observations of families with older children suggest that intermittent pauses in cue mirroring associated with nursing have long term implications. This was illustrated in the study by parents who used the term feeding to name nursing with younger nurslings and also who periodically neglected their older children's signals. This suggests that parents' practices of misnaming children's cues for nursing in infancy impaired their capacity to fully understand their children. It seems that reduced cue reading capacity in infancy impaired their ability to share meaning in future parenting endeavors.

It is interesting that discarding infant and child cues was not always associated with early weaning, and in some cases of decreased sensitivity, parents continued to foster nursing into early childhood. A family in the study who intermittently discarded cues for nursing named as feeding and demonstrated periodic insensitivity to their older child's signals, but who had also allowed their older child to nurse for a few years, exemplified the interesting contradiction. An analysis of this and similar situations demonstrate that although the parents intermittently refuted the multiple physical and emotional aspects of nursing, they accepted that nursing was physiologically essential for children's development over time, and this helped them foster nursing beyond infancy. Thus periodic disregard for nursing as an encompassing relationship might not impair all parents' ability to tolerate nursing beyond infancy in the same way that it obstructs nursing on a daily basis. However, this assertion is made with caution since views of nursing as a means of feeding are also associated with the use of use of objects such as pacifiers that obstruct normal nursing patterns.

Paternal Envy and Misconstrued Themes

Views of nursing as a feeding behavior rather than as an encompassing experience interfered with some parents' ability to support physiologically based nursing patterns over time. Not surprisingly, this pattern was displayed most frequently by fathers who claimed that nursing was a mere feeding behavior void of emotionality and that older children should wean when it was believed that they no longer required nutrition from nursing. Yet it is important to note the significance of unresolved envy in this script - many of the fathers who refuted the emotionality of nursing also displayed behaviors suggesting that they not only acknowledged the special emotional closeness associated with nursing, but they also desired it.

Reverence for Cultural Themes

Questions arise regarding the reasons, other than unresolved paternal envy, that prompted families usually committed to nursing in tune with physiology to intermittently stray. First of all, referring to nursing as feeding means that they had not fully internalized the encompassing qualities of nursing. Second, the view of nursing as a mere feeding behavior is consistent with salient cultural precepts of nursing, suggesting that the families in question were influenced by cultural views. The findings that some families acted in this manner point to the strength of these messages, particularly in light of the family themes that otherwise resound in these systems.

It seems that perceived crisis periods, personal issues such as views of autonomy, independence, envy, and low self-regard tended to render parents more open to cultural influence and views of nursing as feeding. Inexperience with parenting a nursing child, frustration with the demands of parenting, misconceptions about normal infant development, and flawed views of nursing reflecting previous scripts of this behavior, may have also periodically impaired families' views of nursing as encompassing. Interestingly, the last item seemed to be especially true for parents who were healthcare providers, a finding reflecting the predominant view of nursing as merely a means of feeding in the healthcare system. Some of these misconceptions changed with parenting experience and additional knowledge. It seems that it was easier for parents to change cognitively based and incompatible views than it was to remedy views stemming from relational issues.

Fathers were more vulnerable to cultural views of nursing as a means of feeding than mothers were. The discussion on the impact of crisis on fathers in an earlier chapter is one explanation for this discrepancy. In addition, the distinction might have stemmed from parents' discrepant tasks and roles in nursing systems, the different meaning that nursing has for parents' diverse developmental trajectories, and fathers' feelings about the nursing relationship. Fathers' vulnerability to cultural messages negating views of nursing as encompassing were also more prevalent in cases where fathers felt overwhelmed, there was couple strife, and there was unresolved paternal ambivalence.

The finding that unresolved paternal ambivalence impacted conceptualizations of nursing reinforces the concept, discussed in the section on couples, that there was an association between family relationships and nursing behaviors. Similarly, decreased sensitivity to the needs of the nursing child signified unresolved issues at the couple level. This point is illustrated by one of the few families in the case study group that intermittently referred to nursing as feeding, used pacifying tools, and also suffered from couple strife. One might venture that families that coped with internal discord might not have had the emotional strength to internalize novel views, especially when they differed from former scripts or extraneous influences.

Implications of Missed Cues for Nursing for Sensitivity

The behaviors exhibited by parents who intermittently missed cues for nursing suggest that veering from family themes promoting physiological nursing interfered with cue reading for nursing. These parents seemed to have decreased capacity for sensitivity to cues outside of nursing. This pattern reinforces that there is an association between themes and parenting behaviors facilitating physiologically based nursing and the development of sensitive parenting and family styles.

Insensitivity to Cues for Nursing and Siblings

Data suggest that insensitivity to nursing cues may also contribute to conflict between siblings. Earlier it was mentioned that missed cues during nursing seemed to impair parents' capacity to fully understand their children. Consequently, these children experienced intermittent periods of insensitive interactions with their parents. Since attuned responses help children develop positive relational capacities, one might suspect that children with contrasting experiences will express less empathy towards others. One might also propose, therefore, that the transfer of views of nursing as food to older children likely decreased their patience towards ongoing nursing sessions and their lack of sole time with their nursing mothers. Thus views of nursing as food rather than as an encompassing experience might also contribute to discord and rivalry between siblings.

Summary of Themes Supporting the Development of Sensitive Interaction through Physiologically Based Nursing

Reverence for physiology, children, and related behaviors are associated with themes of respect for children's naturally occurring needs and signals, facilitating the development of a cue-based nursing cycle. Consequently, families allowed infants to nurse frequently, helping to establish notions of nursing as an encompassing experience inclusive of several physical and emotional functions. The emotional experience of nursing was evident at all levels of the system. Nursing affected and was influenced by family members' emotional responses. These themes reverberated back to the nursing subsystem and reinforced the practice of cue-based nursing interactions, leading to frequent nursing. Frequent nursing sessions provided parents and children with ample opportunities to fortify themes and practice sensitive interchanges. Veering from salient themes interfered with the establishment of cue-based nursing sessions and subsequently affected the development of sensitivity through breastfeeding. Deviance from physiologically based nursing patterns in families decreeing their desire to nurse indicates that underlying issues likely impaired their ability to fully actualize facilitative themes. Families able to sustain themes internalized sensitive interactions and extended sensitive parenting to areas associated with and outside of nursing.

Extension of Themes Promoting Sensitivity beyond Nursing

Many of the interconnected themes associated with physiologically based nursing extended beyond nursing and evolved to reflect family development. When families internalized themes and practiced behaviors associated with physiology, and acknowledged and implemented nursing as an encompassing experience with emotional facets, they simultaneously internalized tools facilitating sensitive interactions with the nursing child. This factor contributed to family members' capacity to tolerate the frequency of nursing, and this provided more opportunities to practice cue-based interactions with the nursling. Family members' experiences contributed to the development of a sensitive interactional style. Each person's process was unique. Simultaneous internalization processes helped family members reinforce one another's growth.

Families' views and behavioral patterns associated with nursing were transferred to interactions in between nursing. Child-focused nursing patterns were mirrored when parents accepted and supported their children's different rates of development and their unique needs and traits. Parents followed their children's unique rhythms by continuing the patterns of responding to children's needs and signals in between nursing. Thus cue-based nursing relationships laid the foundation for child-led and sensitive communicative patterns in the family.

Sensitivity to Children's Needs for Proximity

Reverence for closeness is a salient family theme as suggested by descriptions of babies who were worn, held, carried, and slept with in between nursing. The central proximity figure was the mother, although in contrast to nursing, several proximity functions were intermittently and increasingly shared by other family members. This behavior implies that families were not only able to tolerate ongoing nursing, but that they were also able to accept that infants remained close to others, especially their mothers.

Families' attitudes towards nursing and perspectives of proximity evolved simultaneously, implying that these trajectories were related. Furthermore, evidence that families did not seem to consider physical closeness as a priority prior to parenting suggests that like with nursing, this internalization stemmed from parents' experience. The likelihood that parents' scripts of closeness developed as they practiced nursing behaviors is suggested by findings that comfort with co-sleeping evolved over time.

Parents' growing consideration for closeness resembled processes associated with nursing. First of all, similar to the way that they nursed, children regulated the degree of closeness to their mothers and to others through cues. Parents' attunement to children's cues for touch and closeness resembled patterns associated with nursing, verifying the influence of interactions associated with nursing on other behaviors.

The data also point to other similarities between processes associated with nursing and proximity behaviors. Since reverence for children's needs for physical closeness stemmed from and was reinforced by parents' sensitive responses to children's needs, one might surmise that parents respect for natural processes and associated naturally occurring needs helped parents learn about this aspect of children's development. One might surmise that since closeness between mothers and children served mainly, but not solely, as an emotional function, families' growing understanding of children's capacity for proximity also contributed to their understanding of the emotionality of nursing. The application of cue-based themes associated with nursing to proximity practices provided parents with a means of gaining feedback for their efforts and reinforced themes of closeness. Thus themes of nursing and proximity were internalized at the same time and supported one another.

It also seems likely that proximity behaviors supported nursing and vice versa due to the relevance of closeness for nursing. One might propose that closeness between nursing mothers and children helped mothers read their infants' cues for nursing with greater ease, increasing the frequency of nursing. By the same token, findings demonstrate that tactile interactions and proximity were integral aspects of mother-infant interaction during nursing, suggesting that nursing helped dyads practice and perfect this style of interaction. First of all, nursing is a physical behavior inclusive of tactile components and facilitating the emergence of touching interchanges between mothers and infants. The positive affect that mothers and infants demonstrated to one another during tactile interactions implied that touch had a positive connotation for them. The view of touch, comfort, and familiarity associated with this interactional component likely facilitated the development of tactile interactions outside of nursing.

Proximity and Transferring Children's Love from the Breast Object to Others

Transferring Love from Breast to Mother

Along with facilitating the expression of mutual regard between nursing couples, proximity behaviors seemed to act as a mediator facilitating interactions between the nursing child and others. The first step in this process was helping infants transfer their feelings from the breast to the mother. Initially, infants' behaviors suggested that they focused all of their emotional energy on the breast, implying that they saw the breast as if it is was a whole and separate object. Older infants interacted with the mother in a more direct manner both during and in between nursing. Closeness in between nursing helped children carry on these mutually satisfying exchanges, and also increased their understanding of their mothers' qualities as an object of interest outside of nursing. Infants' gradual displays of mutual regard and other interactional components towards mothers in between nursing and when they were close to their mothers suggest that they understood and accepted that their mothers were separate beings whom they cared about. Proximity behaviors seemed to help infants develop these images by providing them with a context to practice sensitive interchanges with their mothers.

Children continued to talk about and touch the breast following weaning in some cases, implying that children always retained some sense of the breast as an admired separate entity. However, their growing capacity to rely on mothers for support suggested that children's focus of attention seemed to move at least partially to the actual mother figure. Proximity behaviors seemed to play an important role in this relational process by providing children with a tangible context for transitional interaction. Thus proximity behaviors served as a means of enriching the emotionality of nursing and as a vehicle for transferring emotional bonds from the breast to the mother.

Proximity behaviors facilitated the transfer of children's interactional skills and understanding associated with nursing and mothers to interchanges with others. While mothers continued to function as children's central comfort figure for the first few years of life, other family members were gradually incorporated into children's interactional world. It seems that the good enough feelings that nurslings internalized through nursing and closeness ensured that they contributed to this process by seeking out and engaging in interactions with others.

Transferring Feelings to Fathers through Proximity

The transfer of love from mothers to fathers exemplified how proximity behaviors influenced children's process. Fathers' regard for proximity, reviewed earlier in this discussion, implied that this type of interaction compensated for their feelings of longing and envy of the closeness afforded to nursing dyads through nursing. Fathers used proximity to help them establish relationships with their nursing children. As they engaged in tactile interactions, they practiced their cue-reading skills instilled through nursing, and children subsequently felt heard by their fathers. In addition, children generalized their interactional skills internalized through nursing to their interchanges with father, perpetuating the cycle further. Fathers patiently responded to children's fluctuating needs for closeness, facilitating children's development of views of fathers as trustworthy comfort figures.

Transfer of Attention to All Family Members

Nurslings engaged in close interactions with their siblings, as well as both parents. The extension of close interaction to all family members implies that perspectives of closeness associated with nursing were transferred and accepted by family members. Siblings' actions demonstrated their capacity to match nurslings' needs. The same family techniques that helped instill attitudes related to nursing were relevant in the transfer of messages regarding closeness. Siblings respected and understood physical closeness through their own experiences, ongoing observations, discussions, and tutoring. Infants contributed to these exchanges by seeking out others. Older children were influenced when they saw their parents' model respect for tactile interactions and proximity behaviors by creating family interventions, such as co-sleeping, that perpetuated the message that closeness is good. Proximity strategies, such as co-sleeping, also facilitated the development of interactions between siblings by providing a context for attuned interactions to take place. Thus all members were provided with a means of interacting and establishing a relationship with the nursing child.

The proximity behaviors and mutual tactile exchanges that took place between older siblings indicated that they felt comfortable with this style of interaction. Their experiences as formerly nursing children likely enabled them to relish and partake in tactile interactions and proximity behaviors. Siblings' regard for proximity was apparent in the welcoming attitudes they extended towards their younger brothers and sisters who joined them in their beds. Older siblings comfort with closeness was suggested by practices of co-sleeping with younger siblings. At times, the older sibling acted as the transitional sleeping partner after younger children left the parental bed.

Intense and Ongoing Interactions

Reverence for proximity was illustrated by intense and ongoing interactions between nursing children and their mothers. Joint ownership of this theme was suggested by the calm and accepting behaviors that family members displayed when these interactions took place beside them at all hours. The likelihood that family members felt comfortable with the ongoing interaction during and in between nursing was also suggested by the families' ability to continue with other activities alongside ongoing interaction during and in between frequent nursing sessions.

The capacity of siblings to tolerate and to continue their activities alongside younger nursing siblings is remarkable considering that many of these children were actually quite young and had their own developmental agendas. Children's lack of acknowledgement of nearby close nursing units might be interpreted as attempts to ignore events that disturbed them. Within this perspective, their behavior signified intermittent efforts to block out reminders that another child had replaced them at the beloved breast and with their mothers. The cases of sibling rivalry justify this view. However, older siblings directed most obvious sibling rivalry towards their siblings who were already weaned and close to them in age. Young nurslings, in contrast, seemed to be carefully tolerated. Furthermore, other findings imply that these children who seemed to ignore nursing children also facilitated closeness by calling their mothers' attention to younger children, displaying a calm demeanor when they were close to nursing units, and intermittently engaging in gentle interactions with younger siblings and mothers. The positive affect displayed by children apparently evading siblings indicated that they likely accepted their siblings, and likely ignored them since they were not relevant to their activities at the moment.

Moreover, one might propose that children likely had good enough feelings about themselves in relation to their mothers, the breast, and the nursling, and were thus able to tolerate the interactions that took place beside them. Their feelings were the function of the influence of common experiences with and repeated observations of nursing and proximity on children's developing perspectives of family life. It seemed that the experience of nursing together with ongoing observations and discussions enabled them to internalize the ongoing proximity between their mothers and the nursling as normal. In addition, their sense of being emotionally filled up through nursing contained them as they watched their mother tend to someone else. Their scripts of proximity also provided them with tangible tools that enabled them to actualize proximity behaviors with one another and their parents, endearing family members to one another. Thus the circular impact of observing and experiencing family proximity facilitated the development of themes of reverence for proximity and enhanced siblings' scripts of sensitivity, enabling them to tolerate the persistent presence of their younger siblings, including during interchanges with their mothers.

Parents' Tolerance

The tolerance siblings exhibited for ongoing proximity mirrored the behaviors displayed by parents. However, the issues that parents had to tolerate differed from those that affected children. Mothers displayed an ability to patiently participate in ongoing proximity and nursing. Fathers, like children, tolerated ongoing proximity that deprived them of lone time with their partners. By the same token, mothers' were unable to engage in private couple time with fathers. However, throughout all of this, parents consistently allowed the nursling to remain close to mothers, and at times, fathers. The way that they readily included nursing children in their bed and on family outings, giving up time alone, was testament to their joint ownership of themes of reverence for proximity and sensitivity to their child's needs. Moreover, their ability to reframe possible intrusion in a positive way and to create activities that had meaning for them, including a perceived satisfying level of partner intimacy, suggests that the positivity they displayed was genuine.

The task of internalizing and fulfilling themes of proximity was contingent on the quality of couple interaction, reinforcing the systemic nature of themes.

Processes that facilitated optimal function in other areas were also relevant in this regard. Maternal tutoring and open and validating discourse enabled mothers to transfer and reinforce themes of sensitivity to children's needs for proximity to fathers. Paternal support, encouragement, and mirroring of maternal proximity behaviors likely also played a role in the process of actualizing this theme.

Discrepant View of Closeness

The importance of intact couple process for the transfer of themes of reverence for proximity is demonstrated further by contrasting cases where respect for closeness was not shared consistently and seemed to evoke contention. In line with other similar issues, fathers were the partners demonstrating difficulties accepting proximity. It is important to remember the ambivalent relationship that some fathers had with this interactional component. It is interesting to note that this issue often corresponded with disagreements over themes associated with nursing, especially views of nursing as encompassing. Both of these issues relate to ongoing interaction and closeness and reinforce that there are similarities between themes promoting physiological nursing and proximity behaviors. Earlier discussion on paternal envy and guilt, fathers' sense of being overwhelmed, and associated vulnerability to cultural messages explain the reason that fathers experienced more discomfort with closeness than mothers did. The relevance of autonomy in western culture clarifies why views of nursing as encompassing and proximity behaviors trigger negativity in cases of vulnerability.

Mothers seemed to be less concerned about proximity issues, including their children's independence, suggesting that closeness and intimacy were more central to maternal narratives than they were to fathers' trajectories. Some fathers seemed to be more affected by cultural themes of autonomy and distancing, and this likely also affected their scripts. In addition, the example of parents' diverse understanding of signs of autonomy that was provided in the section on couple development suggest that the increased time that mothers spent with their children enabled them to develop an increased awareness of child development in comparison to their partners, despite high levels of involvement.

Stress, Vulnerability to Cultural Themes, and Distancing

This example is consistent with the concept of maternal leading. Like maternal leading, resolution of this issue was advanced by processes that helped parents reach homeostasis in other difficult situations, especially open communication patterns. Paternal concerns over apparent overdependence were relieved when fathers saw tangible proof of apparent independence in their children. In addition, similar to other instances, fathers with older children were less concerned about young children's apparent dependent behaviors than less experienced parents were. These measures reinforce the important role of experience and tangible proof for paternal scripts. Similarly, the congruence of concerns about independence and cultural reverence for autonomy imply that fathers were likely vulnerable to cultural themes. The data showing that fathers were most likely to disregard themes associated with physiologically based nursing in favor of cultural patterns when they felt stressed, indicates that the same conditions apply in some cases when closeness is discounted. This notion implies that fathers disputing ongoing closeness might have been preoccupied with other emotional issues and were thus unable to integrate novel concepts. That being said, it is fair to suggest that obstructed processes signified underlying problematic issues and that internalizing themes such as proximity behaviors was easier for couples with intact systems, including shared themes and open communication.

Broken Continuum and Reduced Sensitivity

The implication of disregard for ongoing closeness is illustrated by the impact of solitary versus parent-child co-sleeping on function in other areas of sensitivity. The importance of co-sleeping for maintenance of themes associated with physiologically based nursing and corresponding behaviors is suggested by the finding that the majority of families seemed to partake in co-sleeping, albeit in various forms. Thus it seems that solitary sleeping was the exception in this population. The few cases of sole sleeping suggested that reasons for breaks in the continuum of parent-child proximity were inexperience at parenting, themes of couple precedence, and paternal envy of the closeness that the infant experienced with their partners. In this case, the infant was the envied object and the mother was the one the father desired. It is most interesting that sole sleeping often concurred with the use of artificial soothing objects. This behavior points to the concept that physiologically based nursing and proximity behaviors are part of a continuum. Like in the case of solitary sleeping, breaks in the continuum in one area seem to lead to altered behavior in another. In terms of family themes, one might suggest that parents who intermittently veered from themes of proximity also periodically interrupted themes of reverence for physiology and nursing as an encompassing behavior able to meet all of their children's needs. The impact of deviant behaviors on other themes reinforces the likelihood that the development of sensitivity is a continuum commencing with themes promoting physiologically based nursing patterns.

Themes Promoting Sensitive Weaning and Separation Processes

Reverence for Child-Paced Needs and Cues

The continuum of regard for nature and sensitivity to infants' naturally occurring cues for nursing and proximity continued into weaning and reflected children's evolving needs. Despite reverence for proximity in early childhood and although physical closeness was most certainly an important feature of family interaction, findings that children eventually decreased the amount of closeness that they expressed and displayed towards others implied that closeness was not the underlying central component that families valued. As strange as this sounds, it seems that parents did not focus on proximity behavior due to reverence for physical closeness in general. Rather there was something else that they were trying to fulfil when they met needs through proximity tactics. This proposal is reinforced further when one notes that other aspects of early interaction, especially cue-based interchanges, remained constant over time. This pattern suggests that reverence for touch was not a guiding family theme during early interactions. Instead one might venture that parents viewed touch as a transient interactional component that helped families transfer emotional messages which dissipated when other interactional components became more developmentally relevant. While families retained a comfortable attitude towards physical closeness, the locus of interaction changed from touch to other means, while the central theme of responding to children in a manner that reflected their individual pattern and needs remained cogent.

Continued Sensitive Interaction

Children gradually displayed a decreased interest in proximity behaviors and tactile interactions, but continued to interact with their parents in an intimate and responsive manner. The free flowing, intimate, and reciprocal discourse that was observed between parents and children suggests that other forms of intimacy and mutuality replaced early sensual tactile interchanges. This reinforced the notion that family interaction in nursing systems was propelled by the desire to actualize themes of meeting children's needs in a sensitive manner that followed their natural rhythms. Parents remained in tune with their children's changing needs and responded in the same way that they had carefully answered them when they were nursing. The sensitive style remained the salient vestige of the nursing relationship.

Child-Focused Weaning Patterns

Along with altering the degree of tactile interaction, families also respected children's needs for decreased proximity in a manner that reflected their respect for children's needs for intense physical closeness in early childhood. The first steps in the separation process took place when children weaned from nursing. Child-focused weaning processes exemplified the continuation of cue-based processes associated with nursing as children got older.

Respect for children's individual rhythm and needs for nursing and the understanding that nursing is an encompassing behavior with physiological and emotional elements helped parents engage in a variety of child-focused weaning patterns that were described in detail in chapter six. Three salient weaning patterns were demonstrated in this population: mother-led weaning, child-led weaning with maternal contributions, and child-led weaning. The similarity between these different styles is that mothers demonstrated an awareness of children's needs, and these needs were their central consideration. The inability of mothers to fulfil their children's needs through nursing when they perceived that this was what their children required, such as in the case of maternal weaning, caused immense distress to mothers, including feelings of guilt. The centrality of the child and their needs was apparent in the efforts these mothers made to compensate their children. The positive affect displayed by children who weaned with help from their mothers suggests that the cue reading their mothers had internalized through nursing helped them respond effectively to their needs. Another important implication of the weaning styles demonstrated that, left to their own devices, children would likely continue nursing for approximately the first five years of life. Maternal narratives suggesting that some mothers sensed decreased levels of patience for nursing beyond a certain age indicates that this factor might have contributed to the most common style of weaning in this population that took place between the ages of three and five years and was gently augmented by maternal efforts. One might wonder if cultural precepts of early childhood might also contribute to this common weaning pattern.

Shared Processes

Most fathers supported nursing into childhood and demonstrated their shared ownership of the nursing relationship and relevant themes. Fathers and older siblings gently facilitated the process of weaning through non-intrusive means. They gently interacted with nurslings and mirrored the sensitive interchanges associated with nursing, allowing children to gradually transfer their feelings to other comfort objects. These joint efforts reinforced how shared meaning contributed to the sensitive interactions promoting development.

Separation from Mother and Home

The process of child-led weaning from the breast was replicated in the child-paced separation from mother and home. Separation processes in older children were reminiscent of the way young children used their mothers as safe places from which to explore the environment, and boomeranged back and forth from their mother base. Similarly, older children and young adults intermittently turned to their parents and siblings for support and open discussions.

Reverence for Children's Needs and Cues

Separation was not motivated by themes of distancing in these families. Rather families' capacity to support children's separation processes reflected their focus on meeting children's needs. Much like the way they responded to infants' cues for nursing, they answered older children's needs to explore with openness and acceptance. Their immense tolerance can be compared to the patience they displayed when young infants required intense closeness. Both behaviors were difficult and required sacrifice on the part of family members. It seems that family capacity to tolerate separation was due to their respect for natural processes and the belief that it was important to understand and fulfil growing children's needs. In this case, one might venture that themes of reverence for children's naturally occurring needs seemed to help parents and children understand that distancing was part of a normal process. The finding that older children, adolescents, and grown children intermittently reached out to their families for support, continued to interact with them in a responsive manner, and in some cases also engaged in intermittent proximity behaviors also demonstrates that family actions were led by salient family themes.

Respect for Children's Unique Needs, Rhythms, Cues, and Individuality

Themes of sensitivity instilled during nursing remained salient features of parents' scripts and family interaction as children grew, and as nursing became less central to their lives. The concept of supporting young children's unique needs and rhythms during nursing promoted the development of concepts of respect for individuality. Children were allowed to develop at their own rates and to express their individuality. The child-paced processes of closeness, weaning, and separation were all expressions of this theme. The salience of parents' commitment to children as individuals was exemplified by the finding that parents accepted their older and adult children's idiosyncrasies and divergent paths. All of these behaviors were reminiscent of parents' interactions with their young nurslings, implying that cue-based nursing established in infancy facilitated the development of sensitive parenting styles that remained intact long after children weaned.

Recognizing and Meeting Parental Couple Needs

The theme of reverence for children's needs for nursing that evolved into respect for children's individual rhythms was also extended to parents. In contrast with the popular cultural theme of couple precedence, parents' needs were not viewed as more important than their children's needs. Moreover, it seemed that at times their needs might have been considered less valid than their children's requirements. This view contrasts with findings that the quality function in the couple sub-system affected parents' capacity to internalize themes and demonstrate sensitivity to their nursing and other children. In other words, parental capacity for sensitivity was contingent on parents' fulfilling their needs.

Fulfilling Parents' Agendas, Family Themes, and Sensitivity

The data on maternal, paternal, and couple development demonstrates that parents' needs were met at the individual and sub-unit level through the implementation of nursing. Family themes were relevant to parents and fulfilling themes was satisfying. The descriptions of ongoing contact with their young children and the special activities that they created together implied that family activities also met parents' needs. Parents' convictions and capacity to parent against the grain in a culture invested in distancing demonstrated further the importance of family themes to these couples' sense of self over time. The increasing value of these themes for parents' scripts was suggested by the way that parents with more experience disregarded cultural messages with greater ease than parents with less experience. This is most poignantly demonstrated by parents' increased ability to overcome the need to fulfil cultural themes of distancing that conflicted with their desire for ongoing closeness with the baby. Growing capacity for sensitivity to children's needs facilitated by themes, such as reverence for closeness, was solidified over time. These themes not only enriched parenting behaviors, but also seemed to augment individual needs as the sensitive nursing parent increasingly became part of each parents' sense of self.

The connection between family themes associated with sensitive parenting, parenting behaviors, and personal needs is also suggested by the way that parents readily welcomed children into the parental bed at night. The impetus for this practice was meeting children's needs. However, the likelihood that in some cases this also contributed to personal scripts was suggested by findings that some fathers who envied the closeness that mothers' experienced, including those who attempted to obstruct nursing in other ways, seemed to relish co-sleeping with their children. Other narratives suggested that co-sleeping also complied with their needs for sleep. Thus at times behaviors intended as a means of actualizing sensitivity also promoted parents' needs.

Sexual Function

Another indication that parents were able fulfil their needs as individuals and as a couple is suggested by the finding that although there was great variance in sexual function, nevertheless most parents seemed fulfilled by this aspect of their couple interactions. Parental satisfaction was demonstrated by parental narrative implying that intensity of nursing and ongoing proximity stimulated maternal sexual desire and was accompanied by a sense of being womanly. This view makes sense in light of the centrality of reverence for physiology, including the view that nursing was as an essential aspect of the female trajectory, for female scripts.

Views regarding sexual function varied in different families and according to the phase of family development. The phase of family development did not affect sexual desire in the same way for all families. Differences between maternal and paternal libido, and the low intensity of sexual interaction in the establishment phase of family development was described by parents as stemming from maternal exhaustion and a sense of being "all touched out." This feeling concurs with the developmental tasks of the newly formed, intense, and exclusive nursing sub-system. The physicality of this stage of development likely contributed to the fatigue. It seems that exhaustion might have also been due to the extreme emotionality associated with internalizing novel themes and the feelings associated with nursing. These issues might not have only exhausted mothers, but also provided them with a sense of fulfilment that meant they did not require or were unable to engage in additional physical interludes.

Most fathers accepted their partners' varied sexual attitudes and behaviors, including decreased sexual desire. Fathers' reactions to mothers' changing sexual attitudes reinforced the concept that nursing provided fathers with a means of practicing empathetic and responsive interchanges. The repeated attitude that intense parent–child interactions associated with nursing actually enhanced the quality of sexual interchanges exemplified efforts to positively reframe a situation that others viewed as difficult.

Couples' capacity to simultaneously support nursing, associated proximity behaviors, and ongoing intense parenting interactions, and also willingly engage in sexual interchanges with one another suggests that they shared views of the breast as a multifaceted organ, a theme congruent with reverence for physiology. The section on mothers also demonstrated that this view was inherent to mothers' perspectives. The lack of data demonstrating the exact role is another interesting topic for future research.

Along with the similarities, there is a diverse array of sexual attitudes and behaviors. There were differences in the length of time that couples disengaged from sexual activity after birth. This factor not only varied between families, but also in the same family after the birth of different children, regardless of birth order or number of children. Parents seemed to have distinct sexual needs and displayed behaviors that were not gender specific. In addition, couples had assorted means of regaining homeostasis pertaining to sexual function. While open communication patterns reduced dissonance regarding sexual interchanges, sexual intimacy did not seem to be impacted by the couple's communication style. Some couples with closed communication styles used sexual intimacy as a means of restoring homeostasis. The variance in couples sexual behaviors suggest that nursing and associated behaviors might have had an impact on the nature of sexual exchanges between the parenting couple, but other factors, including individuality and couple dynamics, also influenced this area of couple function. Despite all of the differences, this aspect of the couple was relevant in most families.

Processes That Facilitated or Impeded Couple Needs

Open Communication

An important function that seemed to help couples meet their needs as parents and as individuals was open communication. The similarity between open communication patterns in the couple sub-system and sensitive parenting seems to indicate there was an association between communication styles and themes associated with nursing. Open communication helped couples actualize themes, create shared goals in an ongoing manner, receive validation for their efforts, and repair damage when necessary. It seems that this experience facilitated parents' capacity to engage in sensitive processes associated with nursing, such as cue reading. It was as if responding to another person was familiar. By the same token, the feedback that children provided to their parents resembled open discourse between parents and reinforced the system.

Closed Communication

The importance of open communication patterns for couple and parenting function is most evident when one compares the interactions in nursing families with open communication systems to those with contrasting processes. Couples with closed communication systems remained in a heightened state of conflict, suggesting that families who present with ongoing dissension regarding nursing might actually have difficulties discussing their feelings openly. Unresolved tension impaired parents' capacity to consistently answer their children's cues for nursing. This point reinforces the existence of a relationship between interactions at all levels of the system and nursing patterns. Reduced attention to nursing concurred with increased distancing behaviors, inclusive of the use of pacifiers and other distancing devices. Another aspect of this discovery is that the use of tools associated with artificial feeding in families that otherwise attempted to nurse in tune with nature signified underlying unresolved couple dissension. The negative impact of closed communication on nursing explains the small number of parents who demonstrated this style in the study and indicates that the inability to share themes in a validating manner interferes with the internalization of themes associated with nursing that negate common precepts.

Compensatory Measures

The capacity of some parents with closed communication patterns to nurse in a physiological manner, without obstructions, despite difficulties in resolving issues at the couple level, was facilitated by extenuating factors that helped them return to a state of homeostasis despite their incapacity to refine their differences in a verbal manner. Compensatory measures, such as sexual intimacy, temporarily repaired parents' hurt feelings or sense of loss, and increased their capacity to patiently respond to their children. For others, the ability to remain committed to responsive parenting, regardless of obstacles, stemmed from personal ownership of issues related to sensitivity and nursing.

Unresolved Couple Dissonance, Gender Distinctions, and Decreased Sensitivity

Similar to other areas of parenting function, the connection between interactions at the couple level and sensitivity was also more apparent in fathers than in mothers. This additional information adds to evidence suggesting that there was a common pattern in the couple sub-system where most mothers remained focused on family themes and children regardless of the conditions, and fathers, although also committed to family themes, sometimes changed their behaviors. Some fathers reduced their support for nursing when their opposition was not resolved at the couple level, and most mothers remained sensitive to cues for nursing and closeness, despite couple dysfunction. Fathers who reduced support of nursing and proximity behaviors were responding to their relationship with the nursing mother, such as in cases of paternal guilt and envy. In addition, while nursing, like closeness, advances paternal development, it did not seem to be as central for the male trajectory as nursing was for mothers. The findings suggest that in some cases, the lack of relevance of nursing for some fathers impaired their capacity to understand the meaning of nursing from their partners' perspective, causing discord. Furthermore, it is important to remember that mothers led behaviors related to nursing, while fathers followed. In cases of unresolved disagreements, one might propose that fathers simply did not follow as closely.

Mothers seemed to overcome paternal obstructions and managed to remain firmly responsive to their infants' cues better than fathers did when they disagreed with their partners. This behavior is most prominent in mothers of older children who seemed to be less susceptible to their partners' views than were mothers of young infants. This behavior complied with mothers' changing need for support and the trajectory of maternal development. Accordingly, much like the way that experienced mothers ignored cultural obstructions, they also seemed to increasingly prioritize their children's needs over disruptions in the couple relationship.

The data also implied, however, that even though mothers ignored the obstructions that their partners placed in front of nursing and proximity behaviors, the disagreements regarding these issues bothered them, and this increased couple discord. Maternal dissonance is suggested by the finding that some mothers expressed anger and frustration in response to their partners' expressions of negativity towards nursing and subordinate issues. Some mothers altered nursing behaviors to suit their partners. These mothers were the minority, suggesting that nursing-centered themes remained the central force that motivated most maternal behavior, despite obstacles, for most families. The act of altering mothering behavior in order to accommodate the father seemed to exacerbate maternal anger towards the partner that they also tried to appease. The presence of anger for the appeasing mothers suggests that they were also child-centered, but did not have the emotional strength to carry out their themes under all conditions.

Fury, expressed in some cases as walls of silence, resulted when mothers forfeited perceived optimal mothering behaviors and distanced fathers from the nursing dyad. This, in turn, further reduced the fathers' sensitivity towards the nursing child.

The relational function in the couple sub-system had an accumulative and circular impact on the quality of parental sensitivity to nursing and associated behaviors. Unresolved couple discord hindered the parents' capacity to accept the needs of the nursing infant and to internalize fully the sensitive parenting style. One might venture that families who attempted to nurse in tune with physiology, but called nursing feeding, missed cues for nursing, and engaged in distal strategies, might have issues of unresolved couple dissension. And by the same token, parents who actualized themes and demonstrated sensitivity to children's cues were likely able to meet their needs at the couple level.

Sensitive and Free Flowing Communication

The open communication patterns expressed by parents and the cue-based interactions between and with the nursing sub-system prepared members for mutual interactions. At the family level, members' capacity for mutuality was suggested by open communication patterns that mirrored the free flowing discourse between the nursing sub-system, the interchanges between fathers and nursing offspring, and the supportive exchanges between the parental couple unit. Thus the reciprocity instilled through nursing seemed to be a vital means of fostering family development, upholding the nursing system, and perpetuating healthy family interactions.

Families communicated openly with one another in various ways and helped the family retain balance. Similar to interactions between parents, communication between family members included discussions and tutoring. Tutoring enhanced family members' understanding, including children, of the intense nursing situation and related issues. Family discourse enabled members to process new ideas, discuss their interpretations, disclose their feelings, and receive feedback in a validating manner.

Family responsiveness to and support for nursing and systemic development was also enhanced by the same mechanisms that fostered sensitivity for the nursing infant. Members observed one another in a manner that resembled maternal observations of infants' cues for nursing and fathers' observations of the interactions in the nursing system. Sensitive responses were also enhanced when families drew on their own experiences of being responded to and of answering others' needs. Individual experience with themes and patterns associated with nursing provided mothers, fathers, and children with in-depth tools for interaction. Ongoing experience with the nursing sub-system and a sensitive system enabled all members to practice and enhance their existing responsive notions and skills, and to perpetuate themes and patterns associated with nursing. These families demonstrated that the experience of being listened to in one's own nursing experience and of watching others interact with a nursing child, contributes to one's capacity to demonstrate sensitivity to others. The far-reaching implications of themes and behavioral patterns associated with nursing for the family are suggested by findings that these processes were echoed by older and adult offspring.

Summary of Extension of Themes Promoting Sensitivity beyond Nursing

Thus the child-focused, cue-based attitudes instilled through nursing influenced additional family behaviors. Ongoing proximity behaviors and tactile interactions were significant behaviors affected by and influencing the nursing relationship. These behaviors increased regard for emotionality and nursing as encompassing, provided family members with a means of interacting with nurslings, and facilitated infants' efforts to transfer feelings of adoration from the breast to the mother and to others. Older siblings' capacity to tolerate ongoing closeness and nursing stemmed from their own experiences, ongoing practice, and parental interventions, including discussion.

Reverence for proximity and responsiveness to cue-based interactions based on children's individual rhythms established early in the nursing relationship were transferred to family themes regarding weaning and separation. The centrality of respect for children's individuality and rights to develop at their own rate remained salient. Parents altered their interactional components to suit the changing needs of their children, allowing them to separate from the mother, family, and home at their own rate. Intense and reciprocal tactile interactions between parents and children gradually evolved into open and sensitive verbal communication patterns as children grew.

Interactions between the parental couple influenced their capacity to tolerate physically close, ongoing, and intense parenting interactions. Parents were able to fulfil their own agenda as a couple, including engaging in satisfying sexual relations. Closed communication patterns and underlying issues may have interfered with the ability to internalize themes of proximity. Disagreements regarding nursing, associated parenting, and digression from normal nursing patterns and behaviors may have signified unresolved parental dissonance.

Chapter 13
Implications of Family Interactions in Nursing Family Systems

In this chapter, implications of family interactions in systems that nurse in tune with physiologically based patterns will be discussed. Up to this point, interactions in all levels of the family have been reviewed and the associated clinical applications for each unit and the family as a whole have been discussed. Relevant themes fostering sensitivity have been outlined. The review of the implications will demonstrate the significance of family interactions in nursing families for nursing, theories discussed, and for clinical practice.

Implications for Nursing

The Development of Sensitive Interaction through Nursing

An important implication of the discoveries about breastfeeding families is that nursing is far more than a mere means of feeding. Nursing is a complex behavior with physiological, emotional, and relational components, influencing and affected by family interaction. Most importantly, nursing is a context that facilitates the development of sensitive interactions. Mothers internalize sensitivity directly through nursing and associated behaviors. Fathers incorporate sensitive themes through supportive behaviors and by watching and interacting with the nursing unit, and through interactions with nursing mothers. Children learn about sensitivity through their personal experience with nursing and by observing and interacting with their nursing mothers and siblings. Themes promoting sensitivity are reverberated throughout the system. Themes are modified to suit the changing needs of the family and retained over time.

Interconnected themes facilitate the development of physiologically based nursing patterns and sensitive mothering and fathering, contributing to the development of sensitive family style.

The themes include reverence for physiology, enabling families to establish nursing, follow physiological patterns, and note and respond to the occurrence of infants' naturally occurring cues. A connected related theme is that nursing is normal and that it is an encompassing behavior and an emotional experience. Themes associated with nursing are reverence for proximity, individuality, and child-paced development, including weaning and separation. These themes are interconnected with themes associated with nursing and foster their development.

Thus the analysis of family interaction at different levels of individual and subsystemic function clearly indicates that nursing is an optimal context for the development of sensitive interactions that ripple through the system and boomerang back to the nursing unit. The intricate interactions during and between nursing contribute to a sensitive family interactional style with developmental implications for all family members and beyond.

Encompassing and Physiology

Implications of Views of Nursing as an Encompassing Behavior

Views of nursing as encompassing has important implications for the establishment and duration of nursing. Seeing nursing as encompassing reinforces the theme of physiology and contributes to physiologically based nursing patterns in several ways. When nursing is seen as encompassing, breastfeeding becomes the primary source, thus supporting exclusivity. Views of nursing as encompassing also contribute to nursing duration by ensuring that parents turn to the breast frequently. The apparent association between frequency and duration (Vandiver, 1997) indicates that perspectives of nursing as encompassing help parents continue nursing over time.

Encompassing and Nursing as a Love Object

From a psychological perspective, views of nursing as encompassing and comforting enables infants and children to bond to the maternal breast as their only love object. Children continue to turn to nursing over time, ensuring duration. They never require transitional objects to replace the maternal breast. A transitional object is a comforting item other than the mother that helps the child deal with emotional or physical discomfort. Transitional objects take on great meaning for children and are often difficult to replace. It is very important to note that pacifiers, bottles, and other utensils may be considered transitional objects. In some cases, their comfort may be perceived by the child as more worthy than the mother. This implies that the use of pacifiers or other mother replacements interfere with nursing. Green's (2001) findings, implying that children's use of transitional objects, including parts of the mother's body other than the breast, impairs the duration of nursing, reinforces this point. When children's only object is their mother and the maternal breast, they continue to nurse, using the mother and the breast as their central comfort object into early childhood.

Child-Focused Weaning

The different weaning styles demonstrated by children in families nursing in tune with physiology implies that the term child-led weaning commonly used in the literature (La Leche League, 2004) is not applicable in all cases. It seems that in some cases of weaning in early childhood, maternal contributions, albeit minimal, might play a greater role than is implied in the existing literature. Since weaning is a mutual affair, taking children's needs and unique rhythm's into account, a term such as child-focused or child-paced might be a more accurate way to describe full weaning in early childhood.

Implications for Child Development

Good Enough Feelings about Self in Relation to Others

Children and adults from former nursing families display behaviors and attitudes that suggest that nursing contributes to relational development. Nursing is a multifaceted relationship central to children's emotional well being that facilitates children's capacity to interact with others. These concepts contribute to existing theories on children's development, including attachment (Ainsworth et al., 1978; Bowlby, 1987) and object relations theories (Fairbairn, 2002; Klein, 1997, 1998; Weininger, 1989, 1992, 1993; Winnicott, 1957, 1958, 1964). Infants' initial reverence for the breast above all else concurs with object relations theories that suggest that infants' first relational object of interest is the breast. Children's calm attitudes and positive regard for interaction suggest that they internalize good enough feelings through their experiences with the breast and the mother, helping them create a positive world view. Interactions during nursing provide children with a context to experience attuned interactions, demonstrating how attachment behaviors take place between nursing mothers and children. The warm interactions noted between children and their family members suggest that they generalize feelings and relational tools internalized through nursing to their interactions with others, facilitating their integration into the family system.

Proximity behaviors seem to help children transfer their feelings of affection from the breast to the mother. Children's capacity to experience closeness, concurring with maternal sensitivity, likely plays a role in facilitating the comfortable weaning processes. It is most noteworthy that children seem to tolerate weaning from encompassing nursing relationships. Children's developmental capacity to see the maternal breasts as part of the whole mother implies that they are not losing a cherished object when they wean. The mothering object remains salient and tangible. Weaning from an encompassing nursing relationship contrasts greatly with weaning from innate transitional objects that disappear completely when they are taken away or when one outgrows them. Children transfer sensitive and good enough experiences with the breast to the mother through proximity and communicative behaviors.

The sensitive interactions that children experience through nursing are reflected in their interchanges with family members. These experiences enable the young child to internalize further that the world is a good enough place and that interactions with others are beneficial. From a family systems perspective, this facilitates family development and perpetuates the cycle.

There are long term implications of growing up in a sensitive nursing family. Older and adult children are nurturing towards one another and others outside of the family. This suggests that formerly nursed individuals mirror their experiences of being sensitively responded to in their interactions with others and demonstrates the resilience of scripts of interaction instilled through cue-based nursing. One might also venture that the emphasis on connection rather than distancing, including during weaning and separation processes, contributes to the former nursling's positive views of self in relation to others and instills a desire to connect with, rather than distance oneself from others. Regard for others at all levels is also suggested by roles that older children and adults have as activists for social causes. It seems that the experience of being connected to others and the sense of being heard since infancy facilitates altruism, empathy for others, and the capacity to interact and care for others.

Independent, Creative, Responsible, Confident

The responsible, moral, and creative behaviors displayed by older offspring suggest that the offspring are not only independent, but that their autonomy contributes to society, much like their altruism. Early patterns of recognizing and conveying information about one's needs seems to help children learn how to acknowledge their abilities, make decisions, think creatively, and function independently. It seems that when children's cues are listened to, children internalize that they and their interests are valid. They become attuned to their needs much like the way other family members do, respond accordingly, and continue to operate in a self-motivated manner. They learn how to get what they need, much like the way infants cue for nursing. This includes their needs to separate and function independently. Reverence for proximity and child needs seems to contribute to autonomy. This view concurs with McKenna's (1996) suggestion that child-focused processes associated with nursing contribute to the development of autonomy, and disavows the cultural attitude discussed in this paper and evident in some fathers' narratives that distancing is associated with autonomy.

The likelihood that former nurslings function well on their own is also suggested by findings that when children do move away, they tend to adapt well and fit in with great ease to environments that differ from their home context. One might venture that children brought up with cue-based processes gain a sense of confidence that enables them to function in a variety of contexts.

Respect for Physiology

Further signs of autonomy are suggested by evidence that older children support nursing as normal despite strong cultural pressure to think differently. The short term deviation from family themes displayed by teenagers is temporary, and older and adult children continue to regard physiological processes as normal. This behavior implies that children internalize family themes that prevail over cultural views of nursing and peer pressure. In addition, teenagers' comfort around nursing mothers implies that they accept the motherly components of the female breast. This is true even though it appears that children also know that the breast has other meanings. It seems that children from nursing families see the breast as an organ with multiple functions, a view that negates salient cultural conceptions of the breast (Angier, 2000; Saha, 2002). Older children and adult offspring's long standing sense of comfort with nursing, breasts, and other physiological processes points again to the significance of naming these events as normal.

A sign that offspring reverberate themes of respect for nature, nursing, responsiveness, and child-centered notions is apparent in the way that former nursing children parent their own children. For example, they nurse their children in tune with physiological principles, engaging in proximity behaviors and child-led processes. Descriptions of adult children suggest that they are as responsive to their children as their parents were to them, and they continue to engage in open discourse with their families of origin. Their behaviors point to the fortitude of the themes associated with nursing for family members. In addition, their behaviors and attitudes reinforce the concept of circularity and the mutual impact of nursing and the family context. The transfer of family themes and patterns to future generations is consistent with the literature that suggests that family issues are transferred in an intergenerational manner (Kerr &Bowen, 1988), reinforcing that nursing is a family behavior.

Summary

It seems that children's experiences with sensitive parenting and family interchanges established through nursing facilitate the development of scripts that enrich interaction, functional attitudes and behaviors, and positive child outcome, enhancing children's integration into contexts outside of the family. Children mirror the empathy that they experience in caring interactions with others. The trajectory of respect for individual rates of development is apparent in the independent, adaptable, creative, and responsible behaviors they display. Older children and adult's comfort with physiologically based processes, especially nursing, suggests that they internalize and revere the same themes that they experienced as children. Most significantly, adults transfer themes associated with nursing from their families of origin to their interactions with their children.

Implications for Maternal Development

Cue Reading Practice and Perceptions of Nursing

Like earlier research (Epstein, 1993), a review of family interaction demonstrates that nursing helps mothers develop sensitive mothering styles by providing them with frequent opportunities to practice interacting with their children. Nursing also affects maternal perceptions, and these attributions of nursing subsequently affect their behaviors. This concept is salient in the literature on maternal development through nursing (Blyth et al., 2002; Cooke et al., 2003; Dennis, 1999; Epstein, 1993; Kendall-Tackett & Sugarman, 1995; Leff et al., 1994; McLeod et al., 2002; Rich, 1986; Saha, 2002; Schmied & Barclay, 1999; Vandiver, 1997). Mothers' perceptions of the nursing experience also affect their capacity for sensitivity. Maternal perceptions may be influenced by the actual experience of nursing or by what mothers believe that nursing contributes to them or their children.

Fulfills Personal Scripts and Themes

Positive perceptions of nursing enrich maternal capacity for sensitivity, especially when mothers perceive that nursing fulfills their needs. The sense of personal fulfillment seems to help mothers feel more patient towards their children, facilitating sensitive interchanges. Mothers perceive that nursing is compensatory, healing, and positive. Mothers also revere the intimacy that they believe they experience through nursing, a concept that has been noted in the literature (Buckley, 1992; Epstein, 1993; Kendall-Tackett & Sugarman, 1995; Rich, 1986; Saha, 2002; Schmied & Barclay, 1999). Intimacy seems to replenish mothers, filling them up emotionally and increasing their tolerance for mothering. In addition, mothers cherish exclusive interactions during nursing due to their reverence for the physiologically based interdependence of nursing and the sense of uniqueness associated with the task of providing their children with something special. Nursing may be perceived by mothers as an experience that fulfills their personal needs, enhancing their capacity to develop sensitive mothering styles.

Increased Experience Changes Maternal Capacity and Views

The salient family theme of reverence for children's needs is relevant for mothers at the individual level, contributing to their positive perceptions of nursing and the development of sensitivity. It seems that when mothers focus on their children's needs above all else, they display increased tolerance for their children and are able to answer cues in an ongoing manner. Mothers increasingly ignore cultural messages that oppose the style of mothering associated with nursing. This change implies that the ongoing experience of nursing and mothering reinforces the relevance of children's needs above all else for mothers. Mothers' perceptions of children's needs as important contribute to their capacity to nurse in a cue-based manner, enriching the development of sensitive mothering.

Another maternal perspective that seems to help mothers remain attuned to their children's cues for nursing is the view that breasts are multifaceted organs, a perspective discussed in the literature (Angier, 2000; Bartlett, 2000; Saha, 2002). The evidence suggests that an important influence on mothers' views of their breasts stems from their reverence for female processes, a concept related to the family theme of respect for natural processes. In addition, it seems that maternal reverence for children's needs also helps mothers internalize novel views of their breasts. Mothers' views of their breasts as multifaceted organs help them remain attuned their children's cues for nursing, a behavior that evolves into overall sensitive mothering.

Ambivalence

The importance of maternal feelings and attributions for the development of sensitive mothering is illustrated by instances of maternal ambivalence that seem to interfere with the capacity to continually respond to children's cues. Some mothers feel ambivalent about the intensity of the nursing relationship and contemplate the option of intermittently distancing themselves from their children. One explanation for this feeling concurs with the existing literature, suggesting that some mothers have difficulties coping with the lifestyle associated with nursing (Cooke et al., 2003). However, it appears that a far more complex form of maternal ambivalence is more common in this population, especially in first time mothers. This type of ambivalence reflects mothers' overwhelming desire to be close to their infants and their contrasting wish to fulfill culturally condoned concepts of distancing. This form of ambiguity is less prevalent in more experienced mothers, suggesting again that mothers undergo emotional processes while they mother that affect their viewpoints and mothering capacity. Focusing on children's needs might be one strategy that mothers use to overcome their mixed feelings. It seems that the child and mothering become more important than other issues, decreasing ambivalence and increasing the capacity to continually meet needs. While it seems that maternal ambivalence exists, confusion decreases as mothers gain more experience and internalize positive perceptions of nursing, mothering, and their capacity to interact with their children in a sensitive manner.

As mothers internalize the issues associated with nursing, they seem to feel more confident in their role and with their tasks and are able to tolerate the behaviors associated with ongoing cue reading. It seems mothers' sense of self as sensitive and good enough contributes to their cycle of sensitive mothering. Positive perceptions of nursing and associated mothering promote more affirming experiences.

Summary

Hence nursing is a complex experience for mothers and contributes to development in varied ways. Through nursing, mothers fulfill personal scripts and internalize a sense of positive self-regard. These feelings and opportunities to practice cue-based and sensitive interactions with offspring help mothers develop sensitive mothering styles.

Implications for Paternal Development

Supportive Tasks

Supportive tasks are central to paternal scripts, a salient view in the literature (Amper, 1996; Buckner & Matsubara, 1993; Giuglani et al, 1994; Jordan, 1990; Jordan & Wall, 1993; Kessler et al., 1995; Littman et al., 1994; Pollock et al., 2002; Scharff & Savage Scharff, 1991; Sharma & Petrosa, 1997; Stern, 1985; Weininger, 1984; Winnicott, 1957). The review of paternal interaction in nursing families demonstrates that supportive tasks have a unique influence on fathers and contributes to the development of sensitive fathering. Fathers' behaviors and attitudes suggest that when fathers support and care for nursing mothers and children, they are provided with a means of engaging in acts that require them to observe, interpret, and respond to changing cues. Hence, the act of supporting nursing also functions for fathers as a means of facilitating the development of a cue-based fathering style.

Emotional Experience

Fathers in nursing families are emotionally affected by the nursing relationship, and this seems to impact their supportive actions more than cognitive familiarity with nursing. The analysis of fathers' emotions indicates that their feelings affect their capacity to support nursing and to develop sensitive fathering patterns. Paternal capacity to support nursing is facilitated when fathers' needs to protect, feel efficient, and feel closeness are fulfilled. Fathers obstruct nursing when they feel overwhelmed emotionally, perceive that issues associated with nursing contradict their personal agendas, and when they are anxious about their relationship with the mother or child. Fathers experience both positive and negative feelings related to nursing, and these feelings affect and are influenced by their behaviors. It seems that nursing is an emotional experience for fathers, and their actions reflect their emotional interpretation of the situation.

Guilt and Envy

The emotional implications of nursing for fathers are illustrated by fathers' feelings of guilt and envy that interfere with their capacity to adequately fulfil paternal tasks associated with nursing.. Paternal envy is referred to in other literature (Jordan, 1990; Jordan & Wall, 1993; Saha, 2002; Sharma & Petrosa, 1997). Yet, the analysis of fathers' behaviors and attitudes in the study discussed in this text diverges from the concept of paternal envy as it is most commonly espoused in the literature. It is respectfully submitted that fathers envy the closeness between mothers and babies, and although some long to replace their infants, most seem to want to experience what mothers feel. It seems that envy is both a normal and an accepted aspect of paternal development in nursing families. Moreover, paternal envy is growth enhancing when it is resolved. Resolution is facilitated through open communication with mothers and through father-child interactions. Tactile interactions and physical closeness seem to be especially facilitative. These interactions are enhanced by and reinforce themes of sensitivity instilled through nursing. Hence, paternal envy is a natural and integral aspect of paternal development for some fathers in nursing families.

Summary

Paternal development is enhanced when fathers take on distinct roles and tasks associated with nursing. These functions help fathers develop sensitive fathering styles mirroring nursing. Supportive behaviors mirror maternal cue reading during nursing, enhancing fathers' trajectories to sensitive parenting. The quality of paternal behaviors and subsequent sensitive fathering through nursing is contingent on the emotional impact of nursing on fathers and their capacity to resolve ambivalence.

Implications for Couple Processes

Interactions between parental couples affect parents' sensitivity to children's needs associated with nursing. There are several processes that seem to facilitate this task. Significant processes include gender distinct and complementary parenting task allocation and open communication patterns.

Gender Distinct and Complementary Parenting Task Allocation

The gender distinct parenting task allocation seems to play an important role in couple interactions in nursing families. The differences between parents are more evident when infants are young and parents' physiological-based parenting capacities are more relevant than when children are older. Differences in parenting reflect mothers and fathers' distinct gender-based trajectories to parenthood and diverse biologically based capacities, their diverse styles and rates of internalizing knowledge and skills, and the dissimilar ways that parents are affected by their relationship and extraneous events. These notions differ from literature suggesting that a system of equal parenting task allocation facilitates homeostasis at the couple level (Cowan & Cowan, 1999; Goodrich et al., 1988; Held, 1984). Instead, parental function in nursing families is enriched when mothers and fathers engage in a complementary style of task allocation (Beavers, 1977).

In contrast to views reviewed in the introduction to this paper implying that biologically based gender distinctions devalue women and impair their development (Chodorow, 1978; Dinnerstein, 1977; Firestone, 1970), it seems that gender-based and distinct functions reflect the high status of mothers in these families. This view reinforces historically based perspectives showing an association between high regard for women and children, reverence for female physiology, and the increased incidence of maternal nursing reviewed in chapter four. Moreover, fathers benefit developmentally when their own unique issues of support, protection, and feelings of efficiency are fostered by the tasks allocated to them through gender-based parenting associated with nursing. Gender-based parenting in these families is an expression of parental reciprocity, sharing, and mutual respect. The biologically based parenting system is functional, meeting the needs of all family members. Moreover, one might contend that by meeting one another's needs, parents are extending the theme of meeting children's needs to themselves.

Parents' appreciation for their differences is not only expressed by the complementary style, but is also facilitated by this process. This function helps parents support one another as they internalize novel concepts and practice new skills. Mothers transfer the concepts and skills internalized through nursing to fathers who support them in their attuned interactions. This salient pattern is also exemplified by maternal leading and tutoring, and paternal following.

Open Communication

An important tool advancing parents' mutual processes is open communication (Satir, 1967). Open communication helps couples integrate differences into their interactions and parenting tasks. In addition, it is interesting to note the similarity between openness between parents and their responsiveness to their children. The salience of open communication for many families suggests that there might be a connection between communication at the couple level and parents' sensitive interactions with children in some families. A systemic explanation of the similarity implies that some couples' readiness for sensitive dialogue with infants stems from their experiences as a couple, and by the same token, the openness between parents and children resonates back to the couple.

Shared Themes

The validating style of discourse enriches parental sensitivity to children by providing parents with a means of transferring themes to one another. Parents eventually jointly own themes of sensitivity, closeness, reverence for physiology, respect for the dual nature of breasts, and child-centered views. These themes are gradually integrated into couple interactions. The parental couples' capacity to change their tasks to reflect child needs exemplifies the impact of shared themes of sensitivity on couple function. Parental flexibility enables parents to meet their children's needs and nurture them effectively, with important implications for positive child outcome (Volpe, 1989).

Restoring Homeostasis

Open communication also serves as a means of restoring homeostasis for these couples. Parents validate one another's feelings, including those that are difficult to contain. This action seems to enable parents to withstand and resolve disagreements. Parents' ability to tolerate or resolve couple tension affects their capacity to remain attuned to their children. When couples have efficient means of restoring homeostasis, they not only continue to function alongside intense nursing interactions, they also seem to enjoy being with their young children in a continuous manner.

Ongoing Parenting and Couple Relations

Couples in families with physiologically based nursing subsystems rarely leave their children, taking them wherever they go. This behavior has also been described in other literature (Ball, 2002; Bar-Yakov, 2002; Green, 2001; Sears, 1988). It seems that some couples meet their own agendas when they parent in a continuous manner. Some parents perceive that this style of parenting helps them meet their family themes associated with nursing, contributing to a shared sense of fulfillment as a couple. Other issues include those associated with couple interaction, especially mutual respect for difference. Some parents find that meeting children's needs in an ongoing manner enriches the quality of interchanges between the parental couple. Thus ongoing interactions between children and parents are mutually beneficial for everyone.

Sexual Function

The likelihood that many parents continue to function as a couple despite their high degree of ongoing involvement with their children is suggested by the parents' positive perceptions about the quality of their sexual relationship. Most couples indicate that they are pleased with the quality of their sexual relationship. It seems that sexual function and parents' view of this aspect of couple interaction changes over time and is viewed in diverse ways by couples. In addition, sexual behaviors inclusive of frequency and factors affecting sexuality vary greatly. The differences between parents suggest that nursing might not necessarily affect this aspect of couple interaction for all families.

It is interesting to note that couples' positive regard for sexuality suggested by the data used for this book contrasts with findings in other resources (Benson Brown & McPherson, 1998; Rodriguez-Garcia & Frazier, 1995; Sharma & Petosa, 1997). The methodology used in this study, including the qualitative tools, the wide variety of participants, the long period of time, and the capacity to interview couples at different stages of the nursing relationship might have facilitated novel discoveries regarding this aspect of couple function. The variance in the study and the difference between the evidence in the present study and others' work suggests that this aspect of couple interaction might be uncovered further by additional research that includes following couples over time as the nursing relationship changes.

Unresolved Couple Discord

Cases of unresolved couple discord reinforce the importance of open communication as a facilitative measure. Sometimes when parents are unable to reach homeostasis, they present with conflict apparently associated with nursing. Although conflict appears to be related to nursing, breastfeeding is not usually the actual cause. Instead it appears that underlying issues, including a desire to engage in close interactions with a member of the nursing relationship and the inability to resolve issues due to closed communication, are the real reasons for couple conflict. This information implies that parents' apparent conflict over issues related to nursing is merely the presenting symptom that functions as a means of hiding the actual cause of distress. Most importantly, when actual couple issues are not resolved, parents' capacity to engage with their children in an attuned manner, particularly regarding their sensitivity to cues for nursing and associated behaviors, is reduced. Hence, the couple dissension is the root of parents' displays of insensitivity to nursing, including the use of artificial pacifiers and apparatus.

Couples' attitudes and behavior also imply that one parent, usually the mother, might be able to retain sensitivity despite unresolved couple issues. However, when this act does not repair the couple relationship and strife between the parents remains a constant aspect of family life, at least one parent's capacity to sensitively respond to needs for nursing is reduced. Couple interaction and the capacity to return to a state of homeostasis affects the quality of sensitive parenting associated with nursing.

The interactions between the parenting couple affect their ability to sensitively interact with and meet the needs of the nursing child. Positive interactions where couples needs are met enhance sensitivity and contrasting interchanges reduce parents' capacity for sensitivity. The notion that couple interactions affect nursing differs from the results of a study referred to in chapter three that was unable to find an association between the couple relationship and nursing behaviors (Falceto et al., 2004). One might venture that the difference between the findings stems from the distinct methodologies used in each study. The Falceto et al. study observed couples in the early stages of nursing. The data reviewed in this book are based on observations beyond infancy, providing one with a sense of the couple development over time. It seems that couples might have more emotional energy for their relationship when nursing becomes more routine.

Summary

Parents in nursing families meet their needs as a couple while simultaneously engaging with their nursing children in an ongoing manner. Couple mutuality and open discourse are central to their interactions and are displayed by sharing family themes. This sharing leads to the creation of gender-based and complementary task allocation, facilitating nursing with associated behaviors. Mutuality between parents enriches their capacity to interact with nursing children in a sensitive manner. Conflict between parents usually implies there are underlying issues needing resolution, not necessarily related to nursing. Parents' capacity to return to homeostasis enables them to integrate themes of sensitive parenting that evolve into a sensitive family style.

Implications for Family Systems Theory

Nursing is an important relationship that affects interaction at all levels, and interchanges in the family affect the nursing relationship. This information provides insight into the meaning of circularity in these systems, contributing to existing notions of systemic interaction (Bowen, 1978; Goldenberg & Goldenberg, 2007; Kerr & Bowen, 1988; Nichols & Schwartz, 2006). There are families that nurse in tune with physiological principles (WHO, 1981, 2001, 2003), and there are distinct family processes associated with nursing. Families nursing in tune with physiology display unique themes affecting and influenced by their nursing behaviors. The likelihood that there is an association between physiologically based nursing and specific family processes is reinforced further by descriptions of families whose breastfeeding patterns deviate from physiologically based principles and whose family themes and behaviors differ from the families nursing in tune with physiology.

Family themes associated with nursing include reverence for natural processes, respect for children and their unique rhythm, views of nursing as an encompassing relationship, and admiration of nursing and responsiveness. There are obstacles that interfere with some families' capacities to retain essential themes and associated behaviors. Common cultural precepts associated with artificial feeding, such as views of nursing as feeding, appear to impede nursing and associated behaviors. These insights imply that interaction associated with nursing is facilitated by certain themes and hampered by concepts that obstruct nursing.

Families internalize and transfer themes and behaviors associated with nursing through complex processes, including observations, discussions, and tutoring. Additional information showing that families transfer themes to the next generation concurs with theories that family interaction is affected by the intergenerational transmission of family themes and patterns (Bowen, 1978; Kerr & Bowen, 1988). However, this issue was not addressed in depth, suggesting a need for further research in this area.

Our understanding of the interaction in families engaging in physiologically based nursing patterns contributes to existing notions about the family life cycle, especially regarding the stage of transition to parenthood and the parenting of young children (Belsky & Kelly, 1994; Carter & McGoldrick, 2005; Cowan & Cowan, 1999). Families demonstrate that themes associated with nursing affect and are influenced by transitions in the family life cycle. There seems to be specific phases of family development associated with nursing. Movement from phase to phase is associated with child development and related changes in nursing behaviors. Thus nursing families go through unique transitional stages, reflecting themes associated with the changing status of the nursing subsystem.

Themes associated with nursing resonate in the steps that families take to accommodate the changing needs of the nursing unit. Families create boundaries limiting membership in the nursing subsystem to mothers and nursing children, enabling the nursing subsystem to engage in exclusive tasks. Families modify their boundaries, roles, and tasks to mirror the changing nursing system. Boundaries between members of the nursing subsystem and others eventually vanish, as do the distinctions between parents' roles and tasks. Hence, flexibility is an important aspect of the family organization in nursing systems.

Congruent with existing literature, families engaging in physiologically based nursing display specific proximity behaviors (La Leche League, 2004; Liedloff, 1985; McKenna, 1996; Montagu, 1978). It seems there is a unique developmental trajectory of proximity behaviors that concurs with the development of family themes related to nursing. In addition, physical closeness seems to function as a tool, advancing children's relational developmental with the mother and others. Furthermore, proximity behaviors are temporary, reflecting parents' capacity to follow children's leads and implement behaviors suiting their children's individual rhythm.

Parenting based on children's leads is a salient behavior in families nursing in tune with physiology. This behavior is a fundamental aspect of the nursing relationship and facilitates the development of cue-based interactions immediately following children's birth. Nursing, therefore, serves as the initial context for sensitive parenting interactions. Cue-based parenting during nursing evolves into a general style of attuned parenting. Reverence for cue-based nursing is transmitted through the system and evolves into general family themes of responsiveness. Nursing seems to be an important context for the development and enhancement of sensitive parenting and a sensitive family style.

Summary

Interactions in the nursing sub-system are affected by and influence family interchanges. Nursing is associated with specific themes that sustain the development of interchanges in the nursing sub-system. Themes and interaction lead to the development of sensitive interactions in the nursing sub-system that ripple through the family facilitating the development of an attuned family style.

Implications for Existing Literature on Nursing Families

The information presented in this book concurs with many descriptions of nursing in lay literature and research on nursing families discussed in the section on literature in chapter one (Ball, 2002; Bar-Yakov, 2002; Bumgarner, 2000; Granju & Kennedy, 1999; Green, 2001; La Leche League, 2004; Sears, 1988; Stein et al., 2002). This book adds that there are psychological reasons for nursing patterns and associated behaviors. In addition, it seems that several findings on physiologically based weaning processes contribute to existing notions.

Clinical Implications

Throughout the discovery of interactions at different levels of the family system, discussions pertained to interventions specific to the subsystem at hand. It is apparent that work with one unit affects clinical interventions at all levels, reinforcing the interdependence of all family subsystems. This section will provide an overview of clinical interaction, distinguishing between applications for different professional outlooks.

Clinical Work with Families

The information in this section will have relevance for those who see families presenting with breastfeeding, physical, or medical concerns, as well as those presenting with psychosocial issues. The processes are the same, although some of the tools listed might be more appropriate in one context over another. Understanding interactions in nursing families provides clinicians with novel insights about specific family processes associated with physiologically based nursing patterns that are not only functional, but also contribute to the establishment of sensitive and attuned family interactions. These novel discoveries may provide clinicians with new ways of understanding and relating to nursing families.

Misconstrued Views in the Present Findings

In the introduction, it was suggested that the nursing population is a minute faction and that clinicians might be unfamiliar with nursing systems due to their rarity. However, the findings presented in this book are based on a study conducted on a relatively large sample group, especially in light of the qualitative procedures. The similarity of the themes and practices in the relatively large sample group suggest, therefore, that the processes described are relevant for many families. Most of the themes associated with physiologically based nursing and related sensitive family style associated with nursing differ greatly from the salient cultural conceptualizations reviewed earlier. This discrepancy implies that prior to applying knowledge to work with families, one needs to look at one's reaction to the information in this book. Clinical work is advanced when one gains insight into the counter transference issues that disables one from hearing nursing families accurately. Clinicians might discuss these feelings with peers and find ways of incorporating novel concepts into existing scripts.

Along with acknowledging the existence of these salient themes, clinicians will bear in mind the role of individuality in interaction. It is important to understand families' individual styles and the meaning that family themes and processes have for the system at hand. Clinicians would best serve the needs of nursing families by learning about their reality and applying these concepts to clinical practice.

It seems that practitioners who understand and work sincerely with nursing families should focus on restoring homeostasis by referring families to the prominent themes and processes that motivate them. It is important to remember that this book indicates that themes associated with nursing enhance family sensitivity, facilitating homeostasis and growth. Clinicians should optimally help families discover the themes and patterns associated with nursing that have the most relevance for them and use these to enhance family function.

Understanding and helping families from their perspective means incorporating novel concepts of family interaction, including perspectives of family interactions. The findings implying that proximity behaviors and child-focused weaning and separation processes contribute to healthy child development suggest that all practitioners working with children should learn about this style of parenting. It seems especially important for practitioners who work with families at risk for relational difficulties to acknowledge the processes associated with nursing and to find a means of integrating some of these components into their interventions with families. The optimal understanding of nursing families might mean reframing one's view of couple interactions. Since proximity behaviors are important to these families when their children are young and seem to advance positive child outcome, clinical interventions might include helping couples find interesting ways of being together while they remain close to their children.

The clinical implications of the findings that couple and family issues affect the nursing relationship indicate that it is important to assist families that present with issues of family discord to realize the actual source of their conflict rather than scapegoat a healthy process. Although nursing might trigger anxiety, this study shows that for many families the real issues that prompt family strife actually lie beneath the surface. It is relevant to emphasize that this study found that discord related to nursing, the use of objects associated with artificial feeding, and the increased appearance of distancing behaviors, seemed to mask underlying discontent at the individual or couple level. Rather than interfering in the nursing relationship – a gesture that might actually exacerbate family tension – sensitive clinicians might try to help families retain practices that sustain them and focus on resolving the real issues that threaten family homeostasis.

It seems that by supporting this family style, practitioners facilitate optimal family function, individual growth, and healthy child development. This book provides insights that can contribute to clinicians' understanding of the processes associated with nursing. Hopefully, this will lead to more enjoyable and enhanced clinical interaction.

Breastfeeding Education

Clinicians whose focus is on teaching families about nursing may use the novel insights to alter existing teaching plans. The discovery of the themes associated with physiological nursing provides insight into factors facilitating this style of nursing, a significant finding considering that according to statistics many families deviate from physiologically based patterns (Statistics Canada, 2003). The likelihood that these family functions contribute to nursing is reinforced by findings apparent in the descriptions of families who wean early. This evidence shows that the attitudes and practices of families who wean early differ greatly from the themes and patterns associated with physiological nursing. This insight might be used to create educational programs that take families' individuality into account, while at the same time helping them develop themes and behaviors that facilitate physiologically based nursing patterns.

The findings indicate that families undergo specific stages of development associated with nursing. It seems that these stages should be taken into account when counseling parents. This study also emphasizes that there are differences between mothers' and fathers' developmental trajectories, their vulnerability to extraneous influence and couple interaction, and their ways of internalizing novel concepts. These factors should be taken into account in teaching methods. In addition, providing parents with anticipatory guidance about their differences might enrich mutual understanding between the parental couple and alleviate couple strife.

The findings that families use specific language to talk about nursing and that this seems to affect how they implement nursing and associated behaviors reinforces the importance of language use when talking about nursing. In line with existing literature (Smith, 1996; Wiessinger, 1996), this study suggests that in order to enrich family practices associated with physiological nursing, practitioners should use nursing as a term of reference and refer to it as a normal and natural behavior. Moreover, practitioners should refer to nursing as an encompassing behavior rather than as a means of feeding. Discussions regarding the various physical components and roles of nursing, and the emotionality of nursing, will facilitate future dialogue and mutual understanding between parents.

Clinical Work with Families with Risks Impeding Parenting

Nursing offers many protective factors for parents with risks that impede their ability to interact with their children in a sensitive manner. Risks that impede the development of attuned parenting styles include, but are not limited to parental reasons such as a history of impaired interaction, experiences with maltreatment or trauma, physical or mental ailments, addictions, reduced parental support, and teenaged parenting. Child factors include perceived difficult temperament and parents' attributions of child behavior (Landy & Menna, 2006). Socioeconomic status is often listed as an important risk factor (Bronfenbrenner, 1979; Landy & Menna, 2006); however, it is important to note that parents with higher social status might also have any of the listed risk factors. Risk factors impede one's ability to attune to one's child, so it is important to find means of facilitating nursing and associated paths to sensitive parenting for parents enduring risk factors.

Unfortunately, many clinicians abide by the myth that nursing increases parenting risks and is difficult for parents who are already dealing with many stresses. This myth likely stems from a misunderstanding of the physiological and emotional attributes of nursing. In addition, clinicians might perceive nursing as difficult due to the prevalence of nursing problems caused by impediments discussed in chapters three and four. Furthermore, many clinicians are not aware of the contribution of nursing to the development of sensitive parenting styles.

A recent study negates these views. This research indicates that breastfeeding seems to be a protective factor reducing the risk of maternal maltreatment, especially neglect (Strathearn, Mamun, Najman & O'Callaghan, 2009). The researchers suggested that the oxytocin released during nursing helps mothers regulate their behaviors by elevating maternal mood and decreasing maternal stress and anxiety.

The findings that interactions during and associated with physiologically based nursing contribute to the development of sensitivity reinforce that nursing likely plays an important role in reducing the risk of child maltreatment. Nursing provides parents with a tangible means of practicing, observing, reading, interpreting, and responding to infant cues. This built in characteristic of nursing is significant for parents who have never been listened to in their lives, are not cognizant of an empathetic style of interaction, and are not aware that infants display cues. In some cases, clinicians might draw parents' attention to this aspect of nursing, while simultaneously explaining the meaning of infant cues during and beyond nursing. Allowing parents to experience reading cues and to receive feedback might be a new and meaningful experience. Next clinicians may guide parents and use the cues and infant feedback as tools for teaching. For example, therapists might use a Vygotskian approach (Wertsh, 1985) and gently scaffold parents' development as they tutor them about how to observe, read, interpret, and respond to cues for nursing. This teaching concept is similar to existing interventions that use spontaneous interaction as a therapeutic context to enrich parent-infant or child interaction (Cohen et al., 2000; Trad, 1992).

Nursing also facilitates the development of attuned parenting by enriching parents' personal scripts and their sense of self. In circular fashion, parents' internalized sense of efficacy increases parents' capacity to tolerate parenting and enriches their ability to continue to meet needs. One can't emphasize enough how important this factor is for parents who have endured trauma and life events that have reduced their self-esteem. For many, nursing might be an important step towards the development of good enough scripts.

In addition, it is important to remember that children contribute to interaction, and parents' attributions of their behaviors affect their responses. Parents' inability to cope with perceived incessant crying is a salient factor contributing to shaken baby syndrome (AAP, 2001). Bearing this in mind, it is easy to see how the calming effects of nursing on infants and children act as protective factors for parents at risk. In addition, it is important to remember that physiological nursing enables infants to develop normally in contrast with unnecessary illness and accompanying distressful behaviors associated with artificial feeding.

An important clinical intervention regarding work with parents presenting with risks is first of all to alter the existing view that hampers clinical support for nursing. The facilitative components of nursing are significant and important. Clinicians should teach parents about breastfeeding and encourage their efforts to nurse in a physiologically based manner. Naturally, parents presenting with multiple risk factors will require additional support during their nursing experience. By the same token, clinicians will require optimal containing from their colleagues.

Clinical Work with Adoptive Families

Adoptive nursing is referred to on several occasions in this book and case examples are provided. Nursing is a facilitative measure enhancing interaction and family connection. It seems that nursing helps families feel they are getting back on track after experiencing a sense of loss and abnormality associated with infertility or recurrent pregnancy dysfunction.

Nursing seems to be especially important for mothers and has important reparative factors that help mothers fix some of the perceived damage associated with infertility. This theme is associated with reverence for physiological processes. The good enough feelings of repair that mothers internalize through nursing facilitate the development of sensitive interactions with their adopted children.

Once again, primary obstacles in clinical practice are the myths surrounding adoption and nursing. The first step is to realize that this is a possibility for adoptive families. It is important to note that the degree and quality of the physiological nursing relationship may vary from family to family. In all cases, it is important to help families celebrate the parts of nursing that work for them and to acknowledge loss. The role of the clinician is to help families frame the experience in a way that has meaning for them.

Chapter 14
Conclusions

This aim of this book is to provide clinicians with insight into interactions in nursing families as a means of enhancing practice with these families. The data are based on findings from an original study on systemic interaction in nursing families (Epstein-Gilboa, 2006). The study took individuality into account, while also finding some common features in the families. It is apparent that nursing contributes to the systemic interaction in families and vice versa. Mothers and nurslings engage in intricate interactions that affect, and are influenced by, overall family interaction. Interactions associated with nursing are based on children's cues, leading to the development of sensitive mothering and fathering styles. Sensitive parenting associated with nursing facilitates the development of sensitive family interactions that reverberate throughout the system, fortifying interactions in the nursing unit and perpetuating the cycle of sensitive interchanges.

Sensitive interaction in nursing subsystems and in their families is influenced by several interconnected themes circulating in the system. Salient themes include reverence for physiological processes; perspectives of nursing as a normal physiological process; respect for children's needs, individual rhythms, and communication signals; views of nursing as an encompassing behavior inclusive of emotional elements; esteem for reciprocal communication; and mutual respect for individuals' unique characteristics and rates of development. Several of these themes are established prior to nursing, others stem from experiences associated with nursing, and all themes are refined as they circulate throughout the system.

The circularity of family themes and patterns facilitates the establishment of the sensitive family style through nursing. Themes of reverence for physiology enable parents to initiate and establish nursing, seen as a normal step following birth and part of the continuum of naturally occurring processes. Reverence for physiology and related behaviors are associated with themes of respect for children's naturally occurring needs and signals, facilitating the development of a cue-based nursing cycle. Consequently, families allow infants to nurse frequently, helping to establish notions of nursing as an encompassing experience inclusive of several physical and emotional functions. This view reverberates back to the nursing subsystem and reinforces the practice of nursing frequently. Frequent nursing sessions provide parents and children with ample opportunities to fortify themes and practice sensitive interchanges.

Patterns and themes associated with nursing extend to other aspects of interaction with the nursing child and remain salient over time, suggesting that physiologically based nursing is accompanied by specific behaviors that mirror children's needs. Children's needs for proximity are noted and responded to in the same sensitive way that the family responds to nursing. In between nursing, children remain proximal to their mothers, including at night, and family co-sleeping arrangements are common during early childhood. Proximity behaviors help infants learn about relationships and help them transfer feelings about the breast to the mother. The high degree of family tactile and proximity behaviors helps children transfer feelings from the mother to other family members. Thus tactile interactions and proximity behaviors facilitate the development of relationships between children and individuals in the family.

Families alter interactional elements to suit children's novel developmental capacities. This indicates that families remain loyal to the themes established through nursing, namely meeting children's needs and following their unique rhythms. This process helps parents accept children's gradual need for weaning. Although most children nurse into early childhood, the exact timing that weaning takes place depends on the degree of child-led processes and maternal contributions. The most common form of full weaning takes place between the ages of three to five years and is a combination of mainly child-focused processes influenced by minimal maternal contributions.

Nursing and associated behaviors occur frequently alongside additional family activities over long periods of time. Families are able to tolerate, foster, and internalize the themes and patterns associated with nursing due to specific processes. These processes include direct observation of nursing, an act reinforcing one's experience with nursing and contributing to the formation of ideas about relationships. Additional processes include open communication, modeling, discussions, emulating interactions associated with nursing, and flexible systemic interchanges. All of these processes fortify the nursing unit and overall system, and perpetuate themes of sensitivity.

Each family member internalizes sensitivity and other themes associated with nursing differently. Through their sensitive experiences as nurslings, children internalize views of nursing as normal and retain a sense that breasts are relational objects. With these ideas in mind, children contribute to family themes regarding natural processes and nursing. Interactions during nursing also instill a sense of well being and a positive view of self in relation to others. Through nursing and associated behaviors, children are provided with tools for interaction and a sense that relationships with others are worthwhile, enriching children's capacity to contribute to a sensitive family context. The recurring experience of observing nursing helps older children reflect on their own former experiences and reverberate sensitive behaviors in their interactions.

Mothers complement child and family development by engaging with their children in attuned interactions during and beyond nursing. The themes, patterns, and specific behaviors associated with nursing provide mothers with tools for sensitive mothering styles. They learn how to be sensitive to their children's needs by responding to cues for nursing and interacting with their children during nursing. The lessons learned through these interactions help mothers develop attuned mothering styles that they display in between and beyond nursing. The frequency of nursing and associated proximity behaviors provides mothers with ample opportunities to refine their attuned style. The themes of patient and responsive mothering that mothers internalize through nursing are reinforced by family themes, providing additional incentives to practice patient and tolerant interchanges with children over time.

Nursing is also a context that fulfills mothers' emotional and developmental needs, likely due in part to the similarity between mothers' individual scripts and family themes. This factor also contributes to the development of sensitive mothering. For many mothers, nursing provides opportunities to repair negative experiences and to actualize issues associated with their personal philosophy. Many mothers see nursing as an essential part of their natural continuum as women, a theme corresponding to reverence for natural processes. Reverence for physiology and natural processes also contribute to mothers' capacity to accept their bodies. This perspective is associated with views of breasts as multifaceted organs and contributes to mothers' capacity to respond to their children. Mothers' needs for intimacy and positive regard are facilitated through nursing. Through nursing, mothers receive positive feedback for their efforts, increasing their self-confidence and capacity to continue responding sensitively to their children. Experience in mothering also fosters mothers' processes and helps mothers cope with cultural pressure opposing nursing, especially pressure to separate from children. The context of nursing meets mothers' individual needs and when mothers, in turn, feel filled up by nursing and comfortable with the experience, they continue to engage in interactions that contribute to the development of maternal attunement. Interactions during nursing contribute to the development of maternal sensitivity, an important developmental task facilitating children's capacity to see the world in a positive way and to relate to others in a secure manner. Due to their own experiences, mothers perpetuate themes and patterns associated with nursing, and transfer these systemic elements to the system, including to fathers.

Fathers integrate sensitive behaviors by supporting and interacting with the nursing subsystem. They develop attuned responsiveness by matching supportive actions to the needs of the nursing subsystem much like the way mothers internalize sensitivity to children's cues by reading and responding to infant cues regarding nursing. Fathers' supportive behaviors change over time in tune with the evolving needs of the subsystem, and include direct care of the mother and children. Although fathers initially have less direct interactions with their infants than mothers do, they nevertheless engage in some direct interactions right from the start. Opportunities for interaction with babies increase as children grow, and fathers' interactions mirror the sensitive elements of mother-infant interaction associated with nursing.

Fathers also contribute to interactions between the nursing subsystem, and the response of the nursing sub-unit reverberates back to fathers, reinforcing the cycle. Interaction with the nursing subsystem contributes to fathers' understanding and mutual ownership of themes associated with nursing, advancing paternal sensitivity and nursing processes. Like mothers, fathers' emotional needs are fulfilled by their interactions regarding nursing, promoting further the development of paternal sensitivity. The nursing relationship also triggers conflict for fathers and impairs supportive actions when fathers feel overwhelmed by maternal pain, perceive that they are helpless, feel that they are unable to protect members of the nursing unit, and are overcome by feelings of envy. Paternal envy of the relationship between mothers and nurslings is normal, and envy only impairs paternal and family development if it remains unresolved. The resolution of difficult issues advances paternal development and helps fathers reverberate family themes and patterns of sensitivity.

While fathers' and mothers' trajectories are different, they eventually develop similar attuned behaviors promoting sensitive family interchanges. Maternal and paternal function affects and is influenced by their interactions as a couple. An important strength of the parental couple is their ability to integrate, respect, and utilize their distinct biological and gender-based characteristics as a means of reaching mutual family goals associated with nursing. Couple interactions that promote nursing and contingent sensitive patterns are positively affected by open communication, shared reverence for family themes, and mutual respect of each parents' needs and unique features. Associated facilitative couple patterns include their system of gender-distinct and complementary parenting task allocation that changes to reflect children's evolving needs.

Complementary interactions between parents are affected by and reinforce family themes and patterns associated with the establishment of sensitive parenting styles through nursing. Parents' distinct and gender-based development is apparent in their interactions with one another. Mothers transfer themes of sensitivity and attuned practices to the father by modeling and tutoring fathers. Fathers follow their partners and mirror attuned parenting with the children, while at the same time, supporting mothering behaviors.

In contrast, the circularity of themes, patterns, and specific behaviors associated with nursing and sensitive parenting are obstructed when parents' attitudes counter those that support nursing. Salient themes that contradict behaviors associated with nursing are: nursing is a means of infant feeding, couple precedence, discomfort with maternal/child closeness, and emphasis on apparent child independence. These views reflect external cultural themes. Parents are most vulnerable to external influence when they have minimal parenting experience and when there are unresolved issues at the couple level. Fathers are more vulnerable to cultural influence than are mothers. In addition, it is easier to alter dissonance stemming from cognitive sources than it is to resolve issues stemming from relational issues.

Unresolved conflict at the couple level stems from practices associated with couple interaction. Couples with closed communication patterns and without means of repairing conflict are most susceptible to couple strife that impairs nursing. Discord between parents seems to be associated with parental views of nursing as feeding and the use of objects other than nursing to pacify a baby. Disagreements about nursing often mask underlying couple and individual issues that are the real reasons for the conflict.

The capacity of couples to restore homeostasis and to integrate themes and patterns that facilitate physiologically based nursing and contingent responsiveness is dependent on the quality of reparative measures at this level of family interaction. Couples restore homeostasis and return to responsive interchanges by enabling members to communicate and receive validation for their feelings, and also by engaging in compensatory and reparative actions. Couples' capacity to effectively guard and when needed reinstate homeostasis concurs with active parenting. Parents of infants and young children rarely leave their children. Yet parents report that they enjoy satisfying couple interchanges, including sexual intimacy, despite the ongoing presence of their children.

The ongoing closeness between parents, nurslings, and older children contributes to interactions in the sibling subsystem. Much like the way that parents echo and are influenced by themes and patterns associated with nursing, siblings also resonate these systemic elements. Responsive interchanges between siblings reflect each child's individual experiences of nursing, observations of ongoing interactions associated with nursing, parental modeling, and discussions that further reinforce family themes and patterns. Siblings reinforce existing themes and patterns stemming from nursing through their interactions with one another and with the family as a whole.

Themes and patterns associated with nursing enhance individual and subsystemic development and the capacity of members to interact with one another in a sensitive manner. These factors strengthen interactions in the nursing subsystem and the cycle continues. Mothers learn about sensitive and child-paced interactions through their direct experiences with nursing. Fathers and children observe nursing sessions and internalize associated messages. Watching and supporting nursing contributes to the other family members' existing scripts of nursing and interactions that they internalized either as former nurslings or as supportive fathers. These family members reverberate the themes and copy the behaviors, facilitating nursing and reinforcing the system and individual development. This experience contributes to the overall sensitive style.

The cycle of resonating themes and patterns associated with nursing extends beyond infancy, early childhood, and weaning and leads to the establishment and refinement of sensitive family interactions that last over time. Long term observations of older children and adult children of nursing families point to the resilience of associated family themes that reinforce the attuned cycle. Evidence suggests that nursing families reverberate themes of reverence for natural processes when they support natural birth and nursing processes, refer to nursing as a normal behavior, and create family environments that facilitate physiologically based nursing behaviors and patterns. In addition, older children retain views of the breast as a multifaceted organ and not just as a sexual object. Respect for family members' needs resemble reverence for infant and children's needs for nursing. The theme of respect for all family members suggests that present day nursing families resonate the historically based association between respect for women and children and physiologically based patterns of maternal nursing. Reverence for individual rhythm is evident in ongoing family patterns of support for children's individual developmental trajectories, including when older and adult children choose paths that differ from their parents' philosophies. Families' capacity to match their responses to individual needs is also evident in the way that proximity behaviors are reduced and replaced with other means of interaction as children grow. Although family members may continue to engage in tactile interactions, the intensity of these interactions is replaced by open and validating discussions that resemble earlier interchanges between nursing units. Distancing is not a family goal, although it is fostered when it meets children's needs. Children move away gradually, boomeranging back to the family environment much like the way they weaned from the breast.

The long term implications of family interactions are evident in the extension of themes and patterns associated with nursing to realms beyond the nursing relationship and family context. Findings that older and adult children of nursing families are responsible, creative, independent, and nurturing, suggest that themes and patterns associated with nursing contribute to positive child outcome. Patterns of reciprocal communication and reverence for natural processes extend into following generations when grown children replicate themes and patterns associated with nursing with their children.

Interactions between the nursing subsystem are influenced by and affect the development of family themes that are transferred to the entire family system. The development of a sensitive family style is an important implication of this process. Sensitive interactions between the nursing mother and child are supported by the family system and by the same token these interactions generate themes and patterns of attuned responsiveness to the system. All family members and subsystems are shaped by their interchanges with the nursing subsystem, and this facilitates the transfer of sensitive components to their scripts. The themes and patterns associated with nursing facilitate the development of children's relational development, parental sensitivity, mutual couple processes, and overall sensitive family style. Sensitive interactions at the nursing subsystem level of interchange lead to the establishment of an attuned family style that has long term implications for the family, as well as for individual growth. Clinicians optimally support families in accordance with their level of development and individual needs to develop the sensitive family style associated with nursing.

Appendix A
Brief Synopses of Case Studies

Twelve families were followed in the study. This section will present a summary of the prevalent themes that were apparent in the case study analysis. This will give readers a sense of the similarities and individual meaning of themes for different family systems.

Amit Family

Overcoming Infertility, Combining Contrasting Views of Children and Parenting to Form a Cue-Based Parenting Style, Following Children's Rhythms as They Grow, and Enabling the Integration of the New Twin Nursing Subsystem

The Amit family had four children, all of whom had either nursed in the past or were nursing in the present. This family was observed longer and with more intensity than the other families. They were observed during two separate two week periods over four years. In between and after the last two week period, they were contacted by phone. The oldest child in this family, who nursed for the first two years of her life, was followed from age eight to age twelve. Her sister, who nursed for two and a half years, was observed from age four until age eight. The daughters' younger brothers were twin boys who were followed from the age of five and a half months until they were four and a quarter years old. They nursed during this entire period.

Infertility was a salient aspect of the family's history, and all of the children had been conceived through in vitro fertilization. This issue had led to conflicts between the couple regarding the number of children desired. The mother wished for many children. Her children were central to her being, and she believed that it was important to sacrifice everything for the children. The father was ambivalent about his wife's perceived all-giving approach. He often wondered if this approach to child rearing might be detrimental to his children, and at times, he perceived that the "sacrifices" that he made for his children interfered with his love of solitude and privacy. At the same time, the father also revered his wife's interactional style, admired her warm family background that differed from his apparently cold experience, and emulated her sensitivity in his interactions with the children. The couple's open communication style helped them resolve their intermittent disagreements and facilitated the implementation of a child-centered family style. This was established through cue-based nursing relationships that provided the mother with initial tools and the father a context to observe while his wife tutored him in parenting. Although the father had intermittent bouts of frustration with parenting, he gradually began to internalize his wife's child-focused approach and shared child-paced parenting strategies with his wife that were inclusive of continued proximity promoting behaviors. The existence of child-led interventions in the parents' interactions with their older children demonstrated the persistence of cue-based interventions that were established through nursing. This was indicated further by the sensitive way the older children interacted with others, especially their brothers.

Avir Family

Overcoming Difficulties and Establishing Themes of Proximity and Continued Nursing Stemming from Interactions in the Maternal Family of Origin

The Avir family had two children, both of whom had nursed or were nursing during the study. The older child was four years old and had nursed until the age of two and a half years. The younger child was observed from age seventeen to nineteen months and nursed during the study.

The mother had experienced nursing beyond infancy, child-led parenting interventions, and a warm interactional style in her family of origin. This was a salient component of the parents' narrative and both parents, especially the father whose family of origin was described as cold, attempted to emulate the mother's parents. In addition, the couple shared everything and engaged in open and supportive reciprocal interactions with one another. These factors seemed to help the young family as they coped with obstacles, including a mishandled first birthing experience described as "horrible," and most significantly, the results of errors made during a breast surgery procedure that had incapacitated one of the mother's breasts. The trauma to the mother's breast and body had a deep impact on the mother's sense of self, due to her perception that natural birth and nursing were essential components of being a woman. The couple shared the grief and the joys of overcoming obstacles to nursing as they integrated satisfying nursing relationships alongside gentle child-paced and proximity promoting interactions with their children. The sensitive interactions that were displayed by both parents with their children demonstrated the persistence of cue-based interactions commenced at the breast.

Nightingale Family

Parental Strife, Conflicting Issues, and Attempts to Perpetuate a Cue-Based Parenting Style

The Nightingale family had two children, both of whom had nursed or nursed during the study. The older child was three and a half years old and had nursed for three years. The younger child nursed during the study and was observed from four to eleven weeks of age.

Nursing in this family was set in a conflicting environment characterized by parental discord and individual ambivalence about the meaning of nursing. On one hand, the parents revered nursing as a means of optimizing the welfare of their children. They joined together in diverse and complementary roles to ensure the maintenance of nursing into early childhood. In their quest to meet their children's needs, the parents attempted to pay attention to infant-initiated cues for nursing and later to other child-initiated leads. In addition, they were open to their children's needs for physical closeness and sensitively met these needs by promoting a wide variety of proximity promoting behaviors. On the other hand, the parents' interventions regarding nursing reflected an underlying ambivalence about whether nursing constituted a form of nutrition or a mode of soothing. This was more pronounced for the father who usually disregarded the comforting elements of nursing. In addition, the parents' interactions with one another were compacted by deep differences that extended beyond disagreements about parenting. The discord between the parents was often disguised by apparent joining, when in actuality, one partner hampered the efforts of the other. This was exemplified by the way the father displayed his discomfort with the constancy of nursing by interfering with this aspect of nursing. The mother, in turn, displayed subtle gestures of anger while she also tried to appease her husband by going along with several of his measures. This pattern was also evident in the couples' interactions with their older child. Their lack of deep understanding of child development in general, as well as the mother's expressed lack of confidence in her ability to specifically understand her children effectively, seemed to have an impact on the process of child-led rearing. The influence of the confusion on the children was displayed by the way the children sometimes conveyed double messages to their environment that pointed to periodic emotional confusion. However, the capacity of the children to demonstrate confidence and comfort in relation to others indicated that despite all of the upheaval, the children felt confident enough due to the interactions that they had experienced initially at the breast.

Kinor Family

Adoptive Nursing Leads the Way to the Establishment of Intimate and Child-Paced Relationships in the Family

The Kinor family had two adopted children, both of whom had either nursed in the past or nursed during the study. The older child was five years old. He had nursed for the first two and a half years of his life. Part of that time, he had tandem nursed with his then newborn sister. The younger child nursed during the study and was observed from the age of twenty-seven months until just over two and a half years of age.

Lactation had been induced and established in anticipation of the adoption of first the older child and continued after the adoption of the second child. The trials and tribulations of adoptive nursing was facilitated by the warm, free flowing, compassionate, positively reinforcing, and mutually supportive relationship between the parents, who shared everything, including their desire to nurse their children. Although the parents noted that nursing afforded them a biological connection to their children, they downplayed this aspect of nursing and instead focused on the relational aspects of nursing as facilitative factors. The mother emphasized that nursing had provided her with a means of developing intimate and exclusive relationships with her children. Ingredients of the physically intricate nursing relationship were emulated by the father and facilitated his process of emotional attachment to his children. Together, the parents carried the physical intimacy and cue-based parenting established in nursing to other aspects of parenting. Each child's individual rhythm was respected as the parents surrounded the children with warm feedback and active listening. The children, in turn, displayed confidence and reflected their parents' warmth and free flowing communication style in their interactions with others.

Forester Family

Nursing Friendly and Child-Paced Behaviors within an Atmosphere of Ambivalence

The Forester family had two children, both of whom had nursed or were nursing during the study. The older child was six years old during the observational period. She had nursed for the first five years of her life. The younger child was nursing during the study. He was observed from eighteen to twenty-one months of age.

The role of nursing in this family was surrounded by contrasting themes. On one hand, nursing and associated proximity promoting behaviors occurred freely in an atmosphere of acceptance. On the other hand, nursing triggered ongoing disagreements and conflict between the parental couple. Although the couple shared a view that nursing was a natural aspect of life, they were in discord over the apparent long term nursing relationship, closeness between the nursing dyad, maternal preference, and apparent paternal exclusion that was associated with nursing in this family. The father blamed nursing for his apparent lack of equal standing in his children's eyes. He was especially cognizant and distressed by his seeming inability to calm his children. Although he blamed the nursing relationship for this, he concurrently downplayed the unique emotional aspects of nursing. His unresolved envy seemed to lead to contempt for the nursing relationship and associated behaviors, as well as for those who supported nursing. Parental strife regarding these issues persisted due to the closed communication style common to this couple that disallowed the disclosure of genuine feelings. Yet, the mother continued to nurse and engage in proximity behaviors that followed her children's leads. Her individual reasons included her exposure to nursing and like behaviors as a child and her determination to parent her children in a child-paced manner. The father also contributed to the perseverance of behaviors associated with nursing due to his reverence for physical interaction. This was a salient aspect of the couple relationship that contrasted with the lack of open discussions. And like his wife, the father's exposure to the nursing system enabled the development of an attuned parenting style that allowed both parents to enrich their appreciation of children's cues. This, in addition to the warmth that reverberated back to the father from the apparently secure and happy children, reduced some of the floating anxiety. The sensitivity that the children experienced initially in the nursing relationship seemed to lay the foundation for positive shared emotional experiences with others, as well as providing the children with confident outlooks.

Morgan Family

Nursing as a Means of Enriching Child Development

The Morgan family was a nursing family with two children. The older child was ten years old and had nursed for six years. The younger child was observed from four and a quarter years until she was four and a half years old. She nursed during this time.

The parents' open interaction style and joint ownership of nursing as means of enriching child development facilitated the establishment and perpetuation of nursing and associated behaviors in this family. Through nursing, the parents began a pattern of following their children's cues to determine parenting interventions, as was exemplified by child-led weaning. They gently tutored their children through child-focused interactions, as they expressed positive regard, patience, respect, and reciprocity. This style of parenting suited their joint appreciation of personal cerebral advancement, mutual caring, and practical approach to life. The children traveled through their developmental trajectories with ease. In addition to interactive abilities that reflected an underlying positive sense of self in relation to others, the children also displayed advanced developmental tasks that fulfilled family goals of child enrichment.

Florence Family

The Transition to Parenthood and Internalizing Parenting through Nursing

The Florence family had one young infant who nursed during the study and was observed from four to six and a half months of age.

This family demonstrated the complex transition to parenting and the facilitative role that nursing played in the volatile processes that accompany the transformation into a new stage of development. Nursing provided the parents with positive feedback and a sense that they were achieving their central goal of ensuring their child's welfare. Their sense of competence was enhanced by their internalization of a cue-based parenting style associated with meeting cues at the breast. The cue-based parenting style provided them with positive feedback and a sense of efficiency in parenting. This process was reinforced by the couple's open and mutually supportive interaction style. Although at times, the mother's sense of confusion regarding her growing attachment to her infant challenged the system. The strength of the feelings generated through nursing and perpetual mutual support returned the mother to homeostasis. This enabled the parents to patiently withstand the infant's behaviors by corresponding to the baby's needs for frequent contact inclusive of nursing and holding. The system was further reinforced by signs of positive child outcome that met parental goals and enhanced the perpetuation of the system of novel internalization with the inclusion of the new family member.

Ford Family

Nursing as Way of Actualizing Themes of Reverence for Natural Processes and Parenting as a Mission

The Ford family had two children who tandem nursed during the study. The older child was three years old. The younger child was observed from four to nine weeks of age.

The task of shared nursing was facilitated by the parents' highly cooperative style that enabled each partner to engage in complementary but diverse tasks. The parents in this family interacted with an open and supportive communication style. They focused on their joint aspirations to live and raise a family in accordance with natural processes that have perpetuated over time. Their serious outlook to parenting included active research and discussions about this issue. Through nursing, the parents gained additional insight into their children's natural processes, and they developed a means of following their leads accurately. They met their children's needs for physical closeness in a natural and comfortable manner. In addition, they tutored their older child in activities that matched his level of cognitive development and advanced their goal of parenting with purpose. The children approached the breast, their parents, physical interaction, and in the case of the older child, others with comfort. In addition, the older child demonstrated a capacity to cope with periodic frustrations. This seemed to imply that the parents had matched their children's natural rhythms and had tutored them in a balanced and enriching way.

Ginger Family

Overcoming Obstacles amidst a Context of High Regard for Family, Breastfeeding, and Closeness

The Ginger family was a breastfeeding family with three children, all of whom had nursed or nursed during the study. The oldest child was eleven years old. She had nursed for a year. The next child was seven years old and had nursed for two years. The youngest child was three years old and nursed during the study.

The children, like their parents, highly revered nursing and spoke about the current nursing relationship in an admirable manner. The way that all family members joined forces regarding nursing was typical of family behaviors whose ultimate themes were family centrality, reverence for the mother-infant bond, admiration for closeness, and respect for natural processes. Family discourse mirrored function in the parent subsystem and was open and validating. This seemed to enrich the family's capacity to cope with threats to their homeostasis, as was exemplified by nursing difficulties in the first nursing experiences, and most significantly, when the mother fell seriously ill following the birth of the third child. With the father in the leading role, nursing was reinstated following the initial health crisis. Nursing was perceived as a desperately needed relational tool for the mother whose sense of connection to her newly born child had been hampered by her illness. Following joint parental efforts, the newly repaired nursing relationship was interpreted as satisfying and healing as the previous nursing relationships had been. Through nursing, the parents internalized a cue-based parenting style inclusive of immense physical interaction during and in between nursing sessions. Their joy of parenting and family persisted as they raised their children in the same cue-based fashion that they had internalized through nursing. The children's confidence and their interactive qualities in and outside the realm of the family indicated that they retained the sensitive style beyond the folds of the cherished family context.

Mitchell Family

Overcoming Infertility, Medical Challenges, and Developing Warm Nursing Relationships Inclusive of Toddler Nursing and Tandem Twin Nursing

The Mitchell family had three children. The oldest child was five years old and had nursed for three and a half years. The twin boys tandem nursed and were observed from eleven months until just after their first birthdays.

The couple treasured their children, who had all been conceived through various forms of in vitro fertilization after years of infertility. The parents had supported one another during these challenges with their open, supportive, and cooperative style. This facilitated the repair of an initially damaged nursing relationship with the older child. Through this relationship, the parents developed a cue-based parenting style inclusive of child-led weaning and behavior that promoted proximity. The parents were challenged once again when they were provided with devastating and inaccurate information about the twins' health during the pregnancy and following their birth. Initially, this information hampered the function of the parents' mutual support system; however, after they had both assimilated the information, they returned to homeostasis. They shared a process of ensuring optimal development for the twins through the warm child-centered nursing relationship and associated interventions that mirrored the proximity aspects of the first nursing relationship. The tandem-nursed twins responded to their patient environment by developing in an age appropriate manner that surpassed and discounted the ill bill of health they had been given by medical professionals. As the parents withstood the challenges of parenting active nursing twins, they applied the same cue-based parenting style to their interactions with their older child. This child's ability to tolerate feelings of ambivalence towards the twins and to interact with them in a nurturing fashion demonstrated the enduring effects of the former nursing relationship and associated parenting. Similarly, the positive feelings displayed by the twins indicated that they, too, were sustained by the positive essence of the nursing relationship.

Peters Family

Rebuilding Scripts of Parenting, Altering Lifestyles, and Building a Highly Responsive Child-Centered System Inclusive of Tandem Nursing

This family had three children. The oldest child was eight years old during the study and had nursed for four years. The next child was four years old and tandem nursed with her younger sibling, who was observed from eighteen to twenty months of age.

Nursing was a central event in this family that contributed to significant changes in parental scripts and role allocation. The couple's open communication style and shared, but complementary division of labor accompanied family processes. The first nursing experience and associated feelings of closeness generated new found feelings for the mother that led to her eventual departure from her full time high powered job following the birth of the second child. The father, who was influenced by the sensitivity intrinsic to nursing, supported this move. This enabled the mother to fully implement the cue-based parenting style, as well as the proximity behaviors associated with nursing and to respond to her children on a full time basis. The child-led interventions included child-initiated weaning from the breast and the family. While the father played a different role in this process, he proudly worked with his wife to facilitate the integration of tandem nursing and extended co-sleeping into their family lifestyle. Like their parents, the older children actively participated in a system that emulated cue-based nursing and was based on responsiveness to others. The children's relational capacities and the older child's positive outlook and success with developmental tasks outside of the home point to the maintaining elements of the responsive parenting style.

Stevens Family

The Transition to Parenthood and Establishing a Cue-Based Parenting System through Nursing

The Steven's family had one young nursing toddler who was observed from twenty-two to twenty-four months of age.

A prominent theme for this family, especially the mother, was the actualization of a stable and cohesive family system. This was facilitated by the couple's mutual and open communication that was inclusive of task sharing. Nursing fit well into their conceptions of family due to the congruence of nursing with family closeness. In addition, the nursing relationship allowed the mother to actualize her prior dreams of parenting in a cue-based and child-centered manner. The father followed suit, albeit with some initial apprehension, and the family established patterns inclusive of full-time mothering, nursing dyad centrality, mother-child proximity, and child-led weaning from the breast, as well as the mother. These patterns both encouraged and were enhanced by the mother's change of heart and her decision to forfeit full-time employment to take up full time mothering. Similarly, the father underwent changes as he internalized a sensitive fathering style that mirrored his wife's warm and responsive tone. This context nurtured the toddler who demonstrated a high level of positive affect, adept relational tools, and a confident world view.

Appendix B
Example of One Case Study

This family was followed over a four year period and will give the readers an opportunity to see how nursing and associated family themes develop over time.

Description of the Amit Family

Nursing Twins in the Present and the Long Term Trajectory of Children who Nursed in the Past

The Amit family consisted of two parents, Sara and Joseph, and their four children. The older children were Anna and Merry, who were followed from the age of eight until twelve years of age and four until eight years of age, respectively. The two younger children were the nursing twins, David and Adam, who were followed from five and half months of age until they were four and a half years old.

The mother, Sara, was in her forties, with two undergraduate university degrees in related fields of health and social welfare. Until the twins reached one year of age, Sara pursued full time mothering. When the twins were one year old, she commenced a Master's degree in a related field that she fulfilled on a casual basis. When the twins were three years old, Sara also added part-time work to her schedule. Sara insisted that her mothering role was her first priority.

Joseph was the father in the Amit family. He was in his forties and had a post graduate degree in a healthcare field. Joseph was the primary financial provider in this family during the observations.

The Process of Observations and Follow-up

This family was observed for two intensive two week periods while they resided in my home. The first observational period commenced when the twins were five and a half months old, and the second observational period occurred three years later. In between and after the visits, the family was followed up by periodic phone conversations that averaged from once every two weeks to several times a week.

The twins continued to nurse throughout the study. One weaned at four years and four months, and the other twin weaned approximately one month later. In addition, nursing had been a common aspect of family life in this family since the birth of the two older children, who had nursed into their third years of life. The older children had apparently nursed in a similar manner to their brothers, although they weaned much earlier than their brothers. The information about past nursing experiences provided insight into possible trajectories of the nursing relationship in the future. Hence, following this family provided information about the contingent circular relationship between a nursing subsystem and the family system over time.

Family Themes and Patterns

Couple History

Sara and Joseph were a married couple who had been together for sixteen years when the study commenced. Right from the beginning, the couple noted their differences. Sara was warm, friendly, and communicated openly with others, reflecting themes and patterns in her family of origin. Joseph interacted with others in a contrasting manner and wanted to alter the closed communication style that he claimed stemmed from his experiences in his family of origin. Sara matched her partner's wish to change by patiently tutoring him, while also acknowledging his needs for solitude. Free flowing discourse enabled the couple to integrate disjointed parenting themes and continually make compromises for one another that accommodated their partner's changing needs. Evidence that pointed to the efficiency of open communication between the parents during the study, for example, was demonstrated by the similarity in the parents' separate narratives.

Nursing History

First Nursing Experience

The couple's validating communication style helped them endure eight long years of infertility and contingent invasive treatments until Anna was finally born. Sara repeatedly emphasized that she appreciated finally becoming a mother and that nursing was synonymous with motherhood. Anna was exclusively nursed for six months, never had a pacifier or bottle, and continued to nurse until just after her second birthday.

Sara's description of the first nursing experience demonstrated that it set the tone for the style of mother-infant relationships that were typical in this family. "I would never let her be alone for a moment. I nursed her all day and all night long. When she wasn't nursing, I would be with her." Sara claimed that her commitment to follow nature and meet her child's needs enabled her to withstand cultural pressure to distance herself from her baby.

Even though Joseph supported exclusive nursing, he was often skeptical about the intensity of the mother-infant relationship. As was usual for this couple, Sara understood her husband and explained his attitude. She said, "Before Anna was born, Joseph …did not know anything about children…it was very important for him to be very involved, but he did not know how to speak or interact with a baby… he saw the care of a newborn as task oriented. Joseph changed diapers, dressed, and bathed the baby in a precise manner. He was very concerned with completing these tasks properly. He thought that the care of a child should be an orderly and organized event that involved minimal time. He always used to say to me 'I don't understand why it takes so much time and never ends.' It was also very important for Joseph to have time to himself. He enjoyed quiet time reading or working on his own and becoming a parent interfered with that."

Joseph's narrative provided additional insight into his process. "I learned everything I know from Sara…I would see Sara lying beside the babies (meaning the first two children), nursing them, hugging them, and holding them…" Sara's narrative provided insight into the themes that nursing highlighted for Joseph. "Nursing was a serious role model…. (It showed that) you don't leave a child! You are always with your child! You pick the baby up all of the time. You have to meet all of the child's needs…You have to fully devote yourself to the child…You do not go and find someone else to do this…I couldn't let anyone else do this for my child and I think that that is what Joseph saw." Yet, it seemed that Joseph's process was complicated by ambivalence. He said, "I saw how she (Sara) sacrificed as mother and so I learned that to be a parent is to sacrifice. I saw how Sara always answered the babies. I saw how she was always with them and she never went out… You have to sacrifice a lot to bring up children! You always have to do things for them, and there is little time to pursue individual projects…It was very hard for me to not have any time for myself." Despite the difficulties, proof of Joseph's growing ownership of sensitive parenting was illustrated in his stated acceptance of Anna's needs to nurse in a frequent manner, as well as the way that he gradually copied aspects of nursing in his interchanges with her. He held her, carried her, shared his bed with his child, and welcomed Anna on all family outings, including distant travel. Sara claimed that Anna's positive regard for Joseph also enriched the father-daughter relationship. She laughed as she described how Anna often asked her mother to leave her alone with her dad. Joseph smiled as he recalled: "She liked to be with me. She still likes to be with me and to be like me." The child's warm relationship with both parents continued after the nursing relationship ended abruptly just after Anna turned two years old. She suddenly refused to nurse when she succumbed to an acute illness that entailed hospitalization. Sara claimed that the advocacy role that she had developed as a nursing mother had enabled her to protect her child during this ordeal. At this time, Sara also contemplated returning to fertility treatments. When her daughter regained her strength and asked to nurse, Sara gently refused. She explained, "I was afraid that twenty years from now they would discover that fertility treatments had an effect on nursing children, so I did not want to take a chance... I really did not feel that I had a choice...I told Anna that I was taking medicine and that my milk had dried up. As far as I remember, she accepted this with ease. But it is very important that I also stayed near her...I stayed by her to make up for weaning."

Second Nursing Experience: Merry Joined the Family

After a few courses of infertility treatments, Merry was born when Anna was three and a half years old. Even though Joseph continued to yearn for sole time, he was more prepared for the constant nature of parenthood this time around. He efficiently tended to household duties, sensitively looked after his older daughter, assisted with the care of the second child, and provided support to Sara. Joseph's support of nursing was most important when sore and bleeding nipples, as well as two bouts of mastitis, complicated nursing for over a month. Sara emphatically claimed that she had been determined to nurse, although she added, "You know I am not sure that if this was my first child, I would have been able to get through that difficult period and to continue nursing. It was so difficult!" She stated that the most significant factor that enabled her to sustain nursing was her belief that nursing was a necessary component of her optimal role of meeting her children' needs.

The problems eventually cleared up and a satisfying cue-based nursing relationship was established. Like her sister, Merry nursed exclusively until age six months and never used a pacifier or bottle during her entire nursing experience. Sara claimed that this child's needs for closeness were more intense than her sister's needs had been at the same age, and that she nursed and clung to her mother incessantly. According to the mother, Merry retained her strong need for physical contact with her mother, even after she weaned from the breast. As was common for this mother, Sara accepted and fulfilled her daughter's needs willingly. This was illustrated by the way that the Sara wore Merry in a sling until she was at least one year old and took her with her to the university while she completed her second bachelor's degree.

Similar to the first nursing experience, Sara's desire for more children and fear that fertility drugs might harm her child caused her to expedite the weaning process when Merry was two and a half years old. With ambivalence in her voice, Sara recounted that she told her daughter a story that matched the one that was told to her older sister. The mother also emphasized that she continued to hold, co-sleep, and emotionally support her daughter through the weaning process that apparently passed with ease.

Present Nursing Subsystem

Nursing when the Twins were Infants

Sara's decision to start fertility treatments that preceded the birth of the twins was complicated by Joseph's disagreement about this decision. The father explained: "After Anna and then Merry, I didn't want any more children. Two was enough for me. I resisted and then I gave in. I saw that it was very important for Sara." Sara emphasized how much she appreciated her husband's "sacrifice." With humor in her voice, she said, "Imagine Joseph did not even want to have more children and here we found out that we were having twins! I think that he was worried about how we were going to manage with four children." Joseph added that he had also been extremely anxious about the twins' health and the birth throughout the pregnancy. To his relief, the non-medicated birth occurred in a normal fashion with minimal intervention, and the fraternal twins, Adam and David, were healthy. When they were born, Anna was seven years old and her sister Merry was exactly four years old.

This nursing relationship solidified Sara's compassion for nursing. When the twins were a few months old, she said, "Nursing and mothering are connected, and it is hard to separate the two aspects of parenting. The nursing relationship helps mothers love their children and is a special way to form a unique bond with them. Nursing is everything! It is much more than food or immune substance...Nursing is a holistic way of interacting with my children. Nursing is one of the many things that you do... (it) is another link on the chain of events...part of a continuum of sensitive and warm parenting... a wonderful way to meet their (children's) needs. Nursing is an important part of how I parent after the older children weaned. That is why nursing is so important. It is a way that you can meet all of your child's needs when they are small and many of their needs when they get older...No one can meet a child's needs the way a parent can! Parents are responsible for their children's needs!"

Similar to the previous nursing relationships, the twins and their mother remained proximal to one another most of the time and nursed in frequent bouts. Sara's accepting attitude was illustrated in her comments, "I don't know (how often they nurse), I don't time them." Observations indicated that for most of their first year of life, the twins nursed at least once every hour during the day and were slightly more spread out during the night. The length of nursing sessions altered and reflected the infants' cues. Several of the nursing sessions were short quick meetings with mom and other nursing sessions were lengthy. According to Sara, this pattern had been established at birth and resembled the manner in which she had nursed her older children.

Usually Sara tried to nurse her twins separately in order to provide them with individual attention. Joint nursing sessions occurred when one twin cued to nurse before his brother terminated a nursing session or on rare occasions when both infants cued to nurse simultaneously. Shared nursing sessions were most common in the middle of the night.

Also, like with her older children, until the twins were mobile, Sara tended to hold the babies or remain proximal to them in between nursing sessions. She explained the logistics, "I sit on the floor with them. I nurse one and the other twin is beside us on the floor as we all sit together."

Mother-infant proximity included co-sleeping with the babies at night in the parental bed. Sara explained, "Joseph always slept with me and the older children when they were babies. This never interfered with his sleep... Whenever they would wake up, I would move them closer to me and nurse them. This was more difficult with two babies, so we decided that we would all be more comfortable if Joseph left the bed. I thought that he would get more sleep that way. The bed was very crowded. Merry would also sometimes join us in the middle of the night. Joseph easily agreed to sleep on the coach. I think that he likes this arrangement." Joseph confirmed this. "Why should that (sleeping in another location) bother me? I like it. I have space. It is more comfortable that way. I have more room."

This pattern continued until the twins were approximately one year old. At that time, Sara decided that it was unhealthy for the daughters to see their parents sleeping separately. Joseph, reluctantly at first, rejoined his sons and wife in bed. The family placed another mattress by the bed in order to make more room.

The Establishment of Communication through Nursing

Observations of the presenting nursing system provided insight into the way that nursing enriched the open communication pattern in this family. First of all, the majority of early relational experiences between parents and the new child occurred during or pertaining to nursing due to the prominence of this developmental task in early life. This provided the parents with ample experiences at reading, interpreting, and responding to infant-generated cues.

In infancy, the twins often cued for nursing through whining sounds exemplified by "uu uu uu uu" sounds. Sara always responded immediately to the cues with verbal reassurance, a warm smile, visual regard, touch, proficient latching, and expressions of positive regard. For example, in a loving tone, she said, "You are so handsome!" In addition she mirrored their intentions, "Do you want mommy? Do you want tzi tzi (titty)?" The twins reciprocated their mother's positive tone with excited body language, vocalizations that peaked as they approached the breast, and the immediate cessation of whining when they latched onto the breast. The excited tone of the initiation stage of nursing contrasted with the relaxed way the infants terminated their sessions, either by falling asleep at the breast or by calmly letting go of the breast as they looked around.

Interactions during nursing sessions were also characterized by reciprocal expressions of positive affect. Exchanges included mutual regard and touch. Sara frequently groomed her twins as she nursed them. Sara recurrently spoke to, as well as about, her twins in a warm and loving way, mixed with humour. She called her twins by numerous nicknames that she spontaneously made up. She often complimented them on their physical attributes and their behavior. The tone she used was always very calm, and she frequently laughed or smiled as she spoke to them.

Example of Nursing Session at Age Five and a Half Months

A morning nursing session exemplified many of the nursing episodes that occurred during the day and took place after Sara's arms had remained vacant for only fifteen minutes. David awoke from a brief rest beside his mother and cued to nurse. The mother immediately brought him close to her breast as she told him how handsome he was. She reassured the whining baby, "Okay my little bambooni, here is the "tzi tzi" (titty). David muttered quick sounding "uu uu uu" sounds as he was positioned near the breast. He quickly pulled the breast far back into his widely opened mouth. As he began to suckle, he touched his mother's breast and moved his legs in light circular movements against his mother's giving body.

The baby nursed with long deep suckles. His eyes were open and he watched his mother. While he suckled deeply, he moved his hand in jagged movements and tried to touch the glass that his mother drank from as she nursed him. During this session, the little baby periodically pulled off the breast to look around, especially at his mother. She always reciprocated his glance with smiles and warm words. He usually relatched onto the breast on his own. On one occasion, he suckled deeply and placed his hand around his mother's finger. He gently massaged her finger, her breast, and then her arm. She responded by moving her head closer to the baby. David moved his hand back and forth as he purposely touched his mother's hair. Sara looked at him and smiled. He verbalized back 'uuuu' while he continued to suckle.

The couple engaged in ongoing reciprocal interchanges until David pulled off and looked around. After a while, when Sara noted that her son did not glance at the breast or demonstrate an interest in renewing nursing, she placed him in a sitting position on her lap. After a few moments, the other twin cued to nurse through whining signs and the brothers changed places. David was kissed warmly, placed in an infant seat beside his mother, and his brother took his place at the breast.

A similar warm interchange took place between Adam and his mother, although several of the specific exchanges were different and reflected the individual style of this baby. When this session commenced, Sara matched Adam's wide smile with playful gestures that included holding him high above her head. The reciprocity continued when Adam responded to his mother's kiss by pressing his face to his mother's face. Sara kissed Adam warmly on his cheek again. In response to the change in Adam's tone, indicated by the way that Adam uttered a complaining sound "mmmeee" and turned up his nose, his mother moved him into a side lying position for nursing. As Adam moved closer to the breast, he kicked his legs, moved his hands up and down, opened his mouth wide, muttered "uuuu chk," stared at his mother's breast, and opened his mouth wide. Sara said, "Come, come, come" as she helped him latch on by pulling up her breast.

The mother also remained attuned to the non-nursing twin and ensured that he felt comfortable. She retrieved toys for David to suck as she held the nursing twin in her arms and at the breast. She spoke to both babies and turned from one to other to the other as she uttered warm words to each one. For example, at one point, Sara looked at the non-nursing twin, smiled, and said lovingly, "David is also very sweet! You are little and beautiful, little and beautiful." David vocalized and mom imitated the sounds that he made.

Like his brother, Adam also intermittently took short breaks from nursing to look around and briefly engage with others. Also like his brother, he cued to finish this nursing session when he pulled off the breast and remained focused on other objects. In between this nursing session and the next, the mother intermittently held one baby and placed the other twin on a blanket or infant seat beside her. At other times, she held both twins simultaneously until one motioned to nurse again.

Nursing Relationship during the First Few Years

The cue-based nursing relationship, including the reciprocal nature of nursing sessions, reinforced the parents' existing premise of following children's leads that stemmed from the former nursing relationships. The interactions with nursing twins seemed to augment an individualistic approach to child development even further. This was illustrated by the patient way that Sara accepted and responded to the twins' diverse rates of development. For example, she accepted that David enthusiastically integrated solid foods into his diet at the age of six and a half months and that his brother insisted on exclusive nursing until he was approximately eight months of age. The twins also differed in their gross motor and verbal development. For example, Adam quickly graduated from simple crawling to active running, while David seemed content to remain immobile until one year of age when he caught up to his brother.

The twins were also allowed to develop their mutual relationship with one another at their own pace. Nursing played an important role in this trajectory of mutual recognition and influenced, as well as was affected by, the interactions between the brothers. Initially, the twins seemed oblivious to one another as was suggested by the way that they displayed extreme disinterest in one another both during and in between nursing sessions. Their apparent lack of mutual regard not only contrasted with their engrossment with their mother, but also with the way that they engaged with other family members.

At five and a half months of age, for example, the twins rarely looked at one another during shared nursing sessions. In addition, when one twin's spontaneous movements touched the other twin, neither reciprocated the touch. This contrasted with the high degree of mutual tactile interchanges between the mother and her twins. Their lack of regard for one another was also exhibited during single nursing sessions when the non-nursing twin seemed to ignore the sibling at the breast and intermittently fixed his eyes on the mother's face as if in anticipation of his next sole turn at the beloved breast.

The apparent lack of mutual acknowledgement between the twins in between nursing sessions was most poignantly exemplified on one occasion when the twins were placed together on a blanket at six months of age. Adam spontaneously sucked his brother's hand without paying attention to him. Similarly, David seemed unaware that his hand was in his brother's mouth.

The early period of apparent disinterest gradually decreased as the twins neared their first birthday. One might venture that the act of sharing the breast, as well as sucking the other's hand, was an early step towards mutual recognition. This advanced to reciprocal regard, recognition, smiling, and eventually intricate interchanges.

Following their first birthday, the increasingly mobile twins began to follow one another to the breast, initially through crawling and eventually by running. Both twins took turns leading, watching, and following their sibling. They also responded to the same cues for nursing. Both demonstrated incrementing abilities to understand and to react to the language that their mother used during nursing. Initially, the mother had called nursing "tzi tzi" (titty), and the twins had responded to this name when they cued to nurse.

Interestingly, Adam took a leadership role in the creation of new names for nursing that reflected his growing verbal capacities. At approximately sixteen months of age, Adam began calling the breast "et ze" (meaning "that"). His brother followed this example and both twins shouted this out as they approached the breast. With the development of advanced verbal skills, Adam once again initiated a change in the name for nursing and renamed nursing "imi." It is interesting to note the resemblance between the word for nursing "imi" and the word "ima," the name for mommy in the language spoken in the home. The twins differentiated between mother and breast by calling Sara "ibi." The similarity between "imi" and "ibi" seemed to signify the deep emotional meaning that nursing had for them. This became more apparent with the advent of additional verbal skills, and the twins spoke about their love for nursing with one another, their mother, and others in between frequent nursing sessions.

The beloved breast also became a context for interesting games created by the twins, and at times, the interactions between the twins suggested that they were more immersed in one another than they were in their mother. This was illustrated by a pattern that Adam initiated when he was approximately fourteen months old. He poked his sibling and vocalized in a manner that showed his determination to switch breasts part way through a nursing session. Initially, David complied with minimal urging from his brother. Later on, he took turns initiating leading the switching game. Usually, the twins heeded one another's request to exchange breasts. However, there were also instances when the boys bickered when one wanted to switch breasts prior to the other's consent.

The continued influence of their developing relationship on the quality of nursing was evident during the twin's third year of life. At this time, the twins developed a separate nursing pattern and ceased following one another to the breast. David nursed more frequently at night than during the day, while his brother engaged in an opposite routine. This, of course, fluctuated over time. This behavior had many implications and pointed to the boys' need to nurse alone and their capacity to share the breast. One might also venture that the twins' capacity to forego nursing when the other twin nursed suggested that they felt confident in their individual ownership of the nursing relationship. Interestingly, this pattern was also in tune with the family theme of mutual compromise.

Nursing at Age Three and a Half

Nursing remained a central focus for the boys when they were three and a half years old. They continued their pattern of lone nursing sessions and only nursed at the same time on rare occasions. They continued to refer to nursing as "imi," although at times, they added, "I want to nurse." It was fascinating to watch the facial expressions and body language they displayed while they nursed that implied that they experienced deep and pure pleasure. Outside of these actions, there were very few commonalties in the way the twins nursed or in their personalities.

Adam displayed well developed verbal, social, and motor skills that he used to facilitate creative games and outgoing interactions with others. The way that he engaged in deciphering others' thoughts and feelings, making jokes and pulling others' legs, suggested that Adam had a well developed theory of mind that exceeded age appropriate levels of development. His unique capacity and his desire to understand others seemed to contribute to his highly reciprocal and warm interactions.

This very expressive little boy initiated short breaks at the breast almost hourly in between his extremely busy and happy play interludes. He usually approached his mother with the words, "Imi, imi! I want to nurse." He often touched her breast and pulled up his mother's top on his own. At times, he nursed as he stood beside his mother. At other times, he sat on his mother's lap with his head buried in her chest, while his arms gently touched her body. On occasion, he spoke to his mother or others in the room as he held the breast in his mouth. Other times, he intermittently let go of the breast in order to speak, and then immediately returned to nursing. He seemed fully immersed in what appeared to be an extremely pleasurable activity. His feelings were verified one day when he enthusiastically shouted out, "I love tzi tzi (titty), I love imi imi!" He usually nursed at both breasts, and while he switched between breasts, he repeated, "Now I will have some of this one." On one occasion, he explained that he had to have both breasts in order to make sure that the "milk will not become impaired."

Sara usually responded to her son's needs in a patient manner, touching and speaking to him warmly as he nursed. However, dissimilar from observations of the couple during infancy, the mother intermittently initiated the termination of nursing sessions. She said things such as, "Okay Adamy, you have nursed long enough now. It is beginning to hurt mommy. Say thank you to imi and finish up." In addition, she sometimes refused her son's requests for nursing, especially when his requests were seemingly endless. She said, "Come on Adamy, you just nursed, I cannot nurse you now." On the rare occasions when the couple disagreed about the timing of nursing, they resolved their differences through open discourse that resembled their reciprocity at the breast and was characteristic to their relationship. More commonly, Adam withstood his mother's intermittent perceived negative responses. This was illustrated by the way that he compromised with his mother on one occasion and said, "Ok I will cease nursing now, but first I will have a little more of the other breast." After he suckled for a short period on the other breast, he stopped nursing and said, "Ok I have finished. Thank you Imi."

Adam's unique expressions seemed to help him sustain his nursing relationship. This was illustrated on a day when Sara felt extremely exhausted by Adam's incessant nursing and admitted this when she asked him why he continued to nurse so frequently. In a serious tone, Adam answered, "Mommy, I cannot help but nurse when the cute and sweet little tzi tzi (titty) calls me." This naturally warmed Sara's heart, and she stated that she temporarily forgot her frustration.

David's nursing pattern was different from the way his sibling nursed. This was not surprising in light of the brothers' distinct personalities. This twin also displayed well developed verbal and social skills, and actively created interesting games as he interacted with his physical environment in an incessant manner. However, he was much more serious and shyer than his brother. He seemed to engage in more periods of solitary play than his brother did. Although he often complied with his brother's requests for toys, David also stubbornly refuted his brother's demands to give up toys when it did not suit him, and he stood firm when he wanted something from his parents. He showed great initiative and was able to meet his goals in creative ways, including getting the help of others. Furthermore, despite his comparatively quieter demeanor, David seemed to internalize everything in his midst, as was indicated by the way that he recounted intricate details about activities that he had witnessed.

Dissimilar from his brother's persistent daily nursing sessions, David tended to cue to nurse before naps, in the evening, and during the night. Like his brother, he asked to nurse by touching his mother and uttering the words, "Imi! Imi!" in addition to, "I want to nurse." He, too, enjoyed switching between breasts that he touched with longing and deep affection. He often looked up into his mother's eyes with pure adoration. Usually, this little boy's intermittent meetings at the breast were short and often terminated when David fell asleep while nursing. On the few times that he asked to nurse during the day, the sessions were brief and usually lasted less than five minutes. On rare occasions, Sara asked her son to cease nursing when he lingered on the breast for seemingly prolonged periods of time. However, dissimilar from his brother, David appeared insulted by his mother's requests. His perceptive mother attempted to find other ways of gently compensating her son when he infrequently nursed for extremely long periods.

Nursing Contributed to the Development of Scripts of Separateness

The distinct nature of the boys' nursing patterns enabled them to define their boundaries as separate individuals. Nursing also seemed to provide them with a context where they could proclaim their individuality. This was exemplified in a statement that Adam made at age three and a half, "I want to nurse alone. I want to nurse in peace."

Similarly, the boys played games that enabled them to purposely exclude the other twin. This was exemplified by the way that three and a half-year-old David laughed as he told his brother, "There is no room for you in the shower!" As was the common pattern, Adam ignored his brother's warning and joined his brother. Both boys responded with joyous laughter and enthusiastically played together in the shower.

Along with their desire to be alone, the boys also seemed to fully enjoy one another's company. The cooperative nature of their activities increased as they grew. Just like the way that they had followed one another to the breast in an earlier period of development, as three-year-olds, they initiated joint activities together that were creative, vigorous, energetic, often very messy, and usually extremely mischievous. Often, they used games to place well defined boundaries between them and others. This was illustrated by the way they spilled water around them and said, "Only we can play in here. No one else can come in here."

Separation and Access to the Outside World

Sara withstood most of her growing sons' antics and enabled them to investigate their world freely. Similar to the way that she had allowed the twins to dictate the frequency of nursing and their process of partial weaning, she also followed the children's cues for separation. The decision to send them to nursery school at age three reflected their apparent interest in outside stimulation. Also, like their sisters, the path was gradual and momentary regressions were validated.

The twin's varying trajectory was illustrated by the way they simultaneously referred to themselves as "big" and, at other times, referred to themselves as "small." Adam's interest in hearing stories about children who had weaned from nursing suggested that he was interested in this, although he was not yet ready to take the step himself. He was also easily angered by insensitive remarks that others outside of the family made about nursing, and he was irritated when they tried to push the weaning experience on him.

Adam's reaction to the insensitivity of others was illustrated in the way that he refused to return to nursery school after the teacher told him that he was big and no longer needed to nurse. Adam was almost four years old and had enjoyed school previously. He told his mother, "I am still little (meaning young) and I need imi." Sara's capacity to withstand and to resolve her son's intermittent ambivalence was illustrated in the way that she listened carefully to her son and reassured him that he could continue nursing, and that she accepted his need to be "little" and to be close to her. The understanding mother gently reprimanded the teacher and stayed with her son at school until he was ready to let her go again.

Weaning after Age Four: A Gradual Process

Both twins continued to nurse on their fourth birthday. However, one twin was much more interested in nursing than his twin was. Adam nursed more frequently than David. He nursed several times during the day and infrequently at night. He stated clearly that he did not intend on weaning and that he had a need for nursing. Nevertheless, like his brother, he gradually reduced the frequency of nursing. David nursed at night and only infrequently during the day.

Although Sara retained her patient style and endeavored to fulfill her children's needs at all times, she began to tire of nursing, especially at night. She noticed that her twins were busy and happy most of the time. She also noted that they had reduced the frequency of nursing, each twin in their own way. In tune with their changing behaviors, she approached them about the possibility of full weaning from "imi" in the near future. She told them that she did not think that the milk was good anymore in the "imi." In addition, she admitted to her twins that nursing now hurt her sometimes and, therefore, she would like them to nurse for shorter periods of time.

The twins responded to their mother's desire to wean them. David continued to decrease the frequency of his nursing sessions and only nursed for short periods of time, usually at night. Adam followed suit, although he nursed more frequently than his brother. Gradually, the little boys' nursing sessions were shorter and more infrequent. In addition, they copied their mother and said that the milk was "no longer tasty" after they pulled off the breast. They also made funny faces that showed that the milk did not taste good.

The boys continued to nurse for short bursts. They said that they were "testing the milk." This pattern continued for about two months until David fully weaned. Adam continued to nurse for an additional two months. By the time Adam was four and a half, he only nursed about once a week or so. In addition, Sara said that he did not really suckle at that time, but simply played with the breast in his mouth. On the few occasions that Adam attempted suckling, Sara admitted to him that it hurt her now and he immediately stopped.

Both boys continued to talk about nursing and to play with their mother's breasts during their weaning process and after they weaned. Sara said, "They continue to test the breasts to see if there is milk. They also reassure me that the imi milk will become tasty again if I have another baby." They liked to look at the breasts, to touch them, and to include the breasts in their games. For example, they would put the breasts on their heads and laugh.

In this instance as well, Adam, who had nursed more frequently, also played with his mother's breasts more frequently than his brother did. For example, one day he pretended that his mother's breasts were carrots that he pulled up from the ground. As he pulled the breasts, he sang a little song that he had learned in nursery school about carrots. At the age of four and a half, David, who had weaned prior to his brother, proudly declared to his mother, "Mommy I almost never play with your breasts anymore!"

The Nursing Relationship and the Family

Part of the twins' process of spreading their wings included gradually allowing other family members to take over some of the roles formerly associated with nursing, while retaining their mother as their main source of comfort. This was facilitated by the twins' ability to generalize their views of interaction associated with nursing to additional relationships. In circular fashion, family members reinforced the twins' precepts of interchange. Nursing concurred with active family activities, and the proximity between the twins and others also advanced this process. Each subsystem provided, as well as received, distinct feedback that also affected the integration of the twins into the system.

The Parental Couple and the Nursing Subsystem

The parents influenced and were affected by the present nursing system much like in earlier nursing relationships. They continued to view the intense nature of parenting differently. For example, when the twins were infants, Sara said, "This is what is meant when they say that it is a sacrifice, but for me, it is not a sacrifice. It is fun! The joy that I gain from being with my children overrides the sacrifices." In contrast, the transition from two to four children had fortified Joseph's sense of hardship. He openly discussed his ambivalence, while concurrently apologizing for his expressions of frustration. "It's hard for me and I complain. Sara works so hard and she never complains. I want it to pass (looking after newborn twins). Like with Anna. That is what I consider that it has passed. I mean that they will be older like Anna."

In contrast to the previous nursing relationships, the parents' diverse viewpoints affected nursing. Joseph perceived that Sara's dedication to the older children, along with the intensive nursing relationship, was detrimental to her welfare and insisted that she give the twins pacifiers when they were newborns. Sara complied with her husband's request, despite that she had never used a pacifier with her older children and that she felt uncomfortable with this. She stated, "I tried the pacifier in order to appease Joseph and my mother. I know that they were worried about me. Luckily, David refused it, and I only rarely give it to Adam when I am very busy with David." Yet, despite that observations verified that Sara used the pacifier in a minimal fashion, she seemed bothered by the compromise that she had made in order to calm her partner. The angry tone that Sara used later on, when she described how she had rid her son of the pacifier at ten months of age, pointed to the emotional turmoil this had caused for her. In a disdainful manner that was uncharacteristic of the way that she referred to her partner, she remarked, "I never wanted it, he (meaning Joseph) did!"

Common to Joseph's pattern, he admitted that his wife was right. As usual, Joseph provided a perceptive rationale for his behavior that showed that additional reasons had also propelled his actions. He said, "I think it (the desire to reduce the intensity between the nursing triad) comes from what you hear from people around you. They usually say it is not so bad if a baby cries a little. You should not go to a baby immediately... The child will calm down on his own. I am concerned about this, and I think about this a lot because Sara always goes to the babies immediately, right away. Very few people have Sara's patience. Very few people give as much to their children as Sara does. I am not sure that babies need so much attention. I wonder if they need to be alone more." Joseph's reference to babies' needs "to be alone more" seemed to suggest that perhaps the father had displaced his own longing for solitude on his children.

Joseph said that he heard that dependence in early childhood impairs the development of future independence, an issue that was central to Joseph's personal script. At the onset of the study, Joseph's concerns clouded his ability to acknowledge his older child's autonomous behaviors due to his concern that she spent too much time with her parents. Yet, as he watched his daughters become responsible and independent, he changed his view and was more accepting of his twins needs for their mother.

The father's ambivalent definition of nursing also compounded his dilemma. While Joseph firmly believed that nursing enriched children's physiological development, he continued to query the emotional significance of nursing that his wife emphasized. Joseph's ambivalence was heightened when he was overly exhausted and intermittently frustrated by the persistent demands of fathering four children in a needs-focused manner. One might propose that when Joseph was overwhelmed by the functions of parenting and by the sacrifices that were required of him, his long standing themes were triggered and justified by culturally predominant views that promoted parental distancing. This momentarily impaired his process of continually reorganizing his script of responsive interaction.

Despite his mixed feelings, Joseph's reverence for nursing reigned, and he fully supported nursing in response to children's cues. He accepted that his sons nursed at age four and understood that their need for nursing had important emotional elements. Joseph recognized his son's changing cues for nursing and knew the names that his sons called the breasts. Joseph also accepted that his sons needed to nurse at varied times, and he shared his bed with the nursing twins after he returned to the shared bed when the twins were a year old.

Joseph accepted and supported his twins' cues for nursing during family outings. However, he differed from Sara in the way that he felt that nursing should be approached in public settings. Sara's insightful explanation highlighted the complex nature of this issue for the couple. She said, "Even though I was brought up very religious, I am very free with nursing. This is because I do not see breastfeeding as sexual at all. It does not bother me to nurse with my breasts showing when I nurse. I am not bothered at all by what people say or if they are bothered by my nursing openly in public. ....I think that if I cover up my breasts when I nurse, my babies will not be able to breathe. They will not be able to enjoy themselves. They push my top up. I was like this with all of my children. Joseph is very uncomfortable with the way that I nurse very openly. We always argue about this. He tries to cover me when I am nursing in front of people. I think that he might see something sexual in breastfeeding. He is very modest about nudity in general, without any connection to breastfeeding. For example, he puts an undershirt on when he goes out to hang up the laundry."

Functions that Restored Homeostasis when Themes of Dissension Resurfaced

The couple's capacity to contain the aforementioned issues of discord was facilitated by their shared goal of creating a responsive family style and strategies that upheld this objective. Joseph remained determined to father differently than his father and to develop sensitive relationships with his children that emulated his wife and her family. Sara continued to support her husband's efforts and to provide him with ongoing positive reinforcement that reflected her theme of acceptance. She allowed Joseph's progress by not interfering when he took steps on his own and often remained silent as she observed her husband as he interacted with the children. At other times, she reinforced the message that Joseph conveyed to the children. She always seemed extremely pleased by the contact between her husband and the children. This boomeranged back to the father-child system, as well as the couple subsystem, and reinforced the responsive parenting style associated with nursing.

Joseph's trajectory was also advanced by his well developed capacity to question his own motives and his ability to seek out answers to questions regarding relationships, children, their needs, and methods of fulfilling developmental children's requirements. Sara remained his most important source, and he admired her more than anyone else. The tutor and learner relationship that had been established at the onset of this couple's marriage was enriched by the way the couple celebrated the father's change process together.

The pattern of free flowing discourse that had been established during their early marriage helped them integrate disjointed parenting themes and modify ideas. This, too, was affected by Joseph's growth as a communicator.

Sara explained, "Joseph did not always talk about his feelings. Now I think that he does, and he also makes great efforts to listen to me and also the children." Towards the end of the study, Sara added, "I am sure that parenting made Joseph change and open up more than anything else."

Mutuality was also enriched by the couple's capacity to acknowledge one another's needs and make compromises for one another, while consistently retaining the ultimate goal of meeting children's needs as the guiding force. While most of the compromises that Joseph made as a father stemmed from child-centered goals, it also seemed that, at times, he did this in order to please Sara. By the same token, Sara matched Joseph's immense efforts at forgoing his personal needs by ensuring that her husband was provided with time alone whenever possible.

In circular fashion, Joseph supported Sara's efforts to uphold the family system. This was exemplified by the way that he helped her return to a state of homeostasis when she was overwhelmed by ongoing childcare and extreme exhaustion. This was especially true right after the twins' first birthday when their individual needs resulted in almost ongoing nursing sessions without interruption. Interestingly, Sara stated that she felt unsupported when she perceived that her partner disregarded her parenting themes. This was illustrated by the way that Sara angrily refuted her husband's suggestion that she hire outside help for household duties. In contrast, Joseph's help was perceived in a positive way when he validated her mothering goals of meeting their children's needs above all else and joined her in her efforts to meet this goal.

Likewise, the couple complemented one another's parenting tasks in a manner that reflected their individual capacities. Consequently, when the twins were infants, the couple's gender and biological capacities were the guiding force that qualified their task arrangements. The family accepted that initially nursing reinforced a mother-baby alliance that decentralized the father. Sara nursed and focused on the twins while her husband looked after the house and the older children, and engaged in infant care other than nursing. As the children's needs changed, so did the division of parenting tasks in this household. The adaptable nature of the couple subsystem mirrored, as well as likely contributed to, the flexible nature of their parenting style, including nursing.

Yet despite the many compensating measures that this couple managed to instill in their interactions as parents, they continued to disagree about several issues. Their strength as a couple was poignantly demonstrated by the way that they accepted irresolvable discord and comfortably agreed to disagree, while continuing to advance their children's needs in a responsive manner. Sara explained, "Joseph and I realize that we have different views about how parents should respond to children. Joseph thinks that children should be left alone more, and I think that it is important to respond to children. We decided that each parent can do what feels right to them when they are with the children. Since I am with the children more than Joseph, we will do it my way when we are both together with the children. If Joseph is with the children alone, he can do it his way, but I think that he still responds to them a lot."

The Effect of the Nursing Triad on the Couple Relationship Outside of Parenting

In circular fashion, the mutuality between the parents reverberated back to their couple relationship. The couple presented their couple life outside of parenting as rich and fulfilling. This is most interesting in light of the minimal time that they had together alone. The couple rarely went out without their children, who tended to physically surround their parents, even at night. They nevertheless found time for interesting discussions and mutually satisfying activities. In separate interviews, the parents emphasized that couples do not need to go out on their own in order to enjoy themselves and keep their relationship going. For example, they described how much they enjoyed watching television shows together when all four children were asleep for brief periods of time in the late evening.

It also seemed significant that despite the intense physical proximity between the parents and their children, the parents seemed to have a fulfilling, physically intimate relationship with one another. Sara explained that one of her responsibilities was to ensure that all family members' needs were met, and this included meeting her and her husband's needs as couple. She emphasized that physical intimacy was important in a marriage. She added that, "Not just for the marriage, but for me as well. Although now I have less desire than before the babies were born... However, in general, sexual relations with my husband is very important for me personally."

Sara emphasized that the sleeping arrangement in her family did not interfere with meeting the couple's needs, "First of all, many people sleep in the same bed, and they never have sex! For us, it is more exciting. We have to be more creative. This is what makes it very nice. This makes our sex life so much more fun. We make an effort to not forget this part of our life and so we have to find ways to have sex. We make sure that this is a regular part of our life."

"Sex life is more exciting, it is more complicated and more complex. With children you do not have a moment of privacy, so every moment that you have you truly cherish. I also think that every 15 minutes you have together alone becomes more important. You value it more. I think that by having the children around us all the time, including in our bed, we have become more creative and enjoy ourselves as a couple and our intimate times much more than we did when we were alone."

"I would say with the years and the addition of children, our romantic life, not just our sex life, has become more exciting. We have had to become more creative in the ways that we interact with each other, and this has added romance to our marriage. …. Since it has become more difficult for us to be together, it has become more romantic."

"So all of the couple behavior, not just related to sex, has become more exciting, more romantic. The changes that have occurred in Joseph might have also contributed to this change. Joseph who is much more romantic than he used to be, he has learned more how to interact with people and has become more open."

Father's Interactions with the Nursing Twins

The mutual effect of the parents on one another as they traveled through their shared path to parenthood was apparent in the warm interactions between Joseph and his sons. This dad seemed to have moved away from the egocentric approach that he had when he first made the transition to parenthood, and this was indeed remarkable. He seemed to be more cognizant of the important role that nursing played in meeting children's needs and took greater ownership of the nursing relationship than was evident in the couple's portrayal of earlier experiences. This was apparent in the way he confronted those who dared to denigrate nursing and the associated lifestyle. His tone was strong as he said, "I don't have patience for these people. I also don't understand why anyone would not want to nurse their children when it was so much healthier than not nursing." The circular impact of Joseph's convictions was illustrated by the jubilant tone that Sara used when she described her partner's protective tasks, "I think that Joseph is very proud of me that I nurse! He defends me in front of others!"

Like in earlier nursing relationships, the primacy of nursing in the daily life of the twins provided Joseph with vast opportunities to observe Sara modeling mothering through nursing. In this case, he also internalized the way she tended to the twins and their individual rhythms. In Joseph's role as the supportive partner and father, he had opportunities to apply what he had observed to his interactions with the boys in between nursing sessions. This process was also enhanced by Joseph's quest for additional learning, exemplified by his interest in science-based information on breastfeeding, twins, child development, and related issues.

The father demonstrated the effect of watching cue-based interchanges pertaining to nursing when he based his actions on the twins' signs rather than on a set schedule. He spoke to the twins in a gentle manner that resembled his wife's tone and her words. Also like Sara, he used tactile elements and proximity behaviors as a means of calming them. The accepting way that Joseph brought the twins to their mother to nurse when they were infants illustrated his ability to decipher between the twins' needs for general interaction and nursing. Joseph's ability to understand the twins' cues was also suggested when he independently cared for their basic needs. On one occasion, for example, when the twins were infants, he efficiently picked David up from the joint family bed and gave him a bath. The father explained, "The baby looked hot and sweaty. I knew that he had not yet had his morning bath, so of course I bathed him."

Like his wife, the understanding that Joseph gained from following the twins' signals advanced his appreciation of child-paced development. Point in case was Joseph's calm attitude towards the boys' diverse rates of development when they were young toddlers. He said, "I am not worried about David, and we are not taking him to any specialists to ask questions. We know that children develop at different rates and that he will eventually walk just like his brother. I might have thought differently if this was my first child."

The twins provided their father with positive reinforcement that facilitated their interchanges with him. This was particularly true for Adam who smiled and looked at his father from his mother's breast from early infancy onward. While both sons eventually grew extremely fond of their father, Adam continued to demonstrate more interest in his father than his brother did. Importantly, Joseph tended to David with the same great care that he extended to Adam, and this suggested that he accepted this twin's less attentive approach to him.

Joseph's increased capacity to father in a responsive manner was poignantly demonstrated by the way that he forwent his needs for space when his wife asked him to return to the bed that she shared with the twins. He also changed his focus from basic infant care and support of mother-infant centrality in infancy to include novel ways of meeting his sons' needs when this was deemed necessary. Joseph responded to his sons' increasing interest in him by allowing them to follow him around the house much like the way they also pursued their mother. Sara laughed as she described them as "little ducks who follow the mother or father duck." When Joseph noticed the twins' growing interest in imitating him, he purposely created opportunities for joint activities, including gardening and carpentry.

Influence on Nursing Behaviors

The importance of Joseph's flexibility had rippling effects on the nursing routines. The father's interventions changed evening nursing sessions when the twins were approximately one year of age. Sara described the events at that time. "They both refuse to fall asleep at the breast in the evening. They nurse a little and then they want to play with me. I am so tired and so are they. I don't mind it when they wake up in the middle of the night because they nurse and go back to sleep. But in the evening, they don't seem to want to go to sleep at all...Joseph now puts them to sleep in the evening by walking them or by putting them on his chest after I nurse them." This became a constant pattern in this family, and for the next few years, their father put the twins to bed in the evening.

Along with stepping in and taking over some of the comforting tasks originally associated with nursing, Joseph also accepted the twins' continued need to nurse in frequent bouts and to focus on their mother as their central comfort figure. This same patience was evident when the father withstood the twins' increasingly wild antics that often caused chaos in the home. The culmination of Joseph's responsive behaviors increasingly resembled interactions related to nursing and associated parenting, suggesting that the nursing relationship had implications for paternal and maternal development.

The twins' relationship with their dad deepened as they grew, and his role as a direct caregiver and as a comfort figure became more significant. After their first birthday, they often waited for their father to come home from work, and when he did, they immediately followed him around. The twins played with their father and imitated things that he did and said. They loved fixing household items, gardening, and generally accompanying their father whenever possible. Yet, the degree of the boys' interest in their father continued to develop at a different pace, and Adam was still more interested in his father than his brother was. Adam's love for his father was exemplified at age three and a half when he cried angrily after finding out that his father was going away for business and he would not see him for three days.

The Older Siblings and the Nursing Subsystem

The constant nature of nursing in this family provided the girls with opportunities to interact with their brothers and observe the responsive style that accompanied nursing. Ongoing nursing decreased the sole time that the young daughters had with their parents. Yet, most remarkably, despite their preoccupation with the nursing system, the parents seemed to provide their daughters with the same sensitive parenting interventions associated with nursing and, of course, their earlier lives. Evidence that pointed to the influence of nursing on the parenting of older children in this family was the appearance of themes and patterns associated with nursing in the parents' interactions with their daughters.

"Parents must meet all of their children's needs in a way that no one else can!"

The theme of meeting children's needs above all else associated with nursing was also a prominent feature in the interactions between the parents and the older children. The mother emphasized and observations verified that she attempted to meet both Merry and her sister Anna's needs. Sara skilfully responded to her daughters' signals as she concurrently nursed or held at least one of the twins. She was cognizant of the girls' needs to be alone with her and did her best to achieve this goal. The sensitive mothering tools that she had internalized and practiced during each nursing relationship were evident as she interacted with her four children. When the twins were infants, she often engaged in special activities with each daughter while nursing. Frequently, neither the girls nor the twins seemed to acknowledge the presence of the other, and they generated a sense of being fully attended to by their mother. While nursing, Sara enthusiastically played house, read books, helped with homework, spoke with the girls about their daily interests, made them food, and attempted to redirect them when they bickered. Likewise, she accepted and tended to her daughter's full range of their emotions through discussions or warm physical embraces. Sara's capacity to multitask was augmented by Joseph's high degree of involvement in the care of his children. In a manner that resembled the father's interchanges with the twins, he patiently listened to the girls, engaged with them in deep discussions, provided them with genuine feedback, and also met their physical needs. For example, he made special food for Merry that matched her unique appetite. Joseph participated in varied activities that contrasted with his personal script, but that he perceived met his daughter's needs, including attending ballet classes, participating in doll fashion shows, and baking cookies with his older daughter. Joseph's efforts to understand and enjoy these activities pointed to his genuine intent to father in a child-centered manner.

Parenting Interventions Based on Individuality and Child-Led Processes

The parents' support of nursing relationships that reflected children's individual scripts evolved into an appreciation of individuality in child development that was enriched by literature and, most importantly, their experiences as parents. The importance of child-led processes for the parents was illustrated when they overcame personal discomfort in order to advance their children's development. Sara gave a poignant example, "My husband is not that comfortable with nudity or talking about issues related to sex. Yet, he is very accepting of our children's developmental needs and their need to ask questions (about sexuality). He always answers them appropriately and without any embarrassment. I think that he learned that from me."

The parents were particularly sensitive to the developmental tasks of engagement versus separation, a likely remnant of concepts associated with nursing. Much like in nursing, the parents encouraged their daughters' individual rate of readiness for these tasks and disregarded the unsolicited comments of others that negated their view. The daughters started school at their own rate, were allowed to take breaks when they felt the need, and were welcomed into the family bed whenever they signaled a need to be there. At the same time, the parents celebrated their daughters' processes of individuation.

Proof of the ferocity of the concept of individually determined rates of development was illustrated by the tolerant way that the parents accepted Merry's need to remain emotionally closer to her mother than her father, even though this differed from Anna's earlier pattern. The parents also seemed to understand and to encourage their daughters' distinct explorative patterns. Anna progressively included other relationships into her script as she engaged with her environment in a predictable manner, and usually displayed an above age level of maturity inclusive of highly responsive actions. She gradually included many new school peers into her close relational circle, she initiated school projects in a precise manner, and consistently informed her parents of her whereabouts. In contrast, Merry's process reflected her free spirit. Even though she had an intense need for closeness as a young child, she displayed a heightened desire for freedom as she got older. Her actions were often accompanied by wild laughter that pointed to her genuine enthusiasm. From age five onwards, Merry's curiosity mixed with energetic antics often drew her far away from her home base, something that increased as she became more socially competent and increased her peer contacts. At times, she left home unannounced. Even though this often caused her parents great worry, they promoted her independence, while concurrently teaching her about responsible explorations.

Altering Parenting Tasks and Positions

The evolving needs of the older sibling subsystem presented the parents with ongoing challenges that they met by reorganizing their task allocation. They demonstrated an ability to reorganize when they dealt with intermittent displays of sibling rivalry between the sisters. At age nine, Anna exemplified the daughters' attitude towards their rivalry. She said, "I don't know why we fight, but I don't think that we fight that much. It doesn't really bother me." In contrast, Sara reiterated that this issue worried her and threatened her theme of family cohesion. Whereas Sara took the lead in most aspects of childcare, Joseph directed the interventions regarding the girls' fighting. His approach was calm, confident, and reflected his attitude that intermittent fighting between siblings was normal. At times, he allowed the daughters to work out solutions on their own. On other occasions, he guided the girls in a more direct manner.

The modification in parental tasks verified that they reorganized in response to the children's needs. This reorganization reflected the flexibility that was established during nursing and validated that the gender specific tasks, inclusive of maternal centrality that had accompanied nursing, were instated as a means of advancing children's needs. Additional observations of the family showed that the charge that Joseph took with his daughters regarding their rivalry represented an increasing amount of decisive steps that he took in parenting, including with the growing twins. The couple's interactions suggested that Sara's expert stance in child rearing and family interaction was being shared to a greater degree by her husband. Views that had originally belonged to Sara were increasingly owned by Joseph and impacted his capacity to interact with his children in an exceedingly more autonomous manner.

Advancing Children's Internalization of Family Themes and Patterns

Observations of this family over time clearly showed that the children replicated their parents' themes of responsiveness in their interactions with their siblings. It seemed that their personal experience of being responded to in a validating manner, initially through nursing, had instilled positive regard for relationships, as well as a template for interaction. This internal model of interaction was likely enriched by their observations of responsive interactions in their family system. Thus the ongoing nature of the nursing sessions in the midst of family activity enabled the children to consistently view a cue-based parenting intervention and pointed to the important role that nursing had in sustaining revered family themes and patterns.

Sara suggested that nursing augmented her children's capacity to internalize family themes of mutual tolerance. She said, "I think that it (breastfeeding) makes them more understanding because they understand that they were also like that. It makes it easy for me to explain to them because I say, "you were also like that." (Sara emphasized) "You were also like that!" Like in this example, the parents commonly clarified the perspectives of the siblings to one another and transferred their reverence for individuality and mutual understanding to them.

The rippling effect of experiencing, observing, and discussing family themes was evident in the way the children applied these understandings to their interactions with one another. First of all, the salient theme of mutual understanding of other family members' needs, as well as attempts to fulfill others' needs, was apparent in many of their interactions. Like their parents, the children seemed to have an intricate awareness of the role that individual growth and development played in others' scripts. This was exemplified when Anna forgave her sister's mischief and explained that, "This is what children do at her age." Furthermore, she often protected her sister and explained her antics to others with developmental principles in mind. Merry, in turn, increasingly displayed behaviors that suggested she understood her sister had different needs than she did and accepted that they engaged in distinct activities.

Both sisters displayed incredibly insightful behaviors towards their brothers. The capacity of the girls to differentiate between the twins' varied cues, including those specifically designated for nursing, also pointed to the strong effect of watching nursing in action on the children's understanding of one another. The girls' attitudes towards the boys pointed to their understanding of infant development and associated age appropriate needs. This likely contributed to their observed ability to withstand the frequent nursing sessions when the twins were babies and their mother's continued physical preoccupation with the boys as they grew. When the twins' mischievous behavior became more prominent as they grew older, both sisters accepted this and often laughed at their antics. Merry was especially entertained by her brothers' mischief, and, at times, she not only participated in their games, but also instigated some of their lively activities.

Along with genuinely enjoying their brothers, the girls demonstrated sincere nurturing behaviors towards them. Their capacity to effectively care for the twins became increasingly more apparent as the study progressed and the girls developed. Naturally, this talent was most evident for Anna who looked after her brothers in a highly responsible and responsive fashion by the time she turned eleven years old.

In tune with the parents' theme of focusing their actions on the children, the parents seemed to emphasize mutual understanding between the siblings and seemed less centered on increasing their children's understanding of the parents' needs. However, observations over time showed that the children were nevertheless provided with brief insights about their parents' perspectives. Case in point was the way the twins' were sometimes asked to terminate nursing sessions when it hurt mommy.

The daughters' ability to understand their parents became more evident as the study progressed. This was most apparent in Anna's interactions with her parents. She demonstrated intense sensitivity to her parents' viewpoints, and this capacity seemed to increase as she developed. For example, at age eight, Anna explained that her father was very serious and, at times, she tried to humor him. By the time she was eleven years old, she discussed her parents' feelings in great detail and often included her parents' perspectives in her discussions with them.

Mutual Compromise: Capacities and Limitations

Along with expressing an understanding of the other family members, the children often demonstrated a capacity to forfeit their own needs in order to advance the needs of other family members. One might also venture that the daughters' precipitous weaning experiences had provided them with early experience in this regard. The trajectory of mutual compromise continued and was exemplified in the way that the daughters shared their mother, Anna intermittently agreed to tutor her younger sibling, Merry accepted her limitations in comparison to her sister, and eventually both daughters tolerated the needs of their active twin brothers. Observations of the twins' development also pointed to the way that the parents' primed their children to share and to forfeit egocentric desires for one another. The capacity of the children to intermittently forgo their own needs suggested that they had internalized principles of mutual compromise that were also inherent to their parents' scripts. Although the appearance of sibling rivalry that was mentioned earlier and the periodic conflicts between the twins suggested that, at times, the children found it difficult to consistently compromise their needs for others.

Reverence for Open Communication: The Continuation of the Prevalent Family Theme

Transgressions between siblings were often resolved quickly due to the outstanding capacity of each child in this family to express their feelings in a coherent manner and to receive and provide validating feedback. The children seemed to have internalized the family theme of reverence for open and validating communication. The outstanding way that the older children clearly and confidently communicated their needs suggested that the template of free flowing discourse set by nursing extended far beyond weaning. The older daughters and eventually the twins voiced their needs in a manner that suggested that they clearly expected to be heard. This was reminiscent of observations of how the boys expressed their cues for nursing in infancy. The other component of the children's communicative style was their capacity to respond sincerely to others. This seemed to reinforce the system and provided the children with various outlets for expression and validation.

The influence of nursing on the girls' process was suggested by the similarity between their vocal tone, language, and body posture and the actions their mother displayed as she nursed. It also seemed that nursing set the stage for non-verbal communication between the siblings and their family. Although the frequency of tactile interactions between older children and their parents decreased as they developed, touch continued to be a relevant communicative element in this family. This was exemplified by the way the girls occasionally sat close to one another, held hands, and sometimes shared a bed. They readily initiated and accepted warm hugs and comfortably rejoined their parents and younger siblings in the family bed. The daughters also touched and held their brothers with genuine compassion. The twins reciprocated their sisters' warm exchanges, showing the way that young nurslings in this family generalized their experiences of tactile interactions to others outside of the nursing triad.

Another important aspect of communication that seemed to have roots in the nursing system was the way family members were encouraged to express their views, be they negative or positive. This resembled the way that Sara patiently accepted her infants' cues related to nursing without reservation. The parents fortified the system by continually providing their children with a sense of unconditional positive regard similar to the enthusiasm, patience, humor, and extremely positive attitude that Sara showed during nursing. This was demonstrated by extensive mutual complimenting and positive reframing of difficult situations. Positive mutual regard and open communication bounced back to the parental couple and enabled them to fulfill their parenting tasks.

Family themes and patterns that were established at the parental level were observed at the sibling level of interaction. This seemed to reverberate back to the parents and sustain the system further. The children's development as empathetic and happy communicators enriched an ongoing process of growing communication that included periodic bursts of diminished patience that were easily resolved. The capacity for open communication assisted all members in coping with novel challenges and implementing family themes. The circular nature of family interaction sustained the sensitive parenting style and the associated sibling responsiveness, provided ongoing opportunities to observe nursing, and ensured the proliferation of a free flowing and validating communication style in this family system.

Cue-Based, Validating, and Responsive Models with Others outside the Family

The sense of validation and open communication style the children learned during and after nursing influenced their views of interaction with others outside of the family. Observations of the presenting nursing subsystem demonstrated the progressive attention the twins issued to others outside of the triad. The impact of growing up in a sensitive family system was most apparent in the older sibling subsystem.

The daughters' relationships with others suggested that the positive attitude and expressive tools they had internalized in their family allowed them to easily develop meaningful relationships with extended family members and peers. Most significantly, by the time the study was completed, discussion with family members verified that both daughters' peers perceived the girls as important sources for emotional support. The similarity between the girls in this area of development is significant when one recalls that the daughters' paths to separation and their explorative trajectories had been quite distinct. The likelihood that the daughters' peers retained this view is suggested by the constant way that Anna's peer relied on her throughout primary school. The far reaching effects of both girls' empathetic scripts were also indicated by the girls' sensitivity to and warm actions towards the weaker children in their classes. Also important, the daughters were able to cope with intermittent relational crisis, reiterating the existence of healthy models of sense of self in relation to others.

Another important implication of the cue-based parenting strategy that seemed to support the daughters as they ventured out into the world was their strong sense of independence and capacity to function in an autonomous and responsible manner. Anna and later Merry engaged in schoolwork in earnest with minimal intervention from parents or teachers. They resisted increasing peer pressure to engage in activities that were considered unmannerly, cruel, or disruptive. It is interesting that by the end of the study, the father was able to recognize these behaviors in his daughters and this, in turn, reinforced his capacity to sustain the system.

Another telling example of the girl's autonomous thinking was in the way they resisted culturally apparent views of nursing. This was illustrated in the way that both referred to nursing as "normal." At age eight, for example, Anna said, "It is natural and it is normal...it is just what people do." At the same time, she added, "I know that some people don't nurse and I don't understand why." However, she increasingly became aware that breasts had additional connotations that rendered nursing as a deviant behavior. This was suggested in her statement, "I don't want to draw a picture of my mother nursing because then I would have to draw a picture of her breasts, and I don't want to draw breasts." In addition she said, "Some people look at my mother when she nurses and I don't like that." These insights increased as the girls developed and became exposed to cultural disdain for nursing through their friends' expressions. Yet, the strength of their conviction was apparent in the way the girls enjoyed when their friends watched their brothers as they nursed. They answered their friends' questions in an assured manner. Most significantly, their sense of confidence was suggested by the way that both girls proudly and repeatedly proclaimed, "I was also nursed like that when I was a little child!"

Conclusion

The Amit family demonstrated how the nursing relationship is affected by and also impacts family themes and patterns. Salient procedures of open communication and themes of mutually meeting the individual needs of the other were established in the parental couple. Similar processes were reflected and reinforced in the nursing relationship and continued after full weaning.

The nursing relationship enabled the parents to meet their children's needs in a child-led and unique fashion that included forfeiting personal needs. Interactions pertaining to and during nursing were highly reciprocal and mutually satisfying. Behaviors associated with nursing included frequent mother-child contact, holding, and co-sleeping.

The same themes continued following weaning and were expressed by the parents and the older children. The family continued to express physical and emotional closeness and to dialogue freely. These patterns allowed flexibility and enabled the parents to modify their scripts to suit their growing children. It was most significant that family processes generated during nursing had the potential to enrich the children's capacity for autonomy, their ability to engage in mutual discourse, and their evolving sense of empathy. This seemed to affect their relationships in the family and beyond. In turn, their behaviors reverberated back to the nursing system and enabled the continuation of a warm and sensitive family system.

References

Acolet, D., Sleath, K., & Whitelaw, A. (1989). Oxygenation, heart rate, and temperature in very low birthweight infants during skin-to-skin contact with their mothers. Acta Paediatrica Scandinavica, 78, 189-193.

Ainsworth, M.D.S. (1979) Infant-mother attachment. American Psychologist, 34(10), 932-937.

Ainsworth, M.D.S., Blehar, M., Waters, E., & Wall, S. (1978). Patterns of attachment. Hillsdale N.J.: Lawrence Erlbaum Associates.

Aldous, J., Mulligan, G. M., & Bjarnason, T. (1998). Fathering over time: What makes the difference? Journal of Marriage and the Family, 60(4), 809-820.

Alikasifoglu, M., Erginoz, E., Tasdelen Gur, E., Baltas Z., Beker, B. & Arvas, A. (2001). Factors influencing the duration of exclusive breastfeeding in a group of Turkish women. Journal of Human Lactation, 17(3), 220-226.

American Academy of Pediatrics (AAP). (1994). Work group on cow's milk protein and diabetes mellitus: Infant feeding practices and their possible relationship to the etiology of diabetes mellitus. Pediatrics, 94, 752-754.

American Academy of Pediatrics (AAP) Committee on Child Abuse and Neglect. (2001). Shaken baby syndrome: Rotational cranial injuries—technical report. Pediatrics, 108, 206–210.

American Academy of Pediatrics (AAP). (2005). Policy statement: Breastfeeding and the use of human milk. Pediatrics, 115(2), 496-506.

American Academy of Family Physicians. (2007). Breastfeeding (policy statement). Retrieved February 20, 2009, from http://www.aafp.org/online/en/home/policy/policies/b/breastfeedingpolicy.html.

Amper, K. (1996). A new mother learns about breastfeeding from her husband. The Baby Friendly Hospital Initiative Newsletter, March/April 1996.

Anderson, G.C. (1989). Risk in mother-infant separation post birth. Journal of Nursing Scholarship, 21(4), 196-199.

Anderson, G.C., Moore, E., Hepworth, J., Bergman, N. (2003). Early skin-to-skin contact for mothers and their healthy newborn infants. Birth, 30(3), 206-207.

Angier, N. (1991). A potent peptide prompts an urge to cuddle. New York Times, January 22, 1991, C-1, 10.

Angier, N. (2000). Woman: An intimate geography. New York: Anchor Books.

Arms, S. (1994). Immaculate deception II: A fresh look at childbirth. Berkeley, California: Celestial Arts.

Baber, K.M., & Murray, C. I. (2001). A postmodern feminist approach to teaching human sexuality. Family Relations, 50(1), 23-33.

Baby Milk Action. (2006). Hard sell formula: strategies used by the baby food industry in the UK. Retrieved on May 12, 2009, from http://www.babyfeedinglawgroup.org.uk/pdfs/hardsellformula.pdf.

Baby Milk Action & Baby Feeding Law Group. (2009). UK formula marketing practices March 2009. Retrieved on May 11, 2009, from http://www.babyfeedinglawgroup.org.uk/pdfs/bflgmonrepmarch09sm.pdf.

Baddock, S., Galland, B., Bolton, D., Williams S.M., & Taylor, B.J. (2006). Differences in infant and parent behaviors during routine bed sharing compared with cot sleeping in the home setting. Pediatrics, 117(5), 1599-1607.

Ball, H.L. (2002). Reasons to bed-share. Why parents sleep with their infants. Journal of Reproductive and Infant Psychology, 20(4), 207-221.

Bandura, A. (1989). Regulation of cognitive processes through perceived self-efficacy. Developmental Psychology, 25(5), 729-735.

Bartlett, A. (2000). Thinking through breasts: Writing maternity. Feminist Theory, 1(2), 173-88.

Bar-Yakov, L. (2002). The development and evaluation of the attachment parenting scale. [Abstract]. Dissertation Abstracts International: Section B: The Sciences and Engineering, 63(1-B), 562.

Bassin, D. (1994). Maternal subjectivity in the culture of nostalgia: Mourning and memory. In D. Bassin, M. Honey & M.M. Kaplan (Eds.), Representations of motherhood. New Haven: Yale University Press.

Baumslag, N., & Michels, D.L. (1995). Milk, money and madness: The culture and politics of breastfeeding. Westport, Connecticut: Bergin & Garvey.

Beasley, A. (1991). Breastfeeding studies: Culture, biomedicine and methodology. Journal of Human Lactation, 7(1):7-17.

Beavers, W. R. (1977). Psychotherapy and growth: A family systems perspective. New York: Brunner/Mazel.

Beck, C. T., & Watson, S. (2008). Impact of birth trauma on breast-feeding: A tale of two pathways. Nursing Research, 57(4), 228-36.

Beitel, A.H., & Parke, R.D. (1998). Paternal involvement in infancy: The role of maternal and paternal attitudes. Journal of Family Psychology, 12(20), 268-288.

Bell, R.Q. (1974). Contributions of human infants to caregiving and social interaction. In M. Lewis & L.A. Rosenblum (Eds.), The effect of the infant on its caregiver. New York: John Wiley & Sons.

Belsky, J., & Hsieh, K. (1998). Patterns of marital change during the early childhood years: Parent personality, co-parenting and division of labor correlates. Journal of Family Psychology, 12(4), 511-528.

Belsky, J., & Kelly, J. (1994). The transition to parenthood: How a first child changes a marriage. Why some couples grow closer and others apart. New York: Dell Trade Paperback.

Benson Brown, A., & McPherson, K.R. (1998). The reality of breastfeeding. Westport Connecticut: Bergin & Garvey.

Bergman, N. (2005). Kangaroo mother care promotions. Retrieved on Feb. 20, 2009 from http://www.kangaroomothercare.com/.

Blaffer Hrdy, S. (1999). Mother nature: Maternal instincts and how they shape the human species. New York: Ballantine Publishing Group.

Blaffer Hrdy, S., & Carter, C.S. (1995). Mothering and oxytocin or hormonal cocktails for two. Retrieved on February 23, 2009, from http://puffernet.tripod.com/oxytocin.html.

Block, J. (2007) Pushed: The painful truth about childbirth and modern maternity care. Cambridge: De Capo.

Blomquist, H.K., Jonsbo, F., Serenius F., & Persson L.A. (1994). Supplementary feeding in the maternity ward shortens the duration of breastfeeding. Acta Paediatrica Scandanavia, 83, 1122-1126.

Blum, L. (1999). At the breast: Ideologies of breastfeeding and motherhood in the contemporary United States. Boston: Beacon Press.

Blyth, R., Creedy, D.K., Dennis, C.L., Moyle, W., Pratt, J., & De Vries, S.M. (2002). Effect of maternal confidence on breastfeeding duration: An application of breastfeeding self-efficacy theory. Birth, 29(4), 278-284.

Bodnarchuk, J.L., Eaton, W.O. & Martens, P.J. (2006). Transitions in breastfeeding: Daily parent diaries provide evidence of behaviour over time. Journal of Human Lactation, 22(2), 166-173.

Bolton, T., Chow, T., Benton, P.A., & Olson, B.H. (2009). Characteristics associated with longer breastfeeding duration: An analysis of a peer counselling support program. Journal of Human Lactation, 25(1), 18-27.

Bottorff, J.L. (1990). Persistence in breastfeeding. A phenomenological investigation. Journal of Advanced Nursing, 15(2), 201-209.

Bourgoin, G.L., Lahaie, N.R., Rheaume, B.A., Berger, M.G., Dovigi, C.V., Picard, L.M. & Sahai, V.F. (1997). Factors influencing the duration of breastfeeding in the Sudbury region. Canadian Journal of Public Health, 88(4), 238-241.

Bouchet Horwitz, J. (2001). A special gift: Breastfeeding an adopted baby. Mothering, 104, 62-68.

Bowen, M. (1978). Family therapy in clinical practice. New York: Aronson.

Bowlby, J. (1987). Attachment and loss. Great Britain: Penquin Books.

Brady, M. (2009). National breastfeeding awareness week talk – May 2009. (Online video). Retrieved May 11, 2009, from http://www.youtube.com/watchtv=GxPUsbTqa0l.

Brazelton, T.B., & Yogman, M.W. (Eds.). (1986). Introduction: Reciprocity, attachment, effectance: Anlage in early infancy. Affective development in infancy. (pp. 1-10). Norwood, New Jersey: Ablex Publishing.

Breastfeeding Committee for Canada (BCC). (2002). Affordable health care begins with breastfeeding support and the use of human milk. Retrieved on May 10, 2009, from http://breastfeedingcanada.ca/pdf/webdoc47.pdf.

Britton, J.R. & Britton, H. (2008). Maternal self-concept and breastfeeding. Journal of Human Lactation, 24(4), 431-438.

Brodribb, W., Fallon, A., Jackson, C., & Hegney, D. (2009). Breastfeeding knowledge – the experiences of Australian general practice registrars. Australian Family Physician, 38(1-2), 26-29.

Bronfenbrenner, U. (1979). The ecology of human development. Cambridge, MA: Harvard University Press.

Bronner, Y., Barber, T., Vogelhut, J., & Resnik A. K. (2001). Breastfeeding peer counselling: Results from the national WIC survey. Journal of Human Lactation, 17(2), 119-125.

Brooks, A. (2001). Breastfeeding rights challenged. Canadian Lactation Consultant Association/Association Canadienne des Consultantes en lactation News, 15(1), 1-2.

Buckley, K.M. (1992). Beliefs and practices related to extended breastfeeding among La Leche League moms. The Journal of Perinatal Education, 1(2), 45-53.

Buckner, E., & Matsubara, M. (1993). Support network utilization by breastfeeding mothers. Journal of Human Lactation, 9(4), 231-240.

Bugental, D.B., Blue, J., & Cruzcosa, M. (1989). Perceived control over caregiving outcomes: Implications for child abuse. Developmental Psychology, 25, 532-539.

Bumgarner, N.J. (2000). Mothering your nursing toddler. Franklin Park: La Leche League International Inc.

Canadian Paediatric Society. (2004). Maternal depression and child development. Retrieved on March 4, 2009, from http://www.cps.ca/English/statements/PP/pp04-03.htm.

Carter, B., & McGoldrick, M. (1989). The changing family life cycle: A framework for family life therapy. Boston: Allyn and Bacon.

Carter, P. (1995). Feminism, breasts and breast-feeding. New York: St. Martin's Press.

Cassidy, T. (2007). Birth: A history. London: Chatto & Windus.

Ceriani Cernadas, J. M., Noceda, G., Barrera, L., Martinez, A.M., & Garsd, A. (2003). Maternal and perinatal factors influencing the duration of exclusive breastfeeding during the first 6 months of life. Journal of Human Lactation, 19(2), 136-143.

Chamberlain, D. (1997a). Life before birth: Introduction. Retrieved Dec 10, 2004, from http://birthpsychology.com/lifebefore/index.html#intro.

Chamberlain, D. (1997b). Life before birth: Early and very early parenting. Retrieved Dec. 10, 2004, from http://www.birthpsychology.com/lifebefore/early.html.

Cheales-Siebenaler, N.J. (1999). Induced lactation in an adoptive mother. Journal of Human Lactation, 15(1), 41-43.

Chetley, A. & Allain, A. (1998). Protecting infant health: a health worker's guide to the Internation Code of Marketing of Breast Milk Substitutes. Penang, Malaysia: IBFAN.

Chowdorow, N. (1978). The reproduction of mothering. Berkeley: University of California Press.

Christensson, K., Siles, C., Moreno, L., Belaustequi, A., De La Fuente, P., Lagercrantz, H., et al. (1992). Temperature, metabolic adaptation and crying in healthy full-term newborns cared for skin-to-skin or in a cot. Acta Paediatrica, 81, 488-493.

Chung, M., Raman, G., Trikalino, T., Lau, J. & Ip, S. (2008). Interventions in primary care to promote breastfeeding: An evidence review for the US preventive services task force. Annals of Internal Medicine, 149(8), 565-582.

Clarke-Stewart, K.A. (1998). Historical shifts and underlying themes in ideas about rearing young children in the United States: Where have we been? Where are we going? Early Development & Parenting, 7(2), 101-117.

Cohen, N.J., Muir, E., Lojkasek, M., Muir R., Parker C.J., Barwick, M., & Brown, M. (2000). Watch, wait, and wonder: Testing the effectiveness of a new approach to mother-infant psychotherapy. Infant Mental Health Journal, 20(4), 429-451.

Cohen, R., Lange, L., & Slusser, W. (2002). A description of a male-focused breastfeeding promotion corporate lactation program. Journal of Human Lactation, 18(1), 61-65.

Combrinck-Graham, L. & Kerns, L. (1989). Intimacy in families with young children. In D. Kantor and B.F. Okun (Eds.), Intimate environments: Sex, intimacy, and gender in families. New York: Guildford Press.

Cooke, M., Sheehan, A., & Schmied, V. (2003). A description of the relationship between breastfeeding experiences, and weaning in the first 3 months after birth. Journal of Human Lactation, 19(2), 145-156.

Cowan, C.P., & Cowan, P.A. (1999). When parents become partners: The big life change for couples. Mahwah, NJ: Lawrence Erlbaum Associates.

Cramer, B. (1986). Assessment of parent-infant relationships. In T. B. Brazelton & M.W.Yogman (Eds.) Affective development in infancy. Norwood, New Jersey: Ablex Publishing.

Creedy, D.K., Dennis, C.L., Blyth, R., Moyle, W., Pratt, J., & De Vries, S.M. (2003). Psychometric characteristics of the breastfeeding self-efficacy scale: Data from an Australian sample. Research in Nursing & Health, 26, 143-152.

Crockenberg, S., Lyons-Ruth, K., & Dickstein, S. (1993). The family context of infant mental health: II. Infant development in the primary caregiving relationship. In C.H. Zeanah (Ed.), Handbook of infant mental health. New York: The Guilford Press.

Daly, S.E.J., & Hartmann, P.E. (1995a). Infant demand and milk supply. Part 1: Infant demand and milk production in lactation women. Journal of Human Lactation, 11(1), 21-26.

Daly, S.E.J., & Hartmann, P.E. (1995b). Infant demand and milk supply. Part 2: The short-term control of milk synthesis in lactation women. Journal of Human Lactation, 11(1), 27-37.

Davidowitz, E. (1992, June). The breast-feeding taboo. Redbook, 92-114.

Davis-Floyd, R.E. (1994). The technocratic: American childbirth as cultural expression. Social Science Medicine, 38(8), 1125-1140.

DeBeauvoir, S. (1989). The second sex. H. M. Parshley (Trans.) New York: Vintage Books.

Dennis, C.L. (1999). Theoretical underpinnings of breastfeeding confidence: A self-efficacy framework. Journal of Human Lactation, 15(3), 195-201.

Dettwyler, K.A. (1995a). A time to wean: The hominid blueprint for the natural age of weaning in modern human populations. In P. Stuart-Macadam & K.A. Dettwyler (Eds.), Breastfeeding: Biocultural perspectives. New York: Aldine De Gruyter.

Dettwyler, K.A. (1995b). Beauty and the beast. The cultural context of breastfeeding in the United States. In P. Stuart-Macadam & K. Dettwyler (Eds.), Breastfeeding: Biocultural perspectives. New York: Walter de Gruyler Inc. pp 167-216.

Dewey, K.G., Cohen, R.J., & Rivera, L.L. (2001). Effects of exclusive breastfeeding for four versus six months on nutritional status and infant motor development: Results of two randomized trials in Honduras. Journal of Nutrition, 131(2), 262-267.

Dick, M.J., Evans M.L., Arthurs, J.B., Barnes, J.K., Caldwell, R.S., Hutchins, S.S., & Johnson, L.K. (2002). Predicting early breastfeeding attrition. Journal of Human Lactation, 18(1), 21-28.

Dinnerstein, D. (1977). The Mermaid and the minotaur: Sexual arrangements and human malaise. New York: Perennial Library.

Doherty, W.J., Kouneski, E.F., & Erikson, M.F. (1998). Responsible fathering: An overview and conceptual framework. Journal of Marriage and the Family, 60(2), 277-292.

Drazin, P.B. (1991). Should an LC serve in a paid capacity for a formula company breastfeeding hotline? Journal of Human Lactation, 7(2), 82.

Dundaroz, R., Aydin, H.I., Ulucan, H., Baltaci, V., Denli, M., & Gokcay, E. (2002). Preliminary study on DNA damage in non breast-fed infants. Pediatrics International, 44(2), 127-130.

Ehrensaft, D. (1983). When women and men mother. In J. Trebilcot (Ed.), Mothering essays in feminist theory. New Jersey: Rowman & Allanheld.

Elder, S.B., & Gregory, C. (1996). The "lactation game": An innovative teaching method for healthcare professionals. Journal of Human Lactation, 2, 137-38.

Epstein, K. (1993). The interactions between breastfeeding mothers and their babies during the breastfeeding session. Early Child Development and Care, 87, 93-104.

Epstein, N.B., Bishop, D., Ryan, C., Miller, I.W., & Keitner, G.I., (1993). The McMaster model view of healthy family functioning. In F.Walsh (Ed.), Normal family processes. pp. 138-160. New York: The Guilford Press

Epstein-Gilboa, K. (1997a, June). Enhancing future families' ability to breastfeed through appropriate prenatal strategies. Paper presented at Breastfeeding: Creating Support: Seventh Annual National Breastfeeding Seminar Program. Toronto, Canada.

Epstein-Gilboa, K. (1997b, October). Enhancing breastfeeding education during the prenatal stage. The Breastfeeding Network News, 12, 6.

Epstein-Gilboa, K. (1998a, February). Appropriate teaching strategies to promote breastfeeding in a bottle feeding culture. Paper presented at Metro Toronto Breastfeeding Network: Lunch and Learn. Toronto, Canada.

Epstein-Gilboa, K. (1998b). The implications of object relations theory for cognitive/ behavioral perspectives of breastfeeding difficulties in the early post-partum period. Unpublished manuscript.

Epstein-Gilboa, K. (1999). Using language to facilitate breastfeeding. Retrieved on March, 9, 2008, from http://www.infactcanada.ca/FactSheets.htm.

Epstein-Gilboa, K. (2000, Fall). The psychological reality of breastfeeding. Infant Mental Health Project Print, 28, 18-21.

Epstein-Gilboa, K. (2002). Using language to facilitate breastfeeding. Retrieved on April 21, 2009 from http://www.infactcanada.ca/Using%20Language%20to%20 Facilitate%20Breastfeeding%20by%20Keren%20Epstein%20Gilboa.pdf.

Epstein-Gilboa, K. (2003). Gingerbread house theory. The Journal of Perinatal Education, 12(2), v.

Epstein-Gilboa, K. (2006). Systemic interaction in breastfeeding families. Dissertation Abstracts International, 68(01), 669-1088.

Epstein-Gilboa, K. (2008, October). Using language implying that nursing is a normal developmental task. Poster presentation, VELB/European Lactation Consultants Association Conference. Vienna, Austria.

Epstein-Gilboa, K. (2009). Breastfeeding envy: Unresolved patriarchal envy and the obstruction of physiologically based nursing patterns. In R.M. Shaw & A. Bartlett (Eds.), Giving breastmilk. Toronto, Canada: Demeter Press.

Eyer, D.E. (1992). Mother-infant bonding: A scientific myth. New Haven: Yale University Press.

Eyer, D.E. (1996). Motherguilt: How our culture blames mothers for what's wrong with society. Toronto: Random House.

Fairbairn, W.R.D. (2002a). Schizoid factors in the personality. Psychoanlytic studies of the personality (pp.2-27). New York: Routledge.

Fairbairn, W.R.D. (2002b). A revised psychopathology of the psychoses and psychoneuroses. Psychoanlytic studies of the personality (pp.28-58). New York: Routledge.

Fairbairn, W.R.D. (2002c). Object-relationships and dynamic structure. Psychoanlytic studies of the personality (pp.137-151). New York: Routledge.

Falceto, O.G., Giugliani, C.L, & Fernandes, L.C. (2004). Couples' relationships and breastfeeding: Is there an association? Journal of Human Lactation, 20(1), 46-55.

Feldman, R., Weller, A., Sirota, L., & Eidelman, A.I. (2003). Testing a family intervention hypothesis: The contribution of mother-infant skin-to-skin contact (kangaroo care) to family interaction, proximity and touch. Journal of Family Psychology, 17(1), 94-107.

Feldman-Winter, L., Kruse, L., Mulford, C., & Rotondo, F. (2002). Breastfeeding initiation rates derived from electronic birth certificate data in New Jersey. Journal of Human Lactation, 18(4), 373-378.

Field, T., Hernandez–Reif, M., & Feijo, L. (2002). Breastfeeding in depressed mother-infant duos. Early Child Development and Care, 172(6), 539-545.

Fildes, V. (1995). The culture and biology of breastfeeding. In P. Stuart-Macadam & K. A. Dettwyler (Eds.), Breastfeeding: Biocultural perspectives. New York: Aldine De Gruytler.

First, E. (1994). Mothering, hate, and Winnicott. In D. Bassin, M. Honey, & M.M. Kaplan (Eds.), Representatives of motherhood. New Haven: Yale University Press.

Firestone, S. (1970). The dialect of sex: The case for feminist revolution. New Jersey: Cape Publishing.

Fish, M., Stifter, C., & Belsky J. (1993). Early patterns of mother-infant dyadic interaction: infant, mother, and family demographic antecedents. Infant Behavior & Development, 16(1), 1-18.

Fisher, C. (1984). The initiation of breastfeeding. Midwives Chronicle, 97, 39-41.

Fleming, A.S., Ruble, D.N., Flett, G., & Shaul, D.L. (1988). Postpartum adjustment in first-time mothers: Relations between mood, maternal attitudes, and mother-infant interactions. Developmental Psychology, 24(1), 71-81.

Fogel, A. (1993) Developing through relationships: Origins of communication, self and culture. Chicago: The University of Chicago Press.

Forste, R. & Hoffmann, J.P. (2008). Are US mothers meeting the Healthy People 2010 breastfeeding targets for initiation, duration, and exclusivity? The 2003 and 2004 National Immunization Surveys. Journal of Human Lactation, 24(3), 278-288.

Fouts, H.N., Hewlett, B.S., & Lamb, M.E. (2001). Weaning and the nature of early childhood interactions among Bofi foragers in Central Africa. Human Nature, 12(1), 27-46.

Fox, H. (1996). Projective identification. Retrieved July 15, 2005, from http://www.object-relations.com/Projid.doc.
Fox, A., & Schaefer, C. (1999). Pacifier use in young children: Practical research findings. Psychology: A Journal of Human Behavior, 33(1), 30-34.
Fraiberg, S. (1987). The origins of human bonds. In L. Fraiberg (Ed.), Selected writings of Selma Fraiberg. Columbus, Ohio: Ohio State University Press.
Fraiberg, S., Adelson, E., & Shapiro, V. (1987). Ghosts in the nursery: A psychoanlytic approach to the problems of impaired infant-mother relationships. In L. Fraiberg (Ed.), Selected writings of Selma Fraiberg. Columbus, Ohio: Ohio State University Press.
Framo, J.L. (1992). Family of origin therapy: An intergenerational approach. New York: Brunner/Mazel Publishers.
Frank, D. (1989). Commercial discharge packs and breastfeeding counseling: Summary of a study. Journal of Human Lacation, 5(1), 7-10.
Freed, G.L., Fraley, J.K., & Schanler, R.J. (1993). Accuracy of expectant mothers' predictions of fathers' attitudes regarding breastfeeding. Journal of Family Practice, 37(2):148-152.
Friedman, M.E. (1996). Mother's milk: A psychoanalyst looks at breastfeeding. Psychoanalytic Study of the Child, 51, 475-490.
Galinsky, E. (1987). The six stages of parenthood. Reading Massachusetts: Addison-Welsley Publishing.
Galler, J., Harrison, R.H., Biggs, M.A., Ramsey, F., & Forde, V. (1999). Maternal moods predict breastfeeding in Barbados. Journal of Developmental Behavioral Pediatrics, 20(2), 80-87.
Garbarino, J. (1976). A preliminary study of some ecological correlates of child abuse: The socioeconomic stress on mothers. Child Development, 17, 178-185.
Garbarino, J. (1977). The human ecology of child maltreatment: A conceptual model for research. Journal of Marriage and the Family, November, 721-735.
Gerrish, C.J., & Mennella, J.A. (2000). Short-term influence of breastfeeding on the infants' interaction with the environment. Developmental Psychobiology, 36(1), 40-48.
Giles, F. (2003). Fresh milk: The secret life of the breasts. New York: Simon & Schuster.
Gill, S.L. (1998). Being a nursing mother. Dissertation Abstracts International: Section B: The Sciences and Engineering, 59(2-B), 602.
Gilligan, C. (1993). In a different voice: Psychological theory and women's development. Cambridge, MA: Harvard University Press.
Giugliani, E.R.J., Caiaffa, W.T., Vogelhut, J., Witter, F., & Perman, J.A. (1994). Effect of breastfeeding support from different sources on mother's decisions to breastfeed. Journal of Human Lactation, 10(3), 157-161.
Goldberg, S. (1991). Recent developments in the attachment. Canadian Journal of Psychiatry, 36, 393-400.
Golden, J. (2001). A social history of wet nursing in America: From breast to bottle. Columbia: Ohio State University Press.
Goldenberg, I., & Goldenberg, H. (2007). Family therapy: An overview (7th ed.). Florence, KY: Cengage Learning.

Goodrich, T.J., Rampage, C., Ellman, B., & Halstead, K., (1988). Feminist family therapy: A casebook. New York: Norton.

Gorman, K.J. (2002). Breastfeeding and cosleeping: A correlational assessment. Dissertation Abstracts International: Section B: The Sciences & Engineering. 62(9-B), 4273.

Granju, K.A., & Kennedy, B. (1999). Attachment parenting: Instinctive care for your baby and young child. New York: Pocket Books.

Gray, L., Watt, L., & Blass, E.M. (2000). Skin-to-skin contact is analgesic in healthy newborns. Pediatrics, 105(1), e14.

Green, K.E. (2001). Attachment parenting: New ideas, old practices. Dissertations Abstracts International: Section B: The Sciences & Engineering. 61(9-B), 5027.

Greenberg, J.R., & Mitchell, S.A. (2000). Objects relations in psychoanalytic theory. Cambridge: Harvard University Press.

Greenspan, S.I., & Wieder S. (1993). Regulatory disorders. In C.H. Zeanah (Ed.), Handbook of infant mental health. New York: The Guilford Press.

Gribble, K.D. (2006). Mental health, attachment and breastfeeding: implications for adopted children and their mothers. International Breastfeeding Journal, 1, 1-5. Retrieved on February 23, 2009, from http://www.internationalbreastfeedingjournal.com/content/1/1/5.

Griswold, R.L. (1993). Fatherhood in America. New York: Basic Books.

Groër, M.W., & Davis, M.W. (2006). Cytokines, infections, stress, and dysphoric moods in breastfeeders and formula feeders. Journal of Obstetric Gynecologic Neonatal Nursing 2006, 35:599-607.

Groër, M.W., Davis, M.W., & Hemphill, J. (2002). Postpartum stress: Current concepts and the possible protective role of breastfeeding. Journal of Obstetric Gynecologic Neonatal Nursing, 31, 411-417.

Grusec, J.E., Rudy, D., & Martini, T. (1997). Parenting cognitions and child outcomes: An overview and implications for children's internalisation of values. In J.E. Grusec & L. Kuczynski (Eds.), Parenting and children's internalization of values. New York: Wiley.

Guttman, N., & Zimmerman, D.R. (2000). Low income mothers' view on breastfeeding. Social Science and Medicine, 50(10), 1457-1473.

Haiek, L.N., Gauthier, D.L., Brousseau, D., & Rocheleau, L. (2007). Understanding breastfeeding behavior: rates and shifts in patterns in Québec. Journal of Human Lactation, 23(1), 24-31.

Hann, M., Malan, A., Kronson, M., Bergman N., & Huskisson R. (1999). Kangaroo mother care. South African Medical Journal, 89, 37-40.

Happy & Healthy Pregnancy. (2009). Breastfeeding and dads: What men can do. Retrieved on May 19, 2009, from http://www.happyhealthypregnancy.com/info/bow/article.aspx?article_id=2380&s=MyYahoo&_nc=633777888255113634&_nockcheck=true.

Harmon-Jones, C. (2006). Duration, intensity, and exclusivity of breastfeeding: Recent research confirms the importance of these variables. Breastfeeding Abstracts, 25(3), 17-20.

Harper, B. (2005). Gentle birth choices. Vermont: Inner Traditions.

Hauck, Y.L., & Irurita, V.F. (2003). Incompatible expectations: The dilemma of breastfeeding mothers. Healthcare for Women International, 24(1), 62-78.

Hayes, M.J., Roberts, S. M., & Stowe, R. (1996). Early childhood co-sleeping: Parent-child and parent-infant nighttime interactions. Infant Mental Health Journal, 17(4), 348-357.

Health Canada. (2004). Exclusive breastfeeding duration – 2004 Health Canada recommendation. Retrieved on May 21, 2009, from http://www.hc-sc.gc.ca/fn-an/nutrition/child-enfant/infant-nourisson/excl_bf_dur-dur_am_excl-eng.php#ref1.

Hedberg Nyqvist, K., Sjoden, P.O., & Ewald, U. (1999). The development of preterm infants' breastfeeding behavior. Early Human Development, 55, 247-264.

Heinig, M.J. (2001). The cost of breastfeeding support: A primer. Journal of Human Lactation, 17(2), 101-102.

Heinig, M.J. (2003). The "price" of information. Journal of Human Lactation, 19(2), 133-135.

Heinig, M.J., & Dewey, K.G. (1996). Health advantages of breastfeeding for infants: A critical review. Nutrition Research Review, 9, 89-110.

Held, V. (1984). The obligations of mothers and fathers. J. Trebilcot (Ed.), Mothering: Essays in feminist theory. New Jersey: Rowman & Allanheld Publishers.

Henderson, L., Kitzinger, J., & Green, J. (2001). Representing infant feeding: Content analysis of British media portrayals of bottle feeding and breast feeding. British Medical Journal, 322(7278), 90.

Hill, P.D., Hanson, K.S., & Mefford, M.S. (1994). Mothers of low birthweight infants: Breastfeeding patterns and problems. Journal of Human Lactation, 10(3), 169-176.

Hill, P.D., Humenick, S.S., & Tieman, B. (1997). Maternal activities used to soothe crying of 3-week-old breastfed infants. The Journal of Perinatal Education, 6(1), 13-20.

Hop, L.T., Gross, R., Giay, T., Sastroamidjojo, S., Schultink W., & Lang., N.T. (2000). Premature complementary feeding is associated with poorer growth of Vietnamese children. Journal of Nutrition. 130, 2683-2690.

Humenick, S., & Hill, P. (1996). Salespeople and the lactation army: Taking a stand for health and human milk. Journal of Human Lactation, 12(1), 5-8.

Hyde, J.S., DeLamater, J.D., Plant, E.A., & Byrd, J.M. (1996). Sexuality during pregnancy and the year postpartum. Journal of Sex Research, 33(2), 143-151.

Infant Feeding Action Coalition. (1992a, Spring) Breasts, body image and breastfeeding. INFACT Canada Newsletter, 3.

Infant Feeding Action Coalition. (1992b, Spring). Ducking the code: 54th WHA emphasizes applicability of code to follow-up formula. INFACT Canada Newsletter, 4-5.

Infant Feeding Action Coalition. (1992c, Summer). Cow's milk formula trigger in juvenile diabetes? INFACT Canada Newsletter, 1.

Infant Feeding Action Coalition. (1993a, Summer). Formula mishaps and mistakes threaten infant health. INFACT Canada Newsletter, 1, 2.

Infant Feeding Action Coalition. (1993b, Fall). For love & affection & other considerations. INFACT Canada Newsletter, 4, 5.

Infant Feeding Action Coalition. (1993c, Fall). Who cares what you feed your baby? INFACT Canada Newletter, 2, 3.

Infant Feeding Action Coalition. (1994, Winter). Rx: breast only. What difference does it make? INFACT Canada Newsletter, 1, 3.
Infant Feeding Action Coalition. (1995, Winter). Breastfeeding in a bottle feeding culture. INFACT Canada Newsletter, 3, 6.
Infant Feeding Action Coalition. (1996a, Summer). Infant formula companies battle for the breast. INFACT Canada Newsletter, 4.
Infant Feeding Action Coalition. (1996b, Summer). The only food group baby needs. INFACT Canada Newsletter, 5, 7.
Infant Feeding Action Coalition. (1996c, Summer). Women on the frontlines: Breastfeeding and human rights. INFACT Canada Newsletter, 3.
Infant Feeding Action Coalition. (1997a, Winter). Breastfeeding: A human right. INFACT Canada Newsletter, 1, 3.
Infant Feeding Action Coalition. (1997b, Summer). Nutritionists blasted for Nestle sponsorship. INFACT Canada Newsletter, 4, 5.
Infant Feeding Action Coalition. (1998, Fall). Canadian Paediatric Society nutrition advice laced with artificial feeding. INFACT Canada Newsletter, 2.
Infant Feeding Action Coalition. (1999a, Spring & Summer). Formula feeding increases cancer risk. INFACT Canada Newsletter. 1, 3.
Infant Feeding Action Coalition. (1999b, Fall). Complementary feeding "at about six months". INFACT Canada Newsletter. 1, 2.
Infant Feeding Action Coalition. (1999c, Fall). Promotion and labelling of complementary foods violate Canada's laws. INFACT Canada Newsletter, 3.
Infant Feeding Action Coalition. (2002a, Summer/Fall). Optimal duration of exclusive breastfeeding. INFACT Canada Newsletter, 3.
Infant Feeding Action Coalition (2002b). Out of the mouth's of babes: How Canada's infant food industry defies world health organization rules and puts infant health at risk. Retrieved on May 6, 2009 from http://www.infactcanada.ca/200D.PDF.
Infant Feeding Action Coalition. (2003a, Spring). Breastfeeding and intelligence – how a tinkering with deficiencies in formulas cannot replace breastmilk. INFACT Canada Newsletter, 3-4.
Infant Feeding Action Coalition. (2003b, Summer/Fall). Breastfeeding and co-sleeping; Is it safe for babies to sleep alone? INFACT Canada Newsletter, 1-3.
Infant Feeding Action Coalition. (2004, Winter). US breastfeeding campaign sabotaged by corporate pressure. INFACT Canada Newsletter, 5.
Infant Feeding Action Coalition. (2007a, Winter). Breastfeeding and birthing: Do birthing practices affect breastfeeding. INFACT Canada Newsletter, 1-3.
Infant Feeding Action Coalition (2007b). The inner workings of the formula industry. Retrieved on May 7, 2009 from http://www.infactcanada.ca/Newsletters/2007-Winter/inner_workings.htm.
Infant Feeding Action Coalition. (2009a). What is INFACT? Retrieved on March 3, 2009, from http://www.infactcanada.ca/about.htm.
Infant Feeding Action Coalition. (2009b). Kangaroo care. Retrieved on March 3, 2009 from http://www.infactcanada.ca/Kangaroo%20Care.pdf.
International Baby Food Action Network. (1999, January). Nestle Boycott News. What is the problem? IBFAN INFO, 1(1), 7.

Isaacs, S. (1997). The nature and function of phantasy. In D.E. Scharff (Ed), Object relations theory and practice. Northvale, North Jersey: Jason Aronson, Inc. (Original work published in 1948.)

Jordan, P.L. (1990). Laboring for relevance: Expectant and new fatherhood. Nursing Research, 39(1), 11-16.

Jordan, P.L., & Wall V.R. (1993). Supporting the father when an infant is breastfed. Journal of Human Lactation, 9(1), 31-34.

Kaplan, L.J. (1978). Oneness & separateness: From infant to individual. New York: Simon & Schuster.

Karen, R. (1990, February). Becoming attached. The Atlantic Monthly, 35-70.

Karen, R. (1994). Becoming attached: First relationships and how they shape our capacity to love. New York: Oxford University Press.

Kelly, M. (1983). Post-partum document. London: Routledge & Kegan Paul.

Kelly, Y.J., & Watt, R.G. (2004). Breast-feeding initiation and exclusive duration at 6 months by social class – results from the Millennium Cohort Study. Public Health Nutrition, 8(4), 417-421.

Kendall-Tackett, K. A., & Sugarman M. (1995). The social consequences of long-term breastfeeding. Journal of Human Lactation, 11(3), 179-184.

Kendall-Tackett, K. (2005). Depression in new mothers: Causes, consequences, and treatment alternatives. New York: Haworth Maltreatment and Trauma Press.

Kendall-Tackett, K. (2007). A new paradign for depression in new mothers: the central role of inflammation and how breastfeeding and anti-inflammatory treatments protect maternal mental health. International Breastfeeding Journal, 2:6. Retrieved on March 27, 2009 from http://www.granitescientific.com/granitescientific%20home%20page_files/ibj%20new%20paradigm.pdf .

Kennell, J.H., & Klaus, M.H. (1998). Bonding: Recent observations that alter perinatal care. Pediatrics in Review, 19(1), 4-14.

Kerr, M.E., & Bowen, M. (1988). Family evaluation: An approach based on theory. New York: W.W. Norton.

Kessler, L.A., Carlson Gielen, A., Diener-West, M., & Paige, D. (1995). The effect of a woman's significant other on her breastfeeding decision. Journal of Human Lactation, 11(2), 103-109.

Kistin, N., Abramson, R., & Dublin, P. (1994). Effect of peer counsellors on breastfeeding initiation, exclusivity and duration among low income urban women. Journal of Human Lactation, 10(1), 11-16.

Kitzinger, S. (1979). The experience of breastfeeding. Middlesex England: Penguin Books.

Kitzinger, S. (1995). Commentary. In P. Stuart-Macadam & K.A. Dettwyler (Eds.), Breastfeeding: Biocultural perspectives. New York: Aldine De Gruyter.

Klaus, H.M., Kennell, J.H., & Klaus, P.H. (1995). Bonding: Building the foundations of secure attachment and independence. Reading Mass: Addison-Wesley Publishing Company, Inc.

Klaus, M.H., & Klaus, P.H. (1998). Your amazing newborn. Reading Massachusetts: Perseus Books.

Klein, M. (1997a). The psycho-analysis of children (Rev. ed.). London: Vintage Books.

Klein, M. (1997b) Envy and gratitude and other works: 1946-1963. London: Vintage.

Klein, M. (1998). Love, guilt and reparation: and other works 1921-1945. London: Vintage.

Kleinplatz, P. (2001). On the outside looking in: In search of women's sexual experience. Women & Therapy, 24(1-2), 123-132.

Koepke, J.E., & Bigelow, A.E. (1997). Observations of newborn suckling behavior. Infant Behavior and Development, 20(11), 93-97.

Korja, R., Savonlahti, E., Ahlqvist-Björkroth, S., Stolt, S., Haataja, L., Lapinleimu, H., Piha, J., & Lehtonen, L. (2008). Maternal depression is associated with mother infant interaction in preterm infants. Acta Paediatrica. 98(6), 724-730.

Kramer, J.R. (1985). Family interfaces: Transgenerational patterns. New York: Brunner/Mazel.

Kramer, M.S., Barr, R.G., Dagenais, S., Yang, H., Jones, P., Ciofani, L., & Jane, F. (2001). Pacifier use, early weaning, and cry/fuss behavior: A randomized controlled trial. Journal of the American Medical Association, 286(3), 322-326.

Kroeger, M. (2003, Summer). Restoring the mother and baby continuum. Genesis, 5.

Kroeger, M., & Smith, L.J. (2004). Impact of birthing practices on breastfeeding: Protecting the mother and baby continuum. Sudbury MA: Jones and Bartlett.

Kruger, A.C., & Tomasello, M. (1996). Cultural learning and learning culture. In D.R. Olson & N. Torrance (Eds.), The handbook of education and human development. Oxford: Blackwell Publishers.

Kuzela, A.L., Stifter, C.A., & Worobey, J. (1990). Breastfeeding and mother infant interactions. Journal of Reproductive & Infant Psychology, 8(3), 185-194.

Labbok, M. (2008). Exploration of guilt among mothers who do not breastfeed: The physician's role. Journal of Human Lactation, 24(1), 80-84.

Labbok, M., & Krasovec, K. (1990). Towards consistency in breastfeeding definitions. Studies in Family Planning, 21(4), 226-230.

Labbok, M., Wardlaw, T., Blanc, A., Clark, D. & Terreri, N. (2006). Trends in exclusive breastfeeding: Findings about the 1990s. Journal of Human Lactation, 22(3), 272-276.

La Leche League International. (2004). The womanly art of breastfeeding. Franklin Park Illionois: La Leche League International.

Lamb, M.E. (1980). The development of parent-infant attachments in the first two years of life. In F.A. Pedersen (Ed.), The father-infant relationship: Observational studies in the family setting. New York: Praeger Publishers.

Lamb, M.E. (Ed.). (1987). Introduction: The emergent American father. The father's role: Cross cultural perspectives. Hillsdale NJ: Erlbaum.

Lamb, M.E., & Kelly, J.B. (2000). Using child development research to make appropriate custody and access decisions for young children. Family and Conciliation Courts Review, 38(3), 306-307.

Landy, S., & Menna, R. (2006). Early intervention with multi-risk families: An integrative approach. Baltimore, MD: Paul H. Brookes.

Lauwers, J., & Swisher, A. (2005). Counseling the nursing mother: A lactation consultant's guide (4th ed.). Boston: Jones and Bartlett.

Lawrence, R., & Lawrence, R. (2005). Breastfeeding: A guide for the medical profession (6th ed). St. Louis: Mosby.

Leff, E.W., Gagne, M.P., & Jeffries, S.C. (1994). Maternal perceptions of successful breastfeeding. Journal of Human Lactation, 10(2), 99-104.

Levitt, C., Kaczorowski, J., Hanvey, L., Avard, D., & Chance, G. (1996). Breast-feeding policies and practices in Canadian hospitals providing maternity care. Canadian Medical Association Journal, 155(2), 181-188.

Lewis, C. (1986). Becoming a father. Philadelphia: Open University Press.

Li, R., Ogden, C., Ballew, C., Gillespie, C., & Grummer-Strawn, L. (2002). Prevalence of exclusive breastfeeding among US infants: The third national health and nutrition examination survey (phase II, 1991-1994). American Journal of Public Health, 92(7), 1107-1110.

Libbus, M. K., & Kolostov, L.S. (1994). Perceptions of breastfeeding and infant feeding choices in a group of low-income mid-Missouri women. Journal of Human Lactation, 10(1), 17-24.

Libbus, M.K., Bush, T.A., & Hockman, N. M. (1997). Breastfeeding beliefs of low-income primigravidae. International Journal of Nursing Studies, 34(2), 144-150.

Liedloff, J. (1985). The continuum concept: In search of lost happiness. Reading Massachusetts: Addison-Wesley Publishing Company.

Lindberg, L.D. (1996). Women's decisions about breastfeeding and maternal employment. Journal of Marriage and the Family, 58(1), 239-251.

Litton Fox, G., Bruce, C., & Combs-Orme, T. (2000). Parenting expectations and concerns of fathers and mothers of newborn infants. Family Relations, 49(2), 123-131.

Littman, H., Mendendorp, S., & Goldfarb, J. (1994). The decision to breastfeed. The importance of the father's approval. Clinical Pediatrics, 33, 214-219.

Livingstone, V. (1996). In-hospital lactation assessment. Journal of the Society of Obstetricians and Gynaecologists, 18, 45-54.

Losch, M., Dungy, C.L., Russell, D., & Dusdieker, L.B. (1995). Impact of attitudes on maternal decisions regarding infant feeding. Journal of Pediatrics, 126(4), 507-514.

Lothian, J. (2005). The birth of a breastfeeding baby and mother. Journal of Perinatal Education. 14(1), 42-45.

Ludington-Hoe, S.M., Anderson, G.C., Simpson, S., Hollingsead, A., Argote, L.A., Medellin, G., & Rey, H. (1993). Skin to skin contact beginning in the delivery room for Colombian mothers and their preterm infants. Journal of Human Lactation, 9(4), 241-242.

Ludington-Hoe, S.M., & Golant, S.K. (1993). Kangaroo care: The best you can do to help your preterm infant. New York: Bantam Books.

Ludington-Hoe, S.M., Morgan, K., & Abouelfettoh, A. (2008). A clinical guideline for implementation of kangaroo care with premature infants of 30 or more weeks postmenstrual age. Advances in Neonatal Care, 8(3), S3-S23.

Lyons-Ruth, K., & Zeanah, C.H. (1993). The family context of infant mental health: I. Affective development in the primary caregiving relationship. In C.H. Zeanah (Ed.), The handbook of infant mental health. (pp.14-37). New York: The Guilford Press.

Maclean, H. (1990). Women's experience of breastfeeding. Toronto: University of Toronto Press.

Maher, V. (1995). Breastfeeding in cross-cultural perspectives: Paradoxes and proposals. In V. Maher (Ed.), The anthropology of breastfeeding: Natural law or social construct. Oxford: Berg Publishers.

Mahler, M.S., Pine, F., & Bergman, A. (1975). The psychological birth of the human infant. United States: Basic Books.

Main, M. (1995). Recent studies in attachment: Overview with selected implications for clinical work. In S. Goldberg, R. Muir, & J. Kerr (Eds.), Attachment theory: Social development and clinical perspectives (pp. 407-474). Hillsdale N.J.: The Analytic Press.

Marshall, W.M. (1995). Psychophysiological aspects of lactation. Dissertation Abstracts International: Section B: The Sciences & Engineering, 55(7-B), 3055.

Matthews, K., Webber, K., McKim, E., Banoub-Baddour, S., & Laryea, M. (1998). Maternal, infant-feeding decisions: Reasons and influences. Canadian Journal Nurse Research, 30(2), 177-198.

Matthews, M.K. (1991). Mother's satisfaction with their neonates' behaviors. Journal of Obstetrics, Gynecologic and Neonatal Nursing, 20(1), 49-55.

Matthews, M.K. (1993). Assessments and suggested interventions to assist newborn breastfeeding behavior. Journal of Human Lactation, 9(4), 241-246.

Matthiesen, A.S., Ransjo-Arvidson, A.B., Nissen, E., & Uvnas-Moberg, K. (2001). Postpartum maternal oxytocin release by newborns: Effects of infant hand massage and sucking. Birth, 28(1), 13-19.

McBride, B.A., & Rane, T.R. (1998). Parenting alliance as a predictor of father involvement: An exploratory study. Family Relations, 47(3), 229-236.

McKenna, J.J. (1996). Sudden infant death syndrome in cross cultured perspective: Is infant parent cosleeping protective? Annual Review of Anthropology, 25, 201-216.

McKenna, J.J., & Mosko, S. (1993). Evolution and infant sleep: An experimental study of infant-parent co-sleeping and its implications for SIDS. Acta Pediatrics Suppl, 389, 31-36.

McKenna, J.J., Mosko, S., Richard, C., Drummond, S., Hunt, L., Cetel, M.B., et al. (1994). Experimental studies of infant-parent co-sleeping: Mutual physiological and behavioral influences and their relevance to SIDS. Early Human Development, 38, 187-201.

McKenna, J.J., Mosko, S., & Richard, C. (1997). Bedsharing promotes breastfeeding. Pediatrics, 100(2), 214-219.

McLeod, D., Pullon, S., & Cookson, T. (2002). Factors influencing continuation of breastfeeding in a cohort of women. Journal of Human Lactation, 18(4), 335-343.

Mead Johnson. (2009). FAQs – Breastfeeding – Enfamil. Retrieved on May 21, 2009 from http://www.meadjohnson.ca/en/faq/faq_breastfeeding.html.

Merten, S. & Ackermann-Liebrich, U. (2004). Exclusive breastfeeding rates and associated factors in Swiss baby-friendly hospitals. Journal of Human Lactation, 20(1), 9-17.

Mezzacappa, E.S. 2004. Breastfeeding and maternal stress response and health. Nutrition Review, 62(7 Pt 1), 261-268.

Mikiel-Kostyra, K., Mazur, J., & Boltrusko, I. (2002). Effect of early skin-to-skin contact after delivery on duration of breastfeeding: A prospective cohort study. Acta Paediatrica, 91(12), 1301-1306.

Minchin, M. (1998). Breastfeeding matters. Australia: Alma Publications.

Minuchin, S., & Fishman, H.C. (1996). Family therapy techniques. (14th printing). Cambridge Massachusetts: Harvard University Press.

Mohrbacher, N., & Stock, J. (2003) Breastfeeding answer book. 3rd Ed. Schaumburg, IL: La Leche League International.

Montagu, A. (1978). Touching: The human significance of the skin. NewYork: Columbia University Press.

Morton, J.A. (1992). Ineffective suckling: A possible consequence of obstructive positioning. Journal of Human Lacation, 8(2), 83-85.

Nakamura, S., Wind, M., & Danello, M.A. (1999). Review of hazards associated with children placed in adult beds. Pediatrics & Adolescent Medicine, 153(10), 1019-1023.

Neifert, M.R. (1996). Early assessment of the breastfeeding infant. Contemporary Pediatrics, 13(10), 142-166.

Neifert, M.R., Lawrence, R., & Seacat J. (1995). Nipple confusion: Towards a formal definition. Journal of Pediatrics, 126, S125-S129.

Newman, J. (1990). Breastfeeding problems associated with the early introduction of bottles and pacifiers. Journal of Human Lactation, 6, 59-63.

Newman, J. (1992a). The baby friendly hospital initiative. The Canadian Journal of Pediatrics, August, 117-122.

Newman, J. (1992b). Breastfeeding issues and controversies. Contemporary OB/Gyn, July/Aug, 55-60.

Newman, J. (1997, August). Breastfeeding and guilt. Dr. Jack Newman's handouts, Handout 23. Retrieved May 6, 2009, from http://www.breastfeeding.com/advocacy/advocacy_bf_guilt.html.

Newman, J. (1998). Breastfeeding support. Contemporary Pediatrics, 1(3), 6-12.

Newman, J. & Pitman, T. (2009). Dr. Jack Newman's guide to breastfeeding. Revised ed. Toronto: Harper Collins.

Newman, J., & Sterken E. (1992). Establishing breastfeeding: Starting off right. The Canadian Journal of Pediatrics, April, 52-60.

Nichols, M.P., & Schwartz, R.C. (2006). Family therapy: Concepts and methods (7th ed.). New York: Allyn and Bacon.

Nissen, E., Lilja, G., Widstrom, A.M., & Uvnas-Moberg, K. (1995). Elevation of oxytocin levels early postpartum in women. Acta Obstetrics Gynecology Scandinavia, 74(7), 530-533.

Nissen, E., Gustavsson, P., Widstrom, A.M., & Uvnas-Moberg, K. (1998). Oxytocin, prolactin, milk production and their relationship with personality traits in women after vaginal delivery or Cesarean section. Journal of Psychosomatic Obstetrics & Gynecology, 19(1), 49-58.

Oately, K., & Jenkins, J. (1996). Understanding emotions. Cambridge: Blackwell Publishers.

O'Connor, M.E., & Szekely, L.J. (2001). Frequent breastfeeding and food refusal with failure to thrive. Clinical Pediatrics, 40(1), 27-33.

Oddy, W.H. (2001). Breastfeeding protects against illness and infection in infants and children: A review of evidence. Breastfeeding Review, 9(2), 11-18.

Odent, M. (1999, April). Fetal life birth and health. Paper presented at 4th Annual Birth Conference, L & M Associates, Toronto, Ontario.

Okami, P., Weisner T., & Olmstead, R. (2002). Outcome correlates of parent-child bedsharing: An eighteen-year longitudinal study. Developmental and Behavioral Pediatrics, 23(4), 244-253.

Owens, A.M. (2000, Dec. 12). When to wean. National Post online. Retrieved Dec.12, 2000, from http://wysiwyg://Network_page.26/http//...I?f=/stories/20001212/401650.html.

Ozment, S. (1983). When fathers ruled: family life in reformation Europe. Cambridge, Massachusetts: Harvard University Press.

Palmer, G. (1991). Give breastfeeding back to mothers. Journal of Human Lactation, 7(1), 1-2.

Palmer, G. (2009). The politics of breastfeeding: When breasts are bad for business (3rd ed.). London: Printer & Martin Ltd.

Parke, R.D. (1996). Fatherhood. Cambridge Massachusetts: Harvard University Press.

Peddlesen, J. (1998). Can't we just take the money and run? Canadian Lactation Consultant Association News, 12(3), 1,4-5.

Pedersen, F.A. (Ed.). (1980). Research issues related to fathers and infants. The father-infant relationship: Observational studies in the family setting. New York: Praeger Publishers.

Pederson, F.A., Anderson B.J., & Cain R. L. (1980). Parent-infant and husband-wife interactions observed at five months. In F.A. Pederson (Ed.) The father-infant relationship: Observational studies in the family setting. New York: Praeger Publishers.

Persson-Blenow, I., Naslund, B., McNeil, T.F., Kaij, L., & Maimquist-Larson, A. (1984). Offspring of women with non-organic psychosis: Mother-infant interaction at three days of age. Acta Psychiatria Scandinavica, 70, 149-159.

Persson-Blenow, I., Naslund, B., McNeil, T.F., & Kaij, L (1986). Offspring of women with non-organic psychosis: Mother-infant interaction at one year of age. Acta Psychiatria Scandinavica, 73, 207-213.

Petersen, M. (2003, Dec. 4). Breastfeeding ads delayed by a dispute over content. New York Times, C1.

Piper, S., & Parks, P.L. (1996). Predicting the duration of lactation: Evidence from a national survey. Birth, 23(1), 7-12.

Playtex, Canada. (2003). M.O.M.: Mother's Own Milk Program. (Brochure).

Pollard, K., Fleming, P., Young, J., Sawczenko, A., & Blair, P. (1999). Night-time non-nutritive sucking in infants aged 1to 5 months: Relationship with infant state, breastfeeding and bed-sharing versus room-sharing. Early Human Development, 56(2-3), 185-204.

Pollock, C.A., Bustamante-Forest, R., & Giarrantano, G. (2002). Men of diverse cultures: Knowledge and attitudes about breastfeeding. Journal of Obstetric, Gynecologic and Neonatal Nursing, 31(6), 673-679.

Pridham, K.F., Schroeder, M., Brown, R., & Clark, R. (2001). The relationship of a mother's working model of feeding to her feeding behavior. Journal of Advanced Nursing, 35(5), 741-750.

Pruett, K.D. (1997). How men and children affect each other's development. Zero to Three Journal, 18, 1. Retrieved July 20, 2005, from http://www.zerotothree.org/fathers.html.

Quandt, S.A. (1995). Sociocultural aspects of the lactation process. In P. Stuart-Macadam & K.A. Dettwyler (Eds.), Breastfeeding: biocultural perspectives. New York: Aldine De Gruyter.

Rabuzzi, K.A. (1988). Motherself: A mythical analysis of motherhood. Blooomington: Indiana University Press.

Rabuzzi, K.A. (1994). Mother with child: Transformations through childbirth. Bloomington: Indiana University Press.

Ransjo-Arvidson, A.B., Matthiesen, A.S., Lilja, G., Nissen, E., Widstrom, A.M., & Uvnas-Moberg, K. (2001). Maternal analgesia during labor disturbs newborn behavior: Effects on breastfeeding and crying. Birth, 28(1), 5-12.

Reddy, S. (1995). Breast-feeding practices, problems and prospects. Journal of Family Welfare, 41(4), 43-51.

Renfrew, M.J. (1989). Positioning the baby at the breast: More than a visual skill. Journal of Human Lactation, 5(1), 13-16.

Renfrew, M., Fisher, C., & Arms, S. (1990). Bestfeeding. Celestial Arts: Berkeley.

Renfrew, M.J., McFadden, A., Dykes, F., Wallace, L.M., Abbott, S., Burt, S., & Anderson, J.K. (2006). Addressing the learning deficit in breastfeeding: Strategies for change. Maternal and Child Nutrition, 2(4), 239-244.

Reynolds, A. (2001). Breastfeeding and brain development. Pediatric Clinics of North America, 48(1), 159-71.

Rich, A. (1986). Of women born: Motherhood as experience and institution. (10th anniversay ed.). New York: W.W. Norton & Company.

Richter, J. (2002). Holding corporations accountable: Corporate conduct, international codes, and citizen action. London: Zed Books.

Righard, L., & Alade, M.O. (1990). Effect of delivery room routines on success of first breast-feed. Lancet, 336, 1105-1107.

Righard, L. (1998). Are breastfeeding problems related to incorrect breastfeeding technique and the use of pacifiers and bottles. Birth, 25(1), 40-44.

Riordan, J. (2005). Breastfeeding and human lactation. (3rd ed.). Boston: Jones & Bartlett.

Rodriguez-Garcia, R. & Frazier, L. (1995). Cultural paradoxes relating to sexuality and breastfeeding. Journal of Human Lactation, 11(2), 111-121.

Rogers, I.S. (1997). Relactation. Early Human Development, 49, S75-S81.

Rogers, I.S., Emmett, P.M., & Golding, I. (1997). The incidence and duration of breast feeding. Early Human Development, 49(Suppl), S45-S74.

Rosenthal, M.S. (1995). The breastfeeding sourcebook: Everything you need to know. Los Angeles, Ca: Lowell House.

Ryan, K.M., & Grace, V.M. (2001). Medicalization and women's knowledge. The construction of understanding of infant feeding experiences in post WWII New Zealand. Healthcare for Women International, 22(5), 483-500.

Saha, P. (2002). Breastfeeding and sexuality: Professional advice literature from the 1970s to the present. Health Education & Behavior, 29(1), 61-72.

Satir, V.M. (1967). Conjoint family therapy. Palo Alto: Science and Behavior Books.

Scharff, D.E. (Ed.). (1997). The major trends in object relations theory. In Object relations theory and practice. Northvale, New Jersey; Jason Aronson Inc.

Scharff, D.E., & Savege Scharff, J. (1991). Object relations family therapy. Northvale: New Jersey: Jason Aronson Inc.

Schmied, V., & Barclay, L. (1999). Connection and pleasure, disruption and distress: Women's experience of breastfeeding. Journal Human Lactation, 15(4), 325-335.

Scott, J.A. & Mostyn, T. (2003). Women's experiences of breastfeeding in a bottle-feeding culture. Journal of Human Lactation, 19(3), 270-277.

Sears, W. (1988). Developing a parenting style. New Beginnings, 4(2), 35-39.

Sears, W. (1990). Nighttime parenting: How to get your baby and child to sleep. Franklin Park Illinois: La Leche League International.

Segal, J. (1992). Melanie Klein. London: Sage Publications.

Shahar, S. (1990). Childhood in the middle ages. London: Routledge.

Sharma, M., & Petosa, R. (1997). Impact of expectant fathers in breast-feeding decisions. Journal of the American Dietetic Association, 97(11), 1311-1313.

Sheehan, D., Watt, S., Krueger, P. & Sword, W. (2006). The impact of new universal postpartum program on breastfeeding outcomes. Journal of Human Lactation, 22(4), 398-408.

Silverman, D.K. (2003). Mommy nearest: Revisiting the idea of infantile symbiosis and its implications for females. Psychoanalytic Psychology, 20(2), 261-270.

Silverstein, L.B., & Auerbach, C.F. (1999). Deconstructing the essential father. American Psychologist, 54, 397-407.

Slade, P., MacPherson, S.A., Hume, A., & Maresh, M. (1993). Expectations, experiences and satisfaction with labour. British Journal of Clinical Psychology, 32, 469-483.

Slep, A.M.S., & O'Leary, S.G. (1998). The effects of maternal attributions on parenting: An experimental analysis. Journal of Family Psychology. 12(2), 234-243.

Slusser, W.M., & Lange, L. (2002). Breastfeeding in the United States today: Are families prepared? In N. Halfon, K. Taaffe McLearn & M.A. Schuster (Eds.), Child rearing in America: Challenges facing parents with young children. Cambridge: Cambridge University Press.

Slusser, W.M., & Powers, N.G. (1997). Breastfeeding Update 1: Immunology, nutrition, and advocacy. Pediatrics in Review, 18(4), 111-119.

Small, M.F. (1998). Our babies ourselves: How biology and culture shape the way we parent. New York: Anchor Books.

Smith, L.J. (1996). A score sheet for evaluating breastfeeding educational materials. Journal of Human Lactation, 11(4), 307-311.

Smith, L.J. (2007). Impact of birthing practices on the breastfeeding dyad. Journal of Midwifery and Women's Health, 52(6), 621-630.

Snell, B.J., Krantz, M., Keeton, R., Delgado, K., & Peckham, C. (1992). The association of formula samples given at hospital discharge with the early duration of breastfeeding. Journal of Human Lactation, 8(2), 67-71.

Solomon, I. (1995). A primer of Kleinian therapy. Northvale, New Jersey: Jason Aronson.

Statistics Canada. (2003). Health behaviors: Breastfeeding practices. Canadian Community Health Survey. Retrieved on August 2, 2005, from http://www.statcan.ca/english/freepub/82-221-XIE/2004002/nonmed/behaviors4.htm.

Stearns, C.A. (1999). Breastfeeding and the good maternal body. Gender & Society, 13(3), 308-325.

Stein, M.T., Boise, E.G., & Snyder, D.M. (2002). Parental concerns about extended breastfeeding in a toddler. Journal of Developmental and Behavioral Pediatrics, 23(6), 438-442.

Stern, D. (1974). Mother and infant at play. The dyadic interaction involving facial vocal and gaze behaviours. In M. Lewis & L.A. Rosenblum (Eds.), The effect of the infant on its caregiver. New York: John Wiley & Sons.

Stern, D. (1985). The interpersonal world of the infant. United States: Basic Books.

Stratheam, L., Mamum, A.A., Najman, J.M., & O'Callaghan, M.J. (2009). Does breastfeeding protect against substantiated child abuse and neglect? A 15-year cohort study. Pediatrics, 123(2), 483-493.

Stuart-Macadam, P. (1995). Biocultural perspectives on breastfeeding. In P. Stuart-Macadam & K. Dettwyler (Eds.), Breastfeeding: Biocultural perspectives. New York: Aldine De Gruyter.

Sullivan, H.S. (1953). The interpersonal theory of psychiatry. New York: Norton. Quoted in Greenberg, J.R. & Mitchell, S.A. (2000). Objects Relations in Psychoanalytic Theory. (12th printing). Cambridge: Harvard University Press.

Sullivan, H.S. (1972). Personal psychology: Early formulations. New York: W.W. Norton & Company Inc.

Susin, L.R.O. & Giugliani, E.R.J. (2008). Inclusion of fathers in an intervention to promote breastfeeding: Impact on breastfeeding rates. Journal of Human Lactation, 24(4), 386.

Taylor, S.E., Klein, L.C., Lewis, B.P., Gruenwald, T.L., Gurung, R.A.R., & Opdegraff, J.A. (2000). Female responses to stress: Tend-and befriend not fight-or flight. Psychological Review, 107(3), 411-429.

Tender, J.A.F., Janakiram, J., Arce, E., Mason, R., Jordan, T., Marsh, J., Kin, S., Jianping, H., & Moon, R.Y. (2009). Reasons for in-hospital formula supplementation of breastfed infants from low income-families. Journal of Human Lactation, 25(1), 11-17.

Teti, D.M., & Gelfand D.M. (1991). Behavioral competence among mothers of infants in the first year: The mediational role of maternal self-efficacy. Child Development, 62, 918-929.

Thevenin, T. (1976). The family bed: An age old concept in childrearing. Minneapolis, MN: Tine Thevenin.

Thorley, V. (2003). Printed advice on initiating and maintaining breastfeeding in mid-20th-century queensland. Journal of Human Lactation, 19(1), 77-89.

Thurer, S. (1994). The myths of motherhood: How culture reinvents the good mother. New York: Penguin books.

Torres, M.M., Torres, R.R.D., Parrilla Rodriguez, A.M., & Dennis, C.L. (2003). Translation and validation of the breastfeeding self-efficacy scale into Spanish: data from a Puerto Rican population. Journal of Human Lactation, 19(1), 35-42.

Torvaldson, S., Roberts, C.L., Simpson, J.M., Thompson, J.F., Ellwood, D.A. (2006). Intrapartum epidural analgesia and breastfeeding: a prospective cohort study. International Breastfeeding Journal, 1, 1-24.

Trad, P.V. (1992). Interventions with infants and parents: The theory and practice of previewing. NewYork: John Wiley & Sons.

Tronick, E.Z. (1989). Emotions and emotional communication in infants. American Psychologist, 44(2), 112-119.

Tronick, E.Z., Cohn, J. F., & Shea, E. (1986). The transfer of affect between mothers and infants. In T. B. Brazelton and M.W. Yogman (Eds.), Affective development in infancy. Norwood, NJ: Ablex.

Unger, D.G., & Wandersman, L.P. (1985). Social support and adolescent mothers: Action research contributions to theory and applications. Journal of Social Sciences, 41(1), 29-45.

United Nations International Children's Emergency Fund (UNICEF). (1996b, March/April). Experience with adopted child convinces 'fathering expert' that breast is best. Baby Friendly Hospital Initiative News, 2-3.

United Nations International Children's Emergency Fund (UNICEF). (1998a, March). Breastmilk's unique effect on building the brain. Baby Friendly Hospital Initiative News, 2-5.

United Nations International Children's Emergency Fund (UNICEF). (1998b, March). Research in Chile highlights importance of mother-baby interaction. Baby Friendly Hospital Initiative News, 4.

United Nations International Children's Emergency Fund (UNICEF). (1998c, March). Studies show link between breastfeeding and cognitive development in children. Baby Friendly Hospital Initiative News, 1.

United Nations International Children's Emergency Fund (UNICEF) Maharashtra. (2009). Breast crawl: The initiation of breastfeeding by breast crawl. Retrieved on May 21, 2009, from http://breastcrawl.org/.

US Preventive Service Task Force. (2008). Primary care interventions to promote breastfeeding: US Preventive Service Task Force recommendation statement. Annals of Internal Medicine, 149(8), 560-562.

Uvnas-Moberg, K., Widstrom, A.M., Marchini, G., & Winberg, J. (1987). Release of GI hormones in mother and infant by sensory stimulation. Acta Paediatrica Scandinavica, 76(6), 851-860.

Uvnas-Moberg, K., Widstrom, A.M., Werner, S., Matthiesen, A.S., & Winberg, J. (1990). Oxytocin and prolactin levels in breast-feeding women: Correlation with milk yield and duration. Acta Obstetricia et Gynecologica Scandinavica, 69(4), 301-306.

Valaitis, R.K., Sheeshka, J.D., & Fodor O'Brien, M. (1996). Do consumer feeding publications available in physicians' offices protect, promote and support breastfeeding? Journal of Human Lactation, 13 (3), 203-208.

Valsiner, J. (2000). Culture and human development. Thousand Oaks: Sage Publications.

Vandiver, T.A. (1997). Relationship of mothers' perceptions and behaviors to the duration of breastfeeding. Psychological Reports, 80(3), 1375-1384.

Van Esterik, P. (1995). The politics of breastfeeding: An advocacy perspective. In P. Stuart-Macadam & K.A. Dettwyler (Eds.), Breastfeeding : Biocultural perspectives. New York: Aldine De Gruyter.

Verny, T., & Kelly, J. (1981). The secret life of the unborn child. New York: Summit Books.

Volpe, R. (1989). Poverty and child abuse: A review of selected literature. Toronto: The Institute for the Prevention of Child Abuse.

Volpe, R., (1995, Winter/Spring). Another face of child abuse prevention. Connection, 3.

Wagner, M. (1994). Pursuing the birth machine. Australia: Ace Graphics.

Walker, M. (1993). A fresh look at the risks of artificial feeding. Journal of Human Lactation, 9(2), 97-107.

Walker, M. (1998, June 4-5). The hazards of infant formula: New evidence. Paper presented at the conference 'The Cost of Not Breastfeeding': Eighth Annual National Breastfeeding Seminar Program. Toronto, Canada.

Walker, M. (2001). Selling out mothers and babies: marketing breast milk substitutes in the USA. Weston, MA: NABA REAL.

Walker, M. (2006). Breastfeeding management for the clinician. Sudbury MA: Jones and Bartlett.

Walker, M. (2007a). Supplementation of the Breastfed baby: Just one bottle won't hurt or will it? Retrieved on March 4 from http://massbfc.org/formula/bottle.html.

Walker, M. (2007b). International breastfeeding initiatives and their relevance to the current state of breastfeeding in the United States. Journal Midwifery Women's Health, 52(6), 549-555.

Walker, M. (2007a). Still selling out mothers and babies: marketing of breastmilk substitutes n the USA. Weston, MA: NABA REAL.

Weininger, O. (1984) The clinical psychology of Melanie Klein. Springfield, IL: Charles C. Thomas.

Weininger, O. (1989). Children's phantasies: The shaping of relationships. London: Karnac Books.

Weininger, O. (1992). Melanie Klein: From theory to reality. London: Karnac Books.

Weininger, O. (1993). View from the cradle. London: Karnac Books.

Weininger, O. (1996). Being and not being: Clinical applications of the death instinct. London: Karmac Books.

Wertsh, J.V. (1985). Vygotsky and the social formation of mind. Cambridge MA: Harvard University Press.

Widstrom, A.M. (1993). Lessons from Sweden: Aren't babies clever? Retrieved on February 20, 2009, from http://www.birthinternational.com/articles/widstrom01.html.

Widstrom, A.M, Winberg, J., Werner, S., Hamberger, B., Eneroth, P., & Unvas-Moberg, K. (1984). Suckling in lactating women stimulates the secretion of insulin and prolactin without concomitant effects on gastrin, growth hormone, calcitonin, vasopressin or catecholamines. Early Human Development, 10(1-2), 115-122.

Widstrom, A.M., Ransjo-Arvidson, A.B., Christensson, K., Matthiesen, A.S., Winberg, J., & Unvas-Moberg, K. (1987). Gastric suction in healthy newborn infants: Effects on circulation and feeding behavior. Acta Paediatrica Scandinavia, 76, 566-72.

Widstrom, A.M, Winberg, J., Werner, S., Svensson, K., Posloncec, B., & Uvnas-Moberg, K. (1988). Breast feeding-induced effects on plasma gastrin and somatostin levels and their correlation with milk yield in lactation females. Early Human Development, 16(2-3), 293-301.

Widstrom, A.M, Wahlberg, V., Mattiessen, A.S., Eneroth, P., Uvnas-Moberg, K., Werner, S., & Winberg, J. (1990). Short term effects of early suckling and touch on maternal behavior. Early Human Development, 21, 153-163.

Wiessinger, D. (1996). Watch your language. Journal of Human Lactation, 12(1), 1-4.

Winnicott, D.W. (1957). Mother and child. A primer of first relationships. New York: Basic Books, Inc.

Winnicott, D.W. (Ed.). (1958). Collected papers, through pediatrics to psycho-analysis. London: Tavistock.

Winnicott, D.W. (1964). The child, the family and the outside world. Great Britain: Penguin Books.

Winnicott, D.W. (1989). A tribute on the occasion of Hoffer's seventieth birthday. In C. Winnicott, R. Sheppard, & M. Davis (Eds.), Psychoanalytic explorations (pp. 499-505). Cambridge, Mass.: Harvard University Press.

Winnicott, D.W. (1994). What do we know about babies as cloth suckers? Talking to Parents (pp. 15-20). Reading Massachusetts: Addison-Wesley.

Winnicott, D.W. (1997a). The theory of the parent-infant relationship. In D.E. Scharff (Ed.), Object relations theory and practice: an introduction (pp.225- 235). Northvale, North Jersey: Jason Aronson, Inc.

Winnicott, D.W. (1997b). The use of an object and relating through identification. In D.E. Scharff (Ed.), Object relations theory and practice: an introduction (pp 248-245). Northvale, New Jersey: Jason Aronson Inc.

Wolf, J.H. (1999). "Mercenary hirelings" or "a great blessing"?: Doctors' and mothers conflicted perceptions of wet nurses and the ramifications for infant feeding in Chicago, 1871-1961. Journal of Social History, 33(I), 97-113.

Wolf, J.H. (2001). Don't kill your baby: Public health and the decline of breastfeeding in the 19th and 20th centuries. Columbia: The Ohio State University Press.

Woolridge, M. (1986a). The anatomy of infant sucking. Midwifery, 2, 164-171.

Woolridge, M. (1986b). The aetiology of sore nipples. Midwifery, 2, 172-176.

World Health Organization. (1981). International code of marketing of breastmilk susbstitutes. Geneva, Switzerland: WHO.

World Health Organization. (1998a). Breastfeeding. Safe Motherhood. 3, 31-35.

World Health Organization. (1998b). Evidence for the ten steps to successful breastfeeding. Geneva: Division of Child Health and Development.

World Health Organization. (2001). Expert consultation on the optimal duration of exclusive breastfeeding: Conclusions and recommendations. Retrieved March, 2001 from http://.who.int/inf-pr2001/en/note2001-07.html.

World Health Organization. (2003). Global strategy for infant and young child feeding. Geneva Switzerland.

World Health Organization (WHO) and United Nations International Children's Emergency Fund (UNICEF). (1989). Ten steps to promote successful breastfeeding. Geneva: Mother and Child Division, WHO.

World Health Organization (WHO) and United Nations International Children's Emergency Fund (UNICEF). (1990). Innocenti Declaration. WHO/UNICEF policymakers' meeting on "Breastfeeding in the 1990s: A Global Initiative." Florence, Italy.

Zembo, C.T. (2002). Breastfeeding. Obstetrics and Gynecology Clinics of North America, 29(1), 51-76.

Index

A

Abuse 47
Adoptive Families 229
Adoptive Nursing 66
Adoration 174
Adult Centered Attitudes 74
Adult Centered Philosophy 72
Adult-Focused Nursing 159
Adult Focused Parenting Philosophy 72
Adult Precedence 72
Ambivalence 32, 122, 129, 178, 181, 215
Apparent Independence 74
Artificial Apparatus 17
Artificial Baby Milk Companies 54
Artificial Feeding 46, 48, 55
Artificial Feeding As The Norm 74
Attachment 8
Attachment Parenting 73
Attachment Theory 24, 25
Attuned Mothering 103
Authoritarian Figures 48
Autonomy 71
Autonomy 68, 69

B

Bedsharing 23
Behaviors 18
Belittling Behaviors 47
Bidirectional Development 71
Bidirectional Paradigms 69
Bottle Feeding Experience 8
Bottles 182
Breastfeeding 4, 5, 38
Breastfeeding Education 226
Breastfeeding Police 64
Breast Part Object 26
Breast Pump 65, 67
Breast Pump Companies 65
Broken Continuum 187, 197
Broken Nursing Patterns 49
Broken Physiological Continuum 59

C

Carrying 20
Chemists 48
Child Behavior 24
Child Development 58, 102, 152, 178, 211
Child-Focused Environments 18
Child Focused Weaning 211
Child-Focused Weaning Patterns 97
Child-Led Weaning 100
Child-Led Weaning With Maternal Contributions 99
Child-Paced Focus 153
Child-Paced Weaning 154
Child Temperament 24
Circular Causality 39
Clinical Bias 8
Closed Communication 129, 204
Closeness 30
Comfort 173
Communication 206
Communication Style 36, 40
Companies Profiting From Artificial Feeding 53
Compensatory Measures 131
Complementary Interactions 127
Complementary Parenting Task Allocation 78
Complementary Task Allocations 37
Compromised Situations 31
Concepts 13
Confidence 29
Confusion About The Female Breast 74

Contempt 46, 60
Contemptuous Behaviors 47
Contradictory Messages 52
Co-Sleeping 22, 72, 95, 150
Couple Discord 221
Couple Dissonance 205
Couple Needs 201
Couple Precedence 45, 50, 74
Couple Processes 218
CoupLe Relations 220
Couple Relationship 35
Couple Time 132
Cue-Based Interactions 15, 89, 94
Cue-Based Interventions 101
Cue-Based Nursing 94, 112, 171
Cue Names For Nursing 90
Cue Reading 214
Cultural Misnaming 61
Cultural Themes 197
Cultures 44

D

Decisions About Nursing 33
Decreased Parental Sensitivity 129
Depression 16
Desire To Protect 121
Devaluation Of Women's Bodily Experiences 64
Devalued Mothers 50
Devalued Women 44
Development Of Autonomy 144
Deviation 178
Disdain For Natural Female Biology 74
Disregard For Physiological Patterns 59
Distal Strategies 74, 160
Distancing 45, 46, 49, 50, 68, 197
Distancing At Night 72
Distancing Behaviors 68, 160
Distinct Developmental Trajectory 33

Distinct Trajectories 76
Dry Nursing 46
Dysfunctional Closeness 69

E

Early Childhood 43
Educating Mothers 107
Emotional Development 27
Emotional Experience 172
Emotional Messages 91
Emotional Regulation 24
Encompassing Behavior 172, 210
Encompassing Experience 171
Encouragement 108
Enhanced Practice 9
Envy 46, 47, 59, 67, 119, 120, 183, 188, 217
Essentiality Paradigms 37
Establishing Themes 76
Evidence-Based 5
Exclusivity 105, 176, 179
Exclusivity In The Nursing Unit 78
Experts 50
Extreme Disdain 46

F

Families With Risks 227
Family 48
Family Development 75
Family Interaction 149
Family Life Cycle 40
Family Members 193
Family Organization 14
Family Systems Theory 39, 41, 222
Family Themes 40, 74, 201
Fathering 115
Fathers 76, 152, 179, 193
Fears Of Overdependence 122
Feeding 187
Feeding Choice 55, 56, 159
Female Disembodiment 65

Female Processes 175
Female Self-Disdain 47
Feminist Contributions 63
Feminist Theory 71
Feminist Thought 37
Focus On Fathers 118
Free Choice 58
Frustration 178
Full Weaning 73

G

Gender Distinctions 205
Gender-Specific Tasks 73
Germ Theories 49
Good And Giving Breast 60
Good Enough 26
Good Enough Feelings 211
Grief 32
Guilt 182, 217
Guilt Myth 8, 57

H

Healing 176
Healthcare Systems 52
Helplessness 182
Historical Family Themes 51
History Of Nursing 71
Holding 20
Homeostasis 86, 132, 204, 220
Hormonal Feedback Loop 15
Hormonally Based Effects Of Nursing 16

I

Immediate Postnatal Period 78
In Arms Phase 21
Independence 69, 70
Independent 212
Individuation 25, 144
Infant Seats 160
Inflammatory Response 16

Interdependent Nursing Subsystem 18
Intimacy 30, 105
Irreplaceable 177

K

Kangaroo Care 19

L

Lack Of Confidence 50
La Leche League 51
Language Use 3, 59, 227
Loss 32
Love 173, 192, 210

M

Male Envy 46
Maternal Development 28, 32, 214
Maternal Pain 81
Maternal Perceptions 28
Maternal Self-Debasement 50
Maternal Tutoring 168
Medicalization 49
Middle Ages 37, 64
Mislabelling 58
Missed Cues 187, 189
Missed Cues For Nursing 159
Mixed Messages 44, 48
Mother-Led Weaning 98
Motherly Asexual Breasts 62
Multi-Purposed Organ 61
Mutual Influence 35

N

Natural Birthing Processes 163
Next Generation 146
Nighttime Proximity 23
Non-Verbal 7
Normalcy 57
Normalcy Of Artificial Feeding 55

Normalcy Of Nursing 145
Normal Method Of Feeding 57
Normal Nursing Patterns 16
Novel Roles 36
Nursing 3, 4, 55, 56, 58, 214, 227
Nursing Behaviors 51
Nursing Is Normal 166
Nursing Problems 59, 60
Nursing Sessions 17, 92
Nurturing Behaviors 143

O

Object Relations Theory 24, 26
Obstructed Nursing Patterns 44
Open Communication 128, 185, 203, 219
Optimism 143
Over Monitoring 70
Oxytocin 14

P

Parental Couple 38
Paternal Development 33, 35, 216
Paternal Envy 118, 126
Paternal Perceptions 34
Paternal Support 34, 81
Patriarchal Concepts 71
Patriarchy 44, 48
Patronizing Behaviors 47
Perceptions Of Pain 81
Personal Bias 7
Personal Growth 104
Phantasies 26
Physicians 48
Physiologically Based Nursing 73, 186
Physiologically Based Nursing Pattern 13, 24, 43
Positive Feedback 141
Positive Regard 142
Postpartum Period 75

Prenatal Stage 76
Present Day Family Themes 52
Prolactin 15
Protection 181
Protective Tasks 79
Proximal Strategies 18
Proximity 149, 191, 192
Proximity Behaviors 18, 44, 113
Psychotherapeutic Paradigm 7
Pumped Breastmilk 65

R

Reduced Sensitivity 178, 182, 183
Regard For The Infant 30
Repair 176
Research Studies 58
Respect For Children's Needs And Cues 170
Respect For Children's Unique Needs 200
Respect For Gender-Based Processes 167
Respect For Physiology 213
Respecting Exclusive Tasks 83
Reverence For Child-Paced Needs 198
Reverence For Children's Natural Needs And Cues 170
Reverence For Children's Needs And Cues 200
Reverence For Cultural Themes 188
Reverence For Natural Processes 152
Reverence For Nursing 144
Reverence For Parent-Child Closeness 150
Reverence For Physiology 163, 165
Reverence For Science 48
Reverence For Separation 74
Reverence For Women And Children 44

Rights To Natural Processes 51
Rigidity 49, 50
Rocking 20
Roles 40

S

Scientific Form Of Infant Feeding 65
Self 71
Self-Awareness 7
Self-Calming 70
Self-Confidence 104
Self-Control 50
Self-Efficacy 175
Self-Focused 71
Self-Regulation 70
Sense Of Efficacy 29, 181
Sense Of Efficiency 82
Sensitive Behavior 140
Sensitive Cue Reading 31
Sensitive Fathering 111, 118
Sensitive Interaction 139, 209
Sensitivity 175, 180, 186, 187, 189, 191, 197, 201, 205
Separate 155
Separateness 69
Separation 68, 144, 200
Separation-Individuation Theory 24
Separation Processes 198
Sexual Breasts 61
Sexual Function 202, 220
Sexual Intimacy 132
Sexualized Breasts 50
Shared Connection 114
Shared Meaning 36, 173
Shared Ownership Of Nursing 82
Shared Themes 219
Siblings 139, 174, 185, 189
Skin-To-Skin Interaction 14, 19
Social Pressure 134
Solitary Sleeping 160
Solitary Sleeping Arrangements 151
Status 45

Stress 16, 181, 197
Strict Schedules 69
Suckling Difficulties 60
Summary Of Themes 190
Superlative Behavior 56
Supremacy Of Milk Over Relationship 65
Symbiosis 25

T

Tandem Nursing 95, 98
Task Allocation 36, 218
Term Of Reference 3
Themes 48
Themes Develop Over Time 173
Themes Interfering With Nursing 10
Theories 13
Tolerance 180, 195
Touch 19
Tutor 113
Twins 96

U

Unique Features Of Nursing 59
Unspoken Rules 40

V

Validation 180
View Of Closeness 196
Views Of Breasts 169

W

Weaning 9, 32, 67, 75, 98, 101, 117, 160, 198
Weaning Patterns 199
Wet Nursing 45
Withholding And Bad Breast 60
Wrong Terms 58

Y

Young Child Stage 41

Author Bio

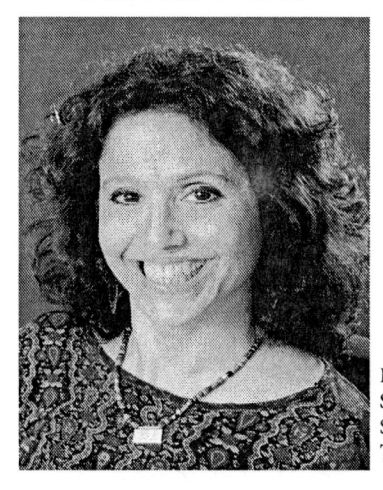

Photo by Doron Sussman, Doron Sussman Photography, Thornhill, ON, Canada

Dr. Keren Epstein-Gilboa PhD, MEd, BSN, RN, FACCE, LCCE, IBCLC, RLC

Keren Epstein-Gilboa is nurse psychotherapist who has been working with families in the transition to parenting and with young children for over twenty-five years. Her professional experience includes individual, group, and family counseling; teaching in university and professional settings; lactation consulting; childbirth education and birth support; and pre-school teaching. She researches and has published material on the psychological aspects of pregnancy, birth, nursing, mothering, and early parenting in peer reviewed journals, newsletters, and online resources. Her chapter on *Breastfeeding Envy: Unresolved Patriachal Envy and the Obstruction of Physiologically Based Nursing Patterns* is published in the book *Giving Milk*.

Dr. Epstein-Gilboa has a Phd in developmental psychology, human development, and family and social relations and a MEd in counseling and applied psychology from the University of Toronto. She has a BSN from the Henrietta Szold Hadassah-Hebrew University School of Nursing. Dr. Epstein-Gilboa has post graduate training in family and couple therapy.

The author is a retired La Leche League Leader and a Fellow in the American College of Childbirth Educators. She has been a Lamaze Certified Childbirth Educator and an International Board Certified Lactation Consultant since 1988.

Ordering Information

Hale Publishing, L.P.

1712 N. Forest Street

Amarillo, Texas, USA 79106

....

8:00 am to 5:00 pm cst

call » 806.376.9900

sales » 800.378.1317

fax » 806.376.9901

....

Online web orders

www.ibreastfeeding.com